# Transforming Healthcare

This comprehensive volume explores cutting-edge technologies, groundbreaking methodologies, and insightful ethical considerations. It brings together leading minds and research across diverse domains, offering readers a glimpse into the future of healthcare. From leveraging AI in diagnostics and personalized treatments to advancing telemedicine and remote patient monitoring, the text addresses real-world challenges and opportunities in the rapidly evolving healthcare industry.

**Key features:**

- Innovative approaches to early disease detection, including Alzheimer's and cancer, using machine learning and deep learning techniques.
- State-of-the-art applications of design thinking, meta-heuristics, and federated learning in healthcare.
- Ethical perspectives on the use of AI technologies and their impact on businesses and patient care.
- A deep dive into the role of IoT, NLP, and AI-driven image processing in revolutionizing healthcare delivery.
- Generalized models analyzing trade credits and their implications for healthcare supply chains.

Whether you're a researcher, healthcare professional, or technology enthusiast, this book serves as an invaluable resource for understanding and shaping the future of health technologies. Packed with diverse perspectives and actionable insights, it's a must-read for anyone passionate about making a difference in healthcare.

## Computational Methods for Industrial Applications

*Series Editor: Bharat Bhushan*

This book series focuses on varied computational methods incorporated within the system with the help of artificial intelligence, learning methods, analytical reasoning and sense-making in big data. Aimed at graduate students, academic researchers and professionals, it covers the most efficient and innovative technological solutions for industrial applications and sustainable smart societies in order to alter green power management, the effects of carbon emissions, air quality metrics, industrial pollution levels, biodiversity and ecology.

**Blockchain for Industry 4.0:** Emergence, Challenges, and Opportunities
*Anoop V.S, Asharaf S, Justin Goldston and Samson Williams*

**Intelligent Systems and Machine Learning for Industry:** Advancements, Challenges and Practices
*P.R Anisha, C. Kishor Kumar Reddy, Nguyen Gia Nhu, Megha Bhushan, Ashok Kumar, Marlia Mohd Hanafiah*

**Sustainability in Industry 5.0:** Theory and Applications
*Edited by C Kishor Kumar Reddy, P R Anisha, Samiya Khan, Marlia Mohd Hanafiah, Lavanya Pamulaparty and R Madana Mohana*

For more information about this series please visit: https://www.routledge.com/Computational-Methods-for-Industrial-Applications/book-series/CRCCMIA

# Transforming Healthcare

## Mode, Technologies, and Implementation

Edited by
Ankush Jain, Vishal Srivastava, Gaurav Singal,
and Mohamed Mosbah

CRC Press
Taylor & Francis Group
Boca Raton London New York

CRC Press is an imprint of the
Taylor & Francis Group, an **informa** business

Front cover image: VZ_art/Shutterstock



First edition published 2026
by CRC Press
2385 NW Executive Center Drive, Suite 320, Boca Raton FL 33431

and by CRC Press
4 Park Square, Milton Park, Abingdon, Oxon, OX14 4RN

*CRC Press is an imprint of Taylor & Francis Group, LLC*



ISBN: 978-1-032-75654-7 (hbk)
ISBN: 978-1-041-06160-1 (pbk)
ISBN: 978-1-003-63408-9 (ebk)

DOI: 10.1201/9781003634089

Typeset in Sabon
by Deanta Global Publishing Services, Chennai, India

# Contents

# About the editors

**Ankush Jain** is an assistant professor in the Department of Computer Science and Engineering at Netaji Subhas University of Technology, Dwarka, New Delhi, India. He completed his MTech and PhD from ABV-Indian Institute of Information Technology and Management (ABV-IIITM), Gwalior, India. Earlier, he worked as an assistant professor at Indira Gandhi Delhi Technical University for Women (IGDTUW), Delhi, India. Dr. Jain has published research articles, patents, and books in internationally acclaimed venues. He serves as a reviewer for various international journals, including *IEEE Transactions on Evolutionary Computation*; *IEEE Transactions on System, Man, and Cybernetics*; *IEEE Transactions on Computational Social Systems*; *IEEE Sensors Journal*; *Information Processing and Management*; *Expert Systems with Applications*; *Soft Computing*; and *JMLC*. His research interests include recommendation systems, evolutionary computation, computer vision, pattern recognition, and machine learning. He is a life member of the ISTE and International Society of Engineers and a professional member of IEEE and ACM.

**Vishal Srivastava** is an assistant professor in the Department of Computer Science and Engineering, Motilal Nehru National Institute of Technology (MNNIT) Allahabad, Prayagraj, India. His main research interests are graphs, complex social networks, image-based computations in AI, pattern recognition, and evolutionary computing. He has published research articles, patents, and books in internationally acclaimed venues.

**Gaurav Singal** received his MTech and PhD from the CSE Department, Malaviya National Institute of Technology, Jaipur, India. He is an assistant professor with the CSE Department, Netaji Subhas University of Technology, New Delhi, India. He has been actively working in research and teaching for the last 12 years and has published in several reputed conferences and journals. His research interests include wireless Internet of Things, edge computing, artificial intelligence, deep learning, and software-defined networks. Singal received a total research grant of approximately 55L from various agencies such as SERB, CST, and DBT on women's security, IoT security, and assistive devices.

**Mohamed Mosbah** is a professor of computer science at the Polytechnic Institute of Bordeaux (Bordeaux INP), France, where he currently serves as vice-president. Previously, he held the position of director of Industrial Partnerships and Innovation in Computer Science and Engineering. Mosbah conducts his research at LaBRI (Laboratoire Bordelais de Recherche en Informatique), a joint research center affiliated with the University of Bordeaux and CNRS, where he also served as deputy director. His research interests span distributed computing, security, sensor networks and their applications, and intelligent transportation systems (ITS). In addition to his academic work, Mosbah is an active member of the scientific community, contributing to numerous technical program committees and organizing international conferences. He is also heavily involved in regional, national, and European research initiatives and projects. Currently, he leads an industrial chair dedicated to new mobilities and intelligent transportation systems, in collaboration with the Bordeaux campus and a consortium of ten partner companies. Mosbah's outstanding contributions have earned him recognition as a distinguished French scientific and academic figure, with his recent inclusion in the *Who's Who in France 2025*.

# Contributors

**Marwa Abdellateef**
UNICAF University
Zambia

**Rohit Agrawal**
Operations Management and Quantitative Techniques
Indian Institute of Management
Bodhgaya, India

**Vidhi Agrawal**
Ajay Kumar Garg
Institute of Management
Ghaziabad, India

**Nidhi Asthana**
School of Technology Management & Engineering
SVKM Narsee Monjee Institute of Management Studies (NMIMS) Deemed-to-be-University
Indore, India

**Khushi Bansal**
Department of Computer Science and Engineering
Ajay Kumar Garg Engineering College
Ghaziabad, India

**Sher Singh Bhakar**
Prestige University
Bhopal, India

**Vansh Budhiraja**
School of Computer Science Engineering and Technology
Bennett University
Greater Noida, India

**Aaquil Bunglowala**
Department of Electronics and TeleCommunication
Sri Aurobindo Institute of Technology
Indore, India

**Abhay Singh Chauhan**
Narsee Monjee Institute of Management Studies
Mumbai, India

**Meghali Das**
Noida Institute of Engineering and Technology
Greater Noida, India

**Lokpriya Gaikwad**
SIES Graduate School of Technology
Navi Mumbai, India

**Divya Gautam**
School of Technology Management & Engineering
SVKM Narsee Monjee Institute of Management Studies (NMIMS) Deemed-to-be-University
Indore, India

**Anindya Ghatak**
School of Computer Science Engineering and Technology
Bennett University
Greater Noida, India

**Ruchira Goel**
Department of Applied Science
Ajay Kumar Garg Engineering College
Ghaziabad, India

**Ram Gopal Gupta**
Department of Computer Science
School of Management Sciences
Varanasi, India

**Ankush Jain**
Department of Computer Science and Engineering
Netaji Subhas University of Technology
Delhi, India

**Biswajit Jana**
School of Computer Science Engineering and Technology
Bennett University
Greater Noida, India

**Shankar Kumar Jha**
School of Commerce & Management Studies
Indus International University
Himachal Pradesh, India

**Sandip Kanase**
Bharati Vidyapeeth College of Engineering
Navi Mumbai, India

**Rohit Kumar**
Department of Computer Science and Engineering
Netaji Subhas University of Technology
Delhi, India

**Sachin Kumar**
Department of Applied Health & Sciences
The University of Aberdeen Medical Statistics
Aberdeen, UK

**Harshita Mathur**
Prestige Institute of Management & Research
Gwalior, India

**Bireshwar Das Mazumdar**
School of Computer Science Engineering and Technology
Bennett University
Greater Noida, India

**Steve McKenna**
Curtin Business School, School of Management and Marketing
Curtin University
Perth, Australia

**Surendra Nagar**
Department of Computer Science and Engineering
Netaji Subhas University of Technology
Delhi, India

**Rashmi Nair**
School of Computing
MIT Art, Design and Technology

University
Pune, India

**R. V. Palanivel**
Berlin School of Business and Innovation
Berlin, Germany

**Gaurav Paliwal**
School of Technology Management & Engineering
SVKM Narsee Monjee Institute of Management Studies (NMIMS) Deemed-to-be-University
Indore, India

**Rahul Sharma**
Information Systems Group
Tallinn University of Technology
Tallinn, Estonia

**Sanjay Sharma**
Department of Applied Sciences & Humanities
Ajay Kumar Garg Engineering College
Ghaziabad, India

**Silky Sharma**
School of Commerce and Management Studies
Dayananda Sagar University
Bengaluru, India

**Vitan Sharma**
Prestige Institute of Management & Research
Gwalior, India

**Tarika Singh Sikarwar**
Prestige Institute of Management & Research
Gwalior, India

**Ashutosh Sirohi**
Department of Computer Science and Engineering
Ajay Kumar Garg Engineering College
Ghaziabad, India

**Ashutosh Srivastava**
School of Computer Science Engineering and Technology
Bennett University
Greater Noida, India

**Divya Srivastava**
School of Computer Science Engineering and Technology
Bennett University
Greater Noida, India

**Garima Srivastava**
Mangalmay Institute of Engineering and Technology
Greater Noida, India

**Nagaraj Subbarao**
School of Commerce & Management Studies
Dayananda Sagar University
Bengaluru, India

**Sudheesh Sudhakaran**
Baxter Healthcare
Illinois, USA

**Vinod Surange**
Symbiosis Institute of Business Management
Symbiosis International Deemed University
Pune, India

**Agung Sutrisno**
Sam Ratulangi University
Manado, Indonesia

**Prashiksha Tiwari**
Prestige Institute of Management & Research
Gwalior, India

**Anand Tyagi**
Department of Applied Sciences & Humanities
Ajay Kumar Garg Engineering College
Ghaziabad, India

**Madhushi Verma**
School of Computer Science Engineering and Technology
Bennett University
Greater Noida, India

Chapter 1

# Innovating health

## Design thinking in emerging technologies

*Gaurav Paliwal, Aaquil Bunglowala, Nidhi Asthana, and Divya Gautam*

### 1.1 INTRODUCTION

Design thinking is one of the user-centred innovation processes: in health, it places the patient, carer, and health professionals at the top of the list of the innovating process (Figure 1.1). By empathizing with these stakeholders, designers get insight into their experience, challenges, and aspirations within the healthcare system. Healthcare innovation is often about tackling complex problems that affect multiple stakeholders and require interdisciplinary collaboration. Design thinking provides a structured way to encourage creativity, collaboration, and iterative prototyping of potential solutions (Figure 1.1). Design thinking does not call for technical solutions. Instead, cross-functional teams work together to pinpoint problems and refine solutions that can meet the diverse needs of their users.

One of the core principles underlying design thinking is the idea of reframing problems as opportunities for innovation. This, in a healthcare perspective, is reframing beyond the symptoms or surface problems to the root cause and unmet needs. Reframing a problem could unlock numerous insights that would drive more meaningful and impactful solutions. Ideation and prototyping hold another principal core aspect in design thinking. With brainstorming sessions and fast prototyping, a team is sure to get a wide range of ideas on board, which can quickly be tested with users for feedback. Fast iteration allows the designers to fail fast and learn quickly in refining their solution based on real-world insights.

Design thinking is for designing experiences—not products or services—so users are empowered and better engaged. In healthcare, this might mean envisioning new patient journey models, driving improved communication between patients and their providers, or designing better intuitive interfaces for healthcare technology. By thinking through the whole healthcare experience, they can solve problems that, while serving functional needs, would raise the quality of care overall.

This book explores the applications of design thinking across dozens of areas of healthcare innovations. The topics of this chapter span

DOI: 10.1201/9781003634089-1

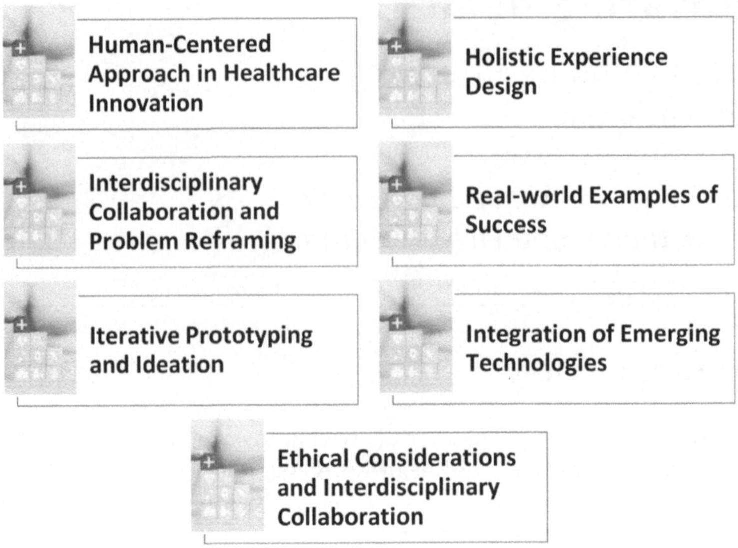


*Figure 1.1* Key themes in human-centred approach of healthcare innovation.

understanding the needs of patients to an integration of rising technologies, inclusive of practical insights, case studies, and best practices in leveraging design thinking to drive positive change in healthcare. The first section introduces this chapter and talks about how to drive innovation in healthcare through design thinking. Section 1.2 delves deeper into so-called key tenets of design thinking by showing them concretely applied in healthcare through the ideas of empathy, iteration, and collaboration to solve complex problems within the healthcare domain. Section 1.3 provides a range of real-life examples on how design thinking initiatives have improved healthcare delivery and patient outcomes. Section 1.4 discusses how emerging technologies are infused into the design thinking process to guide healthcare innovation. Section 1.5 is specifically dedicated to ethical implications and considerations when using a design thinking methodology within healthcare. The regulatory landscape and the standards to be adhered to for implementation of design thinking solutions in healthcare solutions are discussed in Section 1.6. Section 1.7 covers the significance of intersterility collaboration and how it upgrades the effectiveness of approaches of design thinking toward healthcare innovation. In Section 1.8 practice strategies as well as best practices for successful implementation of design thinking in healthcare organizations are covered. Finally, Section 1.9 gives a view of the trends and open opportunity areas that will shape the future of healthcare innovation.

## 1.2 DESIGN THINKING PRINCIPLES IN HEALTHCARE

Design thinking is based on some core principles that enable people to apply it in different domains, including healthcare. These practices centre humans in problem-solving and innovation approaches [37, 71]. It focuses on empathy, creativity, collaboration, and iteration, as indicated in Figure 1.1. At the crux of the design thinking methodology, core practices applied across a wide array of domains, including healthcare, foster innovation and problem-solving. It is, however, a human-centred approach that puts emphasis on empathy, creativity, collaboration, and iteration [8, 10].

Empathy is applied at the most basic heart of design thinking and involves understanding and sharing feelings, thoughts, and experiences with others. In the healthcare system, this means listening to patients, their caretakers, and their providers to comprehensively understand their needs, preferences, and challenges. The essence of design thinking is human-centredness, which puts man at the centre of the innovative process. Without starting from the technological solution, designers undertake to understand the needs, desires, and behaviours of end users in their effort to make solutions relevant, useful, and intuitive [25].

Furthermore, design thinking is highly iterative in the sense that it encourages making frequent cycles of building, testing, and improving prototypes as frequently as possible to determine the problem [11, 43]. The iterative process explicitly promotes relentless learning and improvement, which would lead to the development of user-centred, less bad solutions. Design thinking places a high premium on creativity; it fosters a way to think that allows a divergence of the mind toward idea formulation or thought of something else [11, 60, 64]. Designers use a number of techniques, including brainstorming and sketching, to consider a large number of novel solutions to challenging common assumptions.

Design thinking enforces teamwork and collaboration (Figure 1.2); it is the bringing together of people from different disciplines to tackle a problem jointly. Cross-disciplinary teams work together to find a solution within the process, thereby co-creating solutions out of insights and expertise pooled. In addition, design thinking biases toward action, with an emphasis on real outcomes in the real world. Designers embrace experimentation and learning by making things, prototyping, and testing assumptions in relation to those elements, bringing home functional solutions quickly [12].

Indeed, it will be in this way that the designers will be able to apply design thinking into the incredibly complex healthcare challenges harmoniously and create truly important innovations. We are going to describe some practical applications of this in healthcare with examples and best practices to enhance healthcare outcomes in this book.

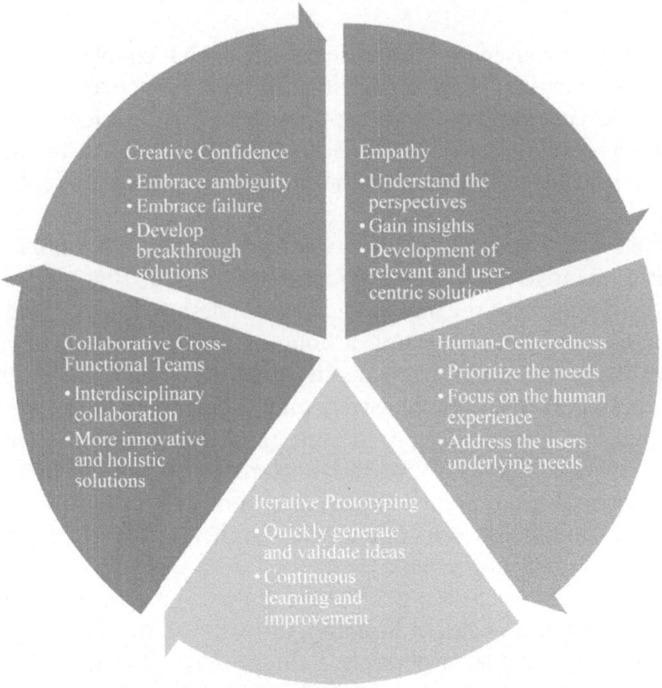


*Figure 1.2* Principles of design thinking.

### 1.2.1 Empathy in healthcare: Putting patients at the centre

Empathy is the key competence in the delivery of healthcare services, and it influences patient–provider interactions and treatment outcome. In healthcare, empathy encompasses more than just an understanding of patients' medical needs; it also involves acknowledging their feelings, worries, and preferences. When a healthcare professional listens to, validates feelings, and is compassionate toward patients, they actively demonstrate empathy. This helps in building trust and collaboration in the care relationship [32, 33].

Healthcare professionals have to be empathetic so that patient-centred care delivery is achieved (Figure 1.3). Although only a very few people are naturally predisposed or sensitive to the feelings of others [34], medical students and doctors can learn to be more empathetic. This would involve using strategies and techniques such as active listening, whereby a provider gives his full attention to the verbal and nonverbal communication cues from the patient, and perspective-taking exercises intended to put one in the patient's shoes to view situations from their vantage point.

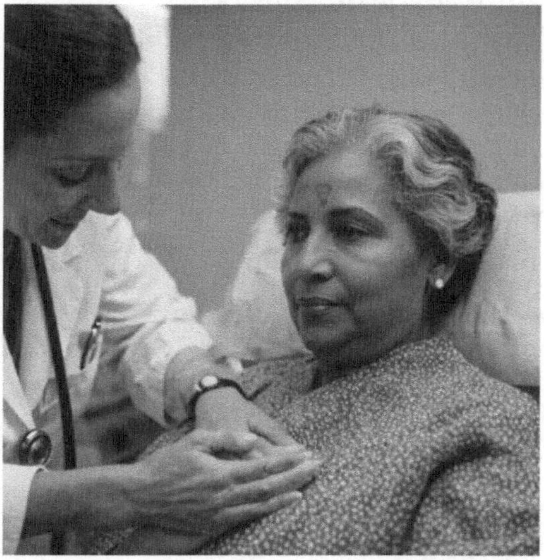

*Figure 1.3* Empathy in patient care clinical service provider.

The development of an atmosphere that preserves patient comfort, dignity, and autonomy is held to be very crucial in the fostering of empathy within health organizations [22]. This can involve physical space arrangements, amenity development, and sign design that may influence the patient's views of being treated with empathy and underpin support. An atmosphere that is warm, inclusive, and considerate responds appositely to the needs of the patient, just as it strengthens the health organizations offer of patient-centred care.

Technology, on the other hand, in most cases, associates health delivery companies with new opportunities to realize empathy and patient engagement. Telemedicine platforms ensure greater access to healthcare from any part of the world, facilitating greater convenience within the reach of patients. For example, patient portals and mobile health applications offer more opportunities and increased convenience for people to access healthcare [13]. Virtual reality and artificial intelligence can be applied to acting out representative activities that evoke empathy and understanding in healthcare encounters [14]. However, maintaining an empathizing role in healthcare is quite challenging for doctors who work in highly pressured and busy scenarios [64]. These are the factors that may be barriers on the side of the providers, such as time constraints, emotional fatigue, and burnout, which shall decrease empathic responses over some time. Understanding the challenges and developing strategies to overcome them by a commitment to provider well-being allows for the organizational cultivation of an empathetic culture in healthcare delivery [45].

### 1.2.2 Ideation: Generating innovative solutions for healthcare challenges

In healthcare innovation, ideation is a critical stage in setting a pathway for the emergence of new solutions to challenging problems. It is typically characterized by processes of brainstorming, creative thinking, and idea generation that particularly addresses healthcare needs. It is, therefore, evident that through the organizational innovation and creativity culture to be developed, the healthcare provider will be capable of sparking varied stakeholder perspectives and ideas from the various disciplines. In these sessions, teams can harness the collective intelligence and creativity potential of their members to ideate and come up with an immense base of diverse possible solutions [73].

Healthcare innovators often begin ideating after many encounters with the problem or challenge they are addressing. By conducting a lot of research with available patients and data, teams can pinpoint key pain points and opportunities for improvement by engaging with patients and healthcare providers. Participants will be encouraged to come up with out-of-the-box ideas by challenging some assumptions that will seem crazy. Techniques like brainstorming, mind mapping, and rapid prototyping provoke creative thinking and help offer innovative solutions [26].

Ideation in healthcare innovation goes far beyond the normal process of brainstorming. It involves the use of state-of-the-art emerging technologies and methodologies like design thinking, co-creation workshops, and hackathons for innovation and collaboration [76]. Feasibility, desirability, and viability are three considerations that teams should bear in mind throughout the process of evaluating prospective solutions. Teams can, therefore, lock into the most promising ideas to develop further and prototype when they assess the factors of, for instance, technical feasibility, user needs, and market demand.

Indeed, ideation eventually triggers healthcare innovation. Being the development arm, healthcare innovation creates solutions that are transformative to answer the new needs of the patients, providers, and the rest of the healthcare system [21]. Human-centred design, a creative culture, and co-creation will bring in new opportunities to drive patient care and patient outcomes.

### 1.2.3 Prototyping and iterative design in healthcare

Prototyping and iterative design play a critical role in healthcare innovation, which is the development of solutions through continuous feedback and improvement. Prototyping, by definition from Faulkner, involves making tangible representations of ideas or concepts for the purpose of testing for feasibility, functionality, and usability. In healthcare, prototypes may take many forms: physical models, digital simulations, or perhaps even interactive prototypes of software applications or medical devices.

Iterative design is the refinement and iteration of prototypes based on user feedback and testing. Refinement and iteration in evolving prototypes, as opposed to following a straight line from concept to final product, means leaving room for the iterative design to be a cycle of testing, learning, and refinement in order to keep on improving the solution in a graduated manner [4]. In essence, prototyping and iterative design in healthcare are the two forms of innovative solutions in response to the needs of patients, providers, and other stakeholders.

For more healthcare teams, prototyping early in the design process allows quick validation of assumptions, identification of any potentially major issues, and obtaining feedback from end users [42]. What is more is that this understanding is made possible for organizations to move from design option to option and solution to solution, deriving real-world insights that improve usability and user experience. Finally, prototyping and iterative design also have the advantage of effective collaboration and communication across the various multidisciplinary teams involved in healthcare innovation. Their specificity can provide tangible prototypes so that stakeholders can experience what the proposed solutions might look like and contribute in a manner that ensures that every individual aligns on project goals.

Prototyping and iterative design are ways in which organizations may reduce risks in healthcare innovation by allowing rapid failure and thereby rapid learning through the process of generation and testing possible failures (Table 1.1). Early identification and consideration of potential problems are undertaken early in the design process, thus minimizing the risk of expensive failure or error on implementation. Ultimately, through such practices, innovation and improvement in healthcare are fostered in ways that an organization can build solutions that are more effective, efficient, and user-friendly. Applying prototyping and iterative design to innovation upgrades the process and yields superior results for patients and providers across the globe [24].

## 1.3 CASE STUDIES: DESIGN THINKING SUCCESS STORIES IN HEALTHCARE

Real-world stories that are brought forth through positive case studies represent a practical way of the use of principles set for design thinking in healthcare innovation. They are concrete examples of how organizations operationalize design thinking methodologies to solve real complex problems towards bettering patient care experiences.

*Table 1.1* Prototyping and iterative design in healthcare

| *Aspect* | *Description* |
|---|---|
| Definition | Prototyping means the ideas turn into feasible, functional, usable, and tangible representations of ideas. Iterative design means refining the prototypes through feedback from users and testing. |
| Forms of prototypes | Physical models, digital simulations of interactive software applications, medical devices. |
| Process | Cycles of testing, learning, and refinement to enhance solutions. |
| Importance in healthcare | Prototyping and iterative design are key development steps in decoding more innovative solutions that meet patients', providers', and stakeholders' needs. |
| Benefits | Early validation of the assumptions, identification of problems, and collection of real-world feedback. Enhance usability and user experience and encourage collaboration. |
| Risk mitigation | Supports decreasing risks by identifying issues earlier and resolving them, therefore avoiding or reducing the chances of expensive mistakes or failures during an implementation. |
| Impact on innovation | Speeds up innovation and produces better results for patients and providers by introducing into circulation more effective, productive, and user-friendly solutions. |

One such important case study is of the Mayo Clinic, one of the world's most famous medical centres, which has been at the forefront of a design thinking project targeting better patient outcomes and satisfaction in the processes and delivery of healthcare [47]. Clinic patients were thoroughly interviewed and observed over a long design process to identify the divergent interests and needs of its patients. Taking an empathetic approach, the Mayo Clinic crafted opportunities for streamlined appointment scheduling, new and fundamentally improved approaches to communication between patients and their providers, as well as redesigning the physical clinic spaces for comfort and access. These design-driven interventions, in turn, showed a visible and measurable rise in the customer satisfaction scores and the operational efficiency at Mayo Clinic [44].

Another example is IDEO, which is an internationally renowned global design and innovation consultancy that worked with the California HealthCare Foundation (CHCF) in re-envisioning the experience of healthcare for people with chronic illness [36]. Figure 1.4 presents IDEO's design thinking methodology that supports innovative solutions for global challenges [75]. IDEO has conducted human-centred design workshops and prototyping sessions, engaging patients, carer service providers, and healthcare providers in co-creating innovative solutions that meet the unique needs of this patient population [40, 58]. The resulting interventions included digital tools for self-management, care coordination platforms, and community-based support networks [28]. Such solutions not only empowered the patients to effectively take part in the management of their health but

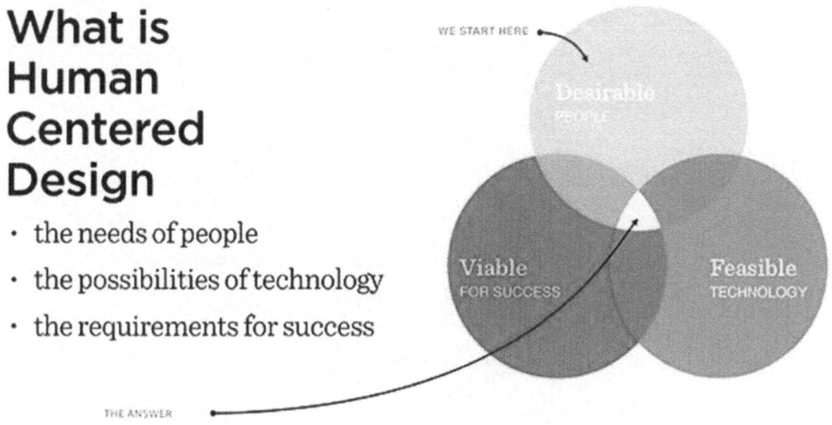


*Figure 1.4* IDEO's design thinking methodology supports innovative solutions to global challenges.

also satisfied collaborative initiatives among the care teams, with regard to healthier individuals moving forward with lower costs in the facility's healthcare system [68, 74].

The success of healthcare comes from individual organizations to concerted activities that are taking place between them. Stanford Medicine X provides a platform that brings patients, providers, designers, and technologists into co-creation of patient-centred solutions through design thinking workshops and hackathons. It has enabled interdisciplinary engagement and innovation, leading to several changing healthcare innovations like mHealth apps and wearable devices by Stanford Medicine X [72].

The design thinking approach to these cases represents how healthcare can see patient-oriented innovation, care delivery process transformation, and increased collaboration among stakeholders. Human-centred design and rapid prototyping have to be embraced in order to bring forth solutions that are relevant and acceptable to the patient and the providers themselves.

## 1.4 INTEGRATING EMERGING TECHNOLOGIES INTO DESIGN THINKING

The areas of design thinking and emerging technologies have recently merged, creating substantial potential to innovate and transform the delivery of healthcare. This section shows how healthcare organizations can leverage emerging technologies with a design thinking framework to take on complex problems and improve the outcomes of their patients (Figure 1.5).

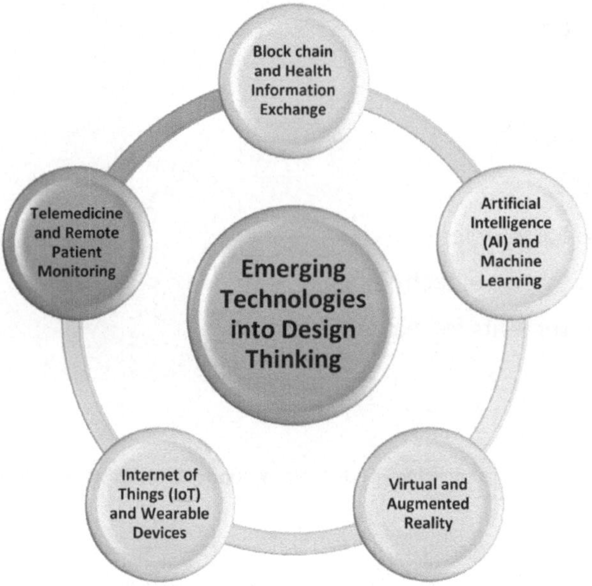


*Figure 1.5* Emerging technologies in design thinking.

### 1.4.1 Artificial intelligence (AI) and machine learning

It has been said that with the advent of cwhanges that can potentially be induced by artificial intelligence (AI) technologies, automation in healthcare for predicting patient outcomes and personalizing treatment plans can be done [57]. Mechanical integration provided by the solution also offers the ability to have decision-making guided based on data insights to improve patient experiences and optimize care delivery workflows [47, 48].

The central enabling factor for which AI is introduced to the mechanics of the solution for enabling design thinking processes is to leverage data-driven insights. AI algorithms can process large amounts of healthcare data—from electronic health records to medical imaging scans—and generate some patterns and meaningful trends [46]. With AI-powered analytics embedded at the design level, organizations obtain deeper insights into patient needs, preferences, and behaviours—critical to more human-centric and efficient development of solutions for healthcare [23].

AI-driven technologies enable predictive analytics, with which one can know in advance what may be a possible outcome with a patient, having identified all potential risks and complications early before their actual occurrence [15]. If predictive analytics and modelling are interwoven into design thinking, it allows the organization to proactively identify opportunities where one can intervene and optimize resource allocation in order to improve patient outcomes. For instance, predictive analytics

*Table 1.2* AI and ML in healthcare

| *Aspect* | *Description* |
|---|---|
| Potential of AI in healthcare | AI can automate tasks, predict patient outcomes, and provide customized treatment plans. |
| Data-driven insights | AI algorithms analyze healthcare data to extract meaningful patterns that inform tailored and effective solutions. |
| Predictive analytics | AI facilitates predictive modelling, anticipating the outcome of patients, so as to identify risks and optimize resource allocation for better patient outcomes. |
| Personalized treatment plans | The analysis AI will do on patient data will provide personalized recommendation concerning treatments, medications, and lifestyle interventions. |
| Automation of routine tasks | AI automates administrative tasks, smoothing workflows and freeing the time of health providers to focus on highly complex, value-added activities. |
| Enhancing patient experiences | AI-driven technologies support patient experiences by informing decision-making and optimizing the care delivery workflow. |
| Revolutionizing healthcare | AI integration into design thinking can change health delivery through the use of data insights, predictive analytics, personalization, and automation. |
| Human-centred approach | AI-driven design thinking contextualizes needs and preference implications of patients, transforming the future of healthcare. |

can help healthcare providers to identify the cases of high-risk readmission or those patients who may have some complications. Such targeted interventions could be done in such a way that the event could be prevented [70, 74].

Beyond that, AI can treat with an increased level of specificity, factoring more patient characteristics and preferences in treatment than ever before possible [6]. Patient data is analyzed by AI algorithms, allowing for the prescription of a treatment plan down to the most granular level of medication dosages, lifestyle changes, and which treatment options are most appropriate. The use of AI in personalization can finally take the overburden of mental iteration by care providers using design thinking to develop care plans that are patient-centred, focusing on individual need and circumstance bound to that person.

AI can thus automate routine activities and workflows, letting healthcare providers focus their efforts on more complex and value-adding jobs in their areas of practice or specialty [50]. Automating the documentation process, data entry, administration workload, and scheduling of appointments with the power of AI technologies in healthcare will enable proper care processes and time management. By this advancement in the use of AI, human health professionals will have time to interact in person, give personal care, and address the needs of a specific patient [5].

Combining AI technologies with the processes of design thinking is going to lead to a change in the healthcare delivery. Insights driven by data, predictive analytics, personalized treatment planning, and workflow automation could work in concert to perfect patient experience, workflows, and ultimately patient outcomes. This AI-driven human-centred approach of design thinking will transform the future of healthcare [67, 77].

### 1.4.2 Virtual and augmented reality (VR/AR)

Virtual reality (VR) and augmented reality (AR) technologies have exceptionally high experience capacity, allowing for full binding and interaction up to the extent they hold the highest promise to revolutionize several aspects of how healthcare is delivered: patient engagement, education, surgical planning, and rehabilitation [30]. In doing so, the technology will enable the experiencing of three-dimensional digital content and blur the line between a real and virtual experience [20].

In patient education, applications of virtual and augmented realities are tools that may be used in the presentation of happening medical matters in a friendly way to patients. In this instance, therefore, virtual representations of the anatomy of the body, medical procedures, and health conditions allow a view that the patient can use in understanding their diagnosis and making a rightful choice of treatment. For example, through VR simulations, the patient can understand how different modalities of treatment or lifestyle alterations could impact health outcomes and thus be better placed to make informed decisions about their care [54].

VR and AR technologies offer critical surgical planning and simulation software that provide visualization of anatomy in three dimensions to help surgeons. Inclusion of patient-specific data like medical images in the VR/AR model has the ability to give surgeons very deep insight into the anatomical structures of a patient before surgery. With this, surgeons is also alerted to many critical scenarios that may arise during the surgery. Such presurgical visualization culminates in overall better surgical outcomes with fewer complications.

The literature indicates the implications of VR and AR applications for rehabilitation and physical therapy. Virtual and augmented realities included in the rehabilitation work stimulate the patient by letting them deal with real-life situations and exercise, hence increasing personal motivation and adherence. Software that would allow additional gamification aspects of VR/AR rehabilitation programs could be developed, as well as the implementation of individual feedback, in order to make these programs more engaging and effective.

It furthermore explores new realms of co-creation for innovative solutions and experiences between healthcare organizations and end users through the integration of VR and AR technologies into the design thinking framework. The methodology guarantees an approach based on empathy, collaboration, and iteration. This application will allow for the development of applications that are more patient-, caregiver-, and provider-oriented in the realm of VR and AR. Sensitive user experiences could be crafted with VR/AR experience refining through iterative prototyping and testing that includes user feedback for the characteristics of accessibility, user convenience, and preference—it will ideally contain the potential reality-user characteristics [51].

### 1.4.3 Internet of Things (IoT) and wearable devices

Continuous real-time monitoring of patient statistics, medication usage, and activity levels is now provided by wearable technologies and IoT devices in healthcare, thus availing valuable insights into the status and behaviour of patient health [2].

IoT and wearables can be integrated into design thinking processes in the activities surrounding healthcare, developing connected health solutions enabling patients to become more proactive in managing their health. Design thinking methodologies are empathetic, collaborative, and iterative, allowing an organization to co-create end-user solutions that meet all of their needs and preferences. This is mainly accomplished through iteratively prototyping and user-testing IoT and wearable solutions, and based on feedback, organizations can refine them to still be intuitive and user-friendly, yet serve goals meaningful to patients [66].

In healthcare, another paramount benefit of IoT and wearables is their support for remote monitoring. A patient can have connected devices for continuous monitoring of health metrics such as pulse, blood pressure, and glucose level. Such real-time data can easily be communicated to the healthcare provider to ensure patients can be continuously monitored from remote areas, with possible timely interventions in case of emergencies or abnormalities. The remote monitoring capabilities in most cases form part of the design thinking process in developing solutions that increase patient engagement, better the coordination of care, and lead to a more personalized and proactive activation of care services delivery.

Additionally, health practitioners can use IoT and wearables to make decisions founded on the data for the best care for their patients, where comprehensive and long-term patient background data are available. In analyzing these trends and patterns in patient health metrics over time, it's also possible to look at potential upcoming risks, disease progression, or treatment plans that will meet patients' individual needs [17]. Design thinking methodologies can assist in designing user-friendly interfaces and decision support tools for organizations using IoT and wearable data, which allow providers to make appropriate care decisions.

*Table 1.3* Internet of Things (IoT) and wearable devices in healthcare

| *Key component* | *Benefits and applications* |
|---|---|
| Continuous monitoring | The vital signs, intake of medicines, and activities are monitored in real time, which gives insight into the health status and behaviours. |
| Connected health solutions | Empower patients for self-management of their conditions through the adoption of IoT and wearables as healthcare solutions through design thinking processes. |
| Empathy and collaboration | Empathy, collaboration, and iterations are central to design thinking methodologies; thus, they will allow co-creation of solutions with end users that fit their needs and preferences. |
| Iterative prototyping | Refine IoT and wearable solutions in line with user feedback to make them intuitive and user-friendly for the benefit of patients. |
| Remote monitoring | Allow for continuous monitoring of health metrics to allow healthcare providers to remotely monitor and intervene if necessary. |
| Enhanced patient engagement | Help integrate remote monitoring in design thinking processes to result in solutions for better patient engagement, coordination in care, and proactive healthcare delivery. |
| Data-driven care decisions | This will provide holistic, longitudinal information about patients, thereby enabling risk profiling, mapping of disease progress, and personalization of treatment. |
| User-friendly interfaces | Design thinking for interfaces and decision support tools to be used. by the provider to know which care decisions to derive from IoT and wearables data. |

### 1.4.4 Telemedicine and remote patient monitoring

Specifically, among the leading issues for modern healthcare, telemedicine platforms and remote patient monitoring technologies have allowed virtual consultations, remote diagnostics, and help with chronic diseases [35]. These technologies have brought patients closer to healthcare providers, allowing them to access these services from the convenience and comfort of their homes, a benefit for those who are far away from their provider or have mobility constraints.

Design thinking methodologies are valuable contributors to reimagining patient and provider experiences with telemedicine and remote patient monitoring. The emphasis on empathy [35], collaboration, and iteration with design thinking allows organizations to co-design solutions with final users that, in principle, could satisfy their needs and preferences [48]. A human-centred approach allows the user experience, accessibility, and usability to take a front-seat approach in the development of telemedicine platforms and technologies for remote monitoring.

The patient experience can be fully reimagined with design thinking for benefits to apply in telemedicine. Knowing the special needs and challenges that patients have when they engage in virtual consultations, organizations can then design friendly interfaces and workflows that increase engagement and satisfaction. Design thinking methodologies, for example, can support the development of an intuitive scheduling system, secure messaging between providers and patients, and virtual waiting rooms that feel as close as possible to an in-person visit.

Design thinking can be used to ensure that telemedicine design is optimized to make the provider experience seamless in workflows and enhance communication. Health providers in an organizational design strategy ensure the practice of design thinking to identify the pain areas and current inefficiencies in the organizational telemedicine workflow for the development of solutions in a co-creation model of innovation [52]. For example, a design thinking approach could guide the development of integrated electronic health record (EHR) systems, telemedicine platforms, and clinical decision support tools that ensure agility in communication and in the documentation of information.

Design thinking can help to ensure the seamless integration of the telemedicine platforms with other remote patient monitoring technologies in the clinical practice [48]. With the help of staff at the frontlines, organizations can be able to identify opportunities for integrating telemedicine along already existing care paths and fine-tuning the work in a manner that ensures seamless patient-care delivery [41]. User feedback is taken to refine telemedicine solutions and ensure they meet the requirements of patients and providers by conducting iterative prototyping and user testing.

### 1.4.5 Blockchain and health information exchange

Blockchain technology is very promising for revolutionizing the way health information is exchanged and has a lot of aspects, including being a secure, decentralized, and immutable platform for storage and exchanging electronic health records. Blockchain technology inherently displays features such as cryptographic hashing, consensus mechanisms, and smart contracts [21]; it, therefore, inherently ensures integrity, security, and interoperability in the care data and hence solves the challenges that have been conventionally suffered by healthcare data management.

Design thinking approaches play a great role in co-designing blockchain-based solutions that empower patients, streamline administrative processes, and reach patient-centred care. Intentional stakeholder engagement with patients, healthcare providers, policymakers, and technologists helps organizations build solutions that truly meet the needs of end users and alleviate pain points [49].

Some of the benefits that result from design thinking applied in blockchain for healthcare include the ability to empower patients, thereby giving them control over health data. Through the decentralized architecture of blockchain, aided by cryptographic techniques, it becomes possible

*Table 1.4* Blockchain and health information exchange in healthcare

| *Key feature* | *Benefits and applications* |
|---|---|
| Blockchain characteristics | Offers an adequately secure, decentralized, immutable platform for the storage and sharing of EHRs. |
| Cryptographic hashing | This helps ensure data integrity and security using cryptographic techniques. |
| Consensus mechanisms | It ensures integrity and consistency of data over the blockchain network. |
| Smart contracts | It automates and enforces the contractual agreements between the parties for every healthcare transaction, increasing efficiency and transparency. |
| Patient empowerment | It helps patients to view, manage, and share their health data in a very safe environment, thus it provides huge control for the owner over the data. |
| User-friendly interfaces | Design thinking helps develop intuitive interfaces for patient consent management and data access. |
| Streamlining administrative processes | Optimizes workflows, enables better interoperability, and automates some manual processes to reduce administrative overhead and improve efficiency. |
| Secure EHR sharing | Facilitate sharing of EHRs between providers, payers, and any authorized person securely yet efficiently to enhance the coordination of care. |
| Stakeholder involvement | It involves users, providers, policymakers, and technologists to design solutions that exactly meet user needs and pain points. |
| Iterative prototyping | Refines blockchain solutions according to the feedback received from users; makes sure that they serve diverse stakeholders. |

to safely access patients' records and manage them by themselves and, if needed, share them with healthcare providers and other parties with authorized access [7]. Design thinking methodologies could usefully inform the user-friendly and dreary consent management interfaces in the development of such systems and thereby empower patients with more control over their health information.

Design thinking can make healthcare administrative processes way more efficient and interoperable. This is possible through engaging healthcare administrators and policymakers in the process, spotting the most apt opportunities for blockchain technology to integrate with existing infrastructure, and implementing solutions to automate manual processes. For example, design thinking can guide the development of blockchain-based solutions for claims processing, credentialing, and supply chain management, thus bringing down the administrative overhead while improving efficiency [53, 59, 61, 62].

Design thinking can also enable the safe sharing of EHRs among stakeholders for better collaboration and coordination in care. It can guide organizations to co-design interoperable blockchain solutions that ensure safety and efficiency in the flow of health data shared among providers, payers, and other authorized parties. Iterative prototyping and user testing will help fine-tune blockchain-based solutions according to user feedback and ensure organizational needs across a diversity of stakeholders [55, 56].

New technologies in design thinking bring additional innovation, collaboration, and patient-centred care opportunities to healthcare organizations. Iterative prototyping enables testing with users for continuous improvement in developing technology-enabled solutions that help meet evolving needs of patients, providers, and healthcare systems [78].

## 1.5 ETHICAL CONSIDERATIONS IN DESIGN THINKING FOR HEALTHCARE

Ethical considerations play a huge role in implementing methodologies of design thinking in healthcare. Therefore, while organizations work toward innovation and change in health using human-centred design, such efforts should keep in focus considerations of ethics and gauge ways that demands of the patient, or other stakeholders, can be met, respecting their well-being (Figure 1.6).

One important ethical consideration is the protection of patient privacy and confidentiality. In most cases, the design thinking process involves the collection of sensitive data or information from the patients to be used in the development of healthcare solutions. Organizations should, therefore, devise appropriate security measures regarding data and adhere to the provisions regarding data protection under regulation so as to prevent unauthorized access or disclosure.

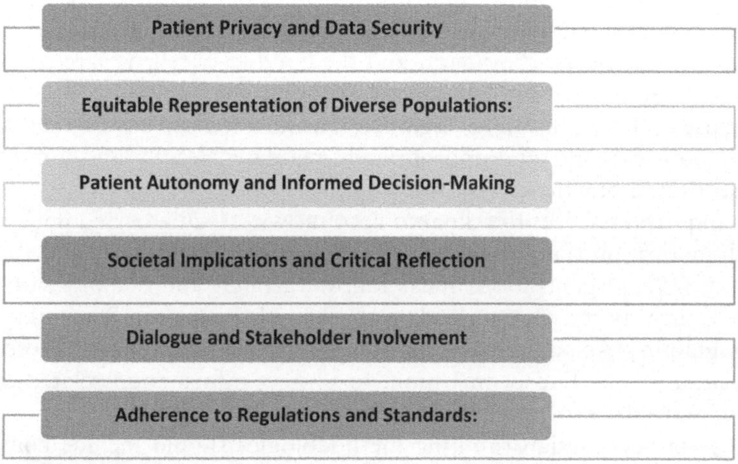


*Figure 1.6* Ethical considerations in design thinking for healthcare.

Another ethical point is the fair representation of diverse patient populations in the design process. There remain many healthcare disparities across various demographic groups, such as race, ethnicity, gender, socioeconomic status, and geographic location. Design thinking methodologies should aim at including richer perspectives and experiences in the process of solving healthcare challenges to ensure an inclusive, culturally sensitive and accessible approach toward all patients.

Organizations should consider such potential for changes in healthcare innovations that influence patient autonomy and decision-making. Although design thinking empowers the patient and increases involvement in healthcare decision-making, individuals have different levels of health literacy, technological literacy, and autonomy. The articulation of healthcare solutions could be designed in a manner that considers the level of autonomy, preferences, and values of the patient for them to make informed choices regarding their care.

At worst, ethical considerations also transcend to issues that might have more social relevance than the products of health innovation using design thinking [79]. Consideration of potential risks and benefits initiated by implementing a new technology or process in general will be for the implementing organizations to consider costs, resource allocation, and social justice in healthcare. Design thinking approaches should include critical reflection among stakeholders and dialogue toward the assessment of potential healthcare innovations and potential harms.

## 1.6 REGULATORY COMPLIANCE AND STANDARDS IN HEALTHCARE INNOVATION

At the root of health innovation, key attributes must be always considered: how to maintain regulatory compliance and standards adherence to ensure the safety of patients, their data, and the good to excellent care provided. In developing pioneering new healthcare solutions, including through the active use of design thinking, organizations now look to ensure such a process is both complex and appropriately regulated legally and among the industry's best practices.

An important aspect to take into account with regulatory compliance in health innovation is to ensure the regulations concerning data privacy and security [29]. Organizations must follow through and comply with provisions, such as those contained in the Health Insurance Portability and Accountability Act in the United States or the General Data Protection Regulation in the European Union, to protect information related to the patient and ensure its availability, integrity, and confidentiality (Figure 1.7). The use of such design thinking methodologies should include considerations for privacy and security right at the beginning of the process to add

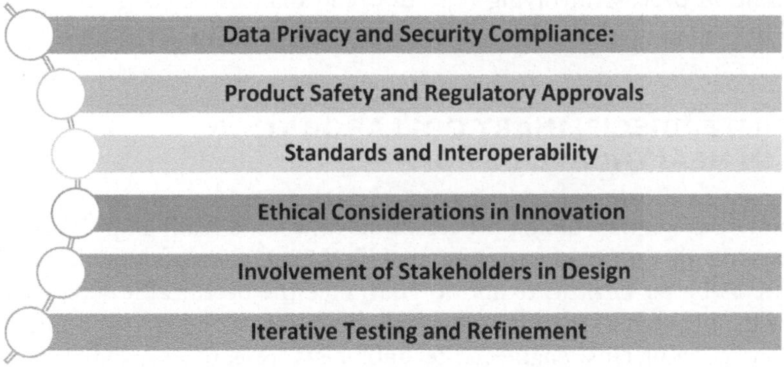


*Figure 1.7* Important points for implementing regulatory compliance and standards.

preventive mechanisms and ensure risk mitigation associated with breaches and unauthorized access.

These healthcare innovations need to comply with regulatory standards ensuring the safety and the efficacy of the product, mainly in the case of medical devices and digital health solutions [3, 81]. Organizations that come up with healthcare-related products or service innovations—be it directly related to patients, doctors, or medical centres—need to have approvals from regulators like the Food and Drug Administration (FDA) in the US or the European Medicines Agency (EMA) in the European Union. Iterative testing and refinement of solutions to address concerns regarding regulatory issues mean the end-user involvement within the design process; therefore, design thinking lays down the pathway in developing products that ensure safety and functioning for end patients.

Organizations integrating EHR systems must look for the standards and interoperability needs that will guarantee that the EHR implementation fits into the present healthcare systems and their workflows seamlessly. For example, Health Level 7 (HL7) is a standard for exchanging data, whereas Digital Imaging and Communications in Medicine (DICOM) is a standard for transferring, viewing, and storing medical images in the interoperations among healthcare ITs. Designing solutions that fit into the already established health systems and their workflows can be achieved through a design thinking approach, which encompasses all stakeholders of the varied backgrounds and specializations associated with the designing process of the solutions.

This also extends to compliance with ethical considerations such as informed consent, patient autonomy, and professional ethics [19]. Designers of health innovations must, therefore, ensure that their solutions respect ethical principles and the dignity and rights of the patients to whom they apply. Design thinking skills can facilitate the determination of ethics in the innovation process involving reflection and dialogue among stakeholders and the incorporation of ethical considerations into the design process.

## 1.7 INTERDISCIPLINARY COLLABORATION IN HEALTHCARE DESIGN

An interdisciplinary design process in healthcare is really important. This brings together a workforce of many with the intention of designing for the future to better healthcare and to guarantee the best health outcomes for patients. Benchmarking a design for health in interdisciplinary cooperation is done by clinicians, engineers, technologists, researchers, and eventually with patients to bring out their clear expertise and perspectives in driving meaningful innovations inside healthcare systems.

Perhaps the most significant benefit of healthcare design through interdisciplinary cooperation is the ability to incorporate different insights and knowledge. The interdisciplinary nature furthers creativity and innovation by possibly questioning convention and pushing limits in search of the different possibility windows for healthcare delivery [45]. Organizations will learn various aspects of healthcare from interdisciplinary professionals, including clinical practice, technology, human factors, and patient preferences.

Interdisciplinary collaboration allows a holistic approach to problem solving and solution development. Health challenges often have many dimensions to them, requiring comprehensive solutions from both a clinical and technological, social, and environmental perspective. The interdisciplinary teams can bring in their aggregated knowledge and skills together to appraise the complex problem from multiple dimensions (Figure 1.8). Through this, they develop solutions that are effective, feasible, and sustainable in real-world settings.

Interdisciplinary practice allows the building of partnerships for co-creation with end users, such as patients, informal carers, and healthcare professionals. This collaboration allows an organization to commit to and

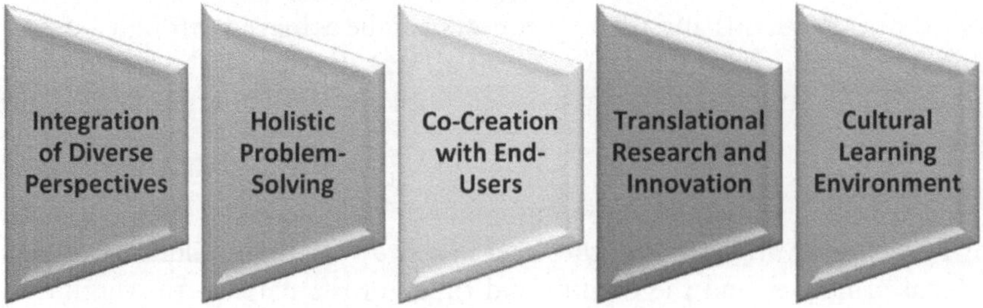


*Figure 1.8* Interdisciplinary collaboration design process in healthcare design.

sustain stakeholders, ensuring health solutions are user-centred and responsive to patient needs and preferences are aligned with clinical workflows. Such a participative approach in the design process creates empathy, trust, and commitment toward the implementation of novel solutions in healthcare settings.

Additionally, interdisciplinary collaboration and work are propelling the translational research movement, which seeks to transform healthcare in general [27]. Interdisciplinary teams bridge the research, practice, and policy worlds in order to allow scientific findings and new innovations to be channelled into benefits for patients and communities. Such innovation-led, translation-driven advancements enforce the evidence-based implementation of practices and intervention methods in clinical settings.

Interdisciplinary collaboration breeds a culture of learning, continuous improvement, and professional development [9]. Healthcare professionals, through their interdisciplinary collaboration, learn about other disciplines' perspectives, methods, and approaches that help in enriching their knowledge and skills. Collaboration encourages critical thinking, reflection, and innovation in healthcare, augmenting quality, delivery, and outcomes. In simple words, the precondition for meaningful innovation to affect the design of healthcare is interdisciplinary collaboration. When professional expertise is combined with the diverse multi-perspective of each participant, it should hence allow companies to be better placed in assisting their clients in addressing complicated health challenges, creating user-centred solutions, driving translational research, and maintaining a learning culture in the environment of improvement. Interdisciplinary collaboration has the power and potential to transform healthcare and drive improved patient outcomes within this increasingly complex, dynamic environment.

## 1.8 IMPLEMENTING DESIGN THINKING: STRATEGIES AND BEST PRACTICES

Design thinking in healthcare is a way of solving human-centred problems through step-by-step, iterative problem-solving activities so that all stakeholders are involved. Figure 1.3 illustrates the strategies and best practices, also discussed next, in implementing design thinking for health settings:

- Leadership support: Leaders should support a culture of innovation and design thinking in an organization. Leadership support will help set priorities for the allocation of resources and even ways to get over resistance to change (Figure 1.9).
- Cross-functional teams: Build interdisciplinary teams of clinicians, designers, engineers, technologists, and—where appropriate—patients.

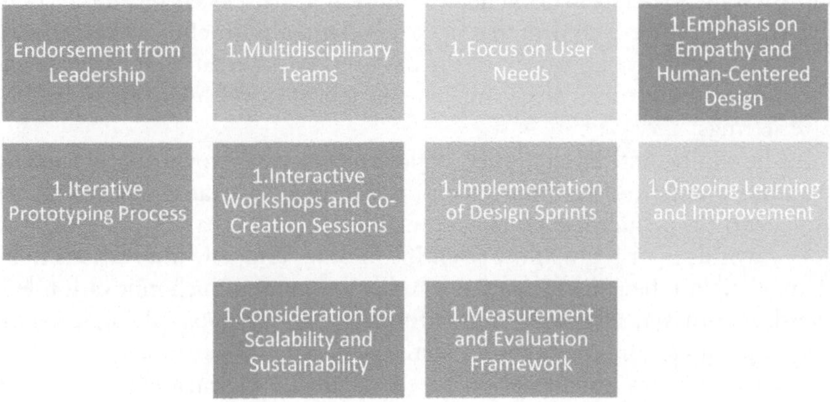


*Figure 1.9* Strategies and best practices for effectively implementing design thinking in healthcare settings.

They operate at the intersection of varied approaches and solutions to complex health problems.

- User-centred approach: Ensure that user needs and preferences and the user experience are the top priority during design. This knowledge comes from the patients, the caregivers, and the healthcare providers. Conduct user research through interviews and observations to better understand their needs and pain points.
- Empathy and human-centred design: Instil an empathic attitude towards end users by immersing team members in their environments and experiences. Human-centred design principles emphasize understanding the emotions, motivations, and behaviours of end users to develop solutions that resonate with their needs and aspirations.
- Iterative prototyping: Develop a culture of experiment with iterations through a rapid prototyping approach, with early and constant feedback from users. This way, with iterative prototyping, teams can test and validate their assumptions, thus shaping the solution in a user-centric way to make the design more effective for users.
- Collaborative workshops and co-creation sessions: Organize interactive workshops and co-creation sessions where stakeholders could come up with ideas, explore new opportunities, co-design solutions, and hence be in an innovative mood. This can be done through engagement with team members so that active participation, creativity, and an open mind combine in the process of ideation, which supports innovation.
- Design sprints: Introduce design sprints, which involve time-boxed sessions built to solve particular, defined problems or challenges within just a number of days. Such sprints will often have a structured approach of activities including problem framing, ideation,

prototyping, and testing in the indulgence of providing accelerated design capable of driving actionable insights.

- Continuous learning and improvement: Create a forum for a habitual culture of continuous learning and improvement for the reflection of every task and feedback, through sharing knowledge among members of the team. Ensure that failure is taken as a source of learning and growth, whereas success and milestones are celebrated.
- Scalability and sustainability: Create strategies to scale and sustain design thinking within an organization. Develop a framework, tools, and processes to embed design thinking into current workflows and practices, and cultivate champions and advocates who will drive the adoption and momentum of design thinking [31].
- Measurement and evaluation: Define key performance indicators and metrics to track the impacts and effectiveness of the design thinking effort. Continuously measure the outputs, such as user satisfaction, adoption rates, and patient outcomes, to enable needed decisions and course corrections.

Using such strategies and best practices, healthcare organizations can fully leverage design thinking to bring innovation and improved patient experiences, providing solutions for complex health challenges.

## 1.9 FUTURE DIRECTIONS: TRENDS AND OPPORTUNITIES IN HEALTHCARE INNOVATION

The future of innovation in healthcare is the new and emerging trends and opportunities, which have tremendous potential for changing care delivery, improving patient outcomes, and tackling new healthcare challenges (Figure 1.10). Embracing these trends, leveraging technological advancement within the healthcare ecosystem, allows a shift toward innovative and transformational care.

The salient trend is that most patients are already using digital health technologies and telemedicine. Telemedicine overall experienced rapid growth—a booster was the COVID-19 pandemic [35, 80, 82]. This trend is believed to continue, as telemedicine offers the ability to extend care access, ensure better care coordination, and engage more patients in the pool of care located in rural or sparsely populated areas [1].

Artificial and machine learning are driving innovation in health workflows. AI algorithms are entering health workflows for the interpretative part of medical imaging, predictive analytics, decision support, and clinical. In that way, they will help in improving diagnostic accuracy, treatment personalization, and efficient resource usage, which will manifest in more effective and efficient healthcare service delivery [63].

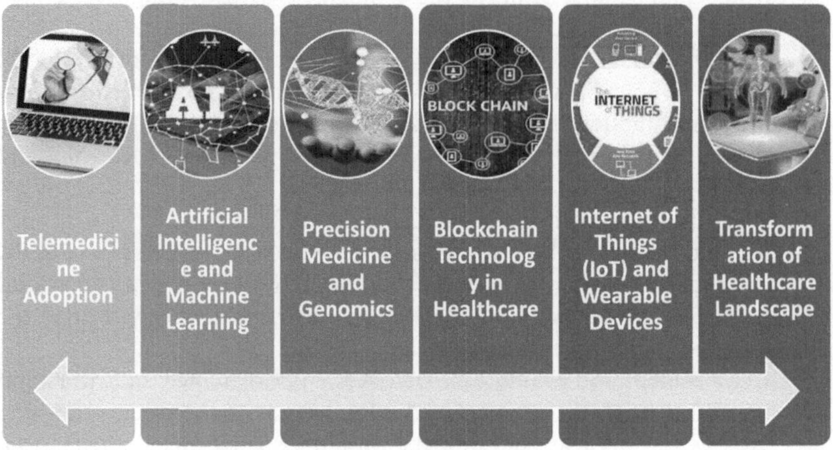


*Figure 1.10* Domains having opportunities in healthcare innovation.

Another area of great advance in the healthcare field is precision medicine and genomics. Genomic advances, biomarker identification, and molecular diagnostics have powered the development of targeted therapies and precision treatment directions [38]. Through precision medicine, costs are going down, with better results for patients and care specifically designed around each patient through the consideration of their genetic makeup, lifestyle, and environmental factors [16].

Research in the application of blockchain technology is underway to secure health information interchange. Blockchain-based solutions generally provide a basis for establishing leverage with respect toward the integrity of data, the privacy of patients, and interoperability—a way of enhancing the smoothness and efficiency of healthcare delivery. The secure sharing of electronic health records and transparent transactions provided by blockchain technology can transform healthcare data management and governance [65, 69].

The IoT and wearable sensors have revolutionized patient healthcare in that it has made it possible to monitor important health metrics, drug adherence levels, and activity patterns continuously [18]. All these make it possible for the very early detection of the onset of a disease, remote patient monitoring, enabling care tailored to the specific needs of the particular patient, to be able to self-manage better [39]. In conclusion, the future of innovation in healthcare harbours many emerging trends and opportunities that can change the way care is given and transform the outcomes of healthcare for patients. Trends in healthcare organizations can be embraced and taken up a few notches through the use of technology, thereby being innovative, increasing quality of care, and ultimately changing healthcare.

## REFERENCES


1. American Medical Association. (2021). *8 digital health trends that will shape the future of care delivery*. Retrieved from https://www.ama-assn.org/practice-management/digital/8-digital-health-trends-will-shape-future-care-delivery
2. Banaee, H., Ahmed, M. U., & Loutfi, A. (2013). Data mining for wearable sensors in health monitoring systems: A review of recent trends and challenges. *Sensors*, 13(12), 17472–17500.
3. Bashshur, R. L., Doarn, C. R., Frenk, J. M., Kvedar, J. C., Woolliscroft, J. O., & Wootton, R. (2018). Beyond the COVID pandemic, telemedicine, and health care. *Telemedicine and e-Health*, 24(5), 367–372.
4. Baxter, K. (1995). *Product design: A practical guide to systematic methods of new product development*. CRC Press.
5. Beam, A. L., & Kohane, I. S. (2018). Big data and machine learning in health care. *JAMA*, 319(13), 1317–1318.
6. Beaulieu-Jones, B. K., Orzechowski, P., Moore, J. H., & Grebe, T. A. (2018). Machine learning for patient risk stratification: standing on, or looking over, the shoulders of clinicians? *NPJ Digital Medicine*, 1(1), 1–4.
7. Benchoufi, M., & Ravaud, P. (2017). Blockchain technology for improving clinical research quality. *Trials*, 18(1), 335.
8. Birkenmaier, J., Umlas, A., & Grothaus, M. C. (2015). *Application of human-centered design to improve health system performance*. U.S. Agency for International Development.
9. Bleakley, A. (2006). Broadening conceptions of learning in medical education: the message from teamworking. *Medical Education*, 40(2), 150–157.
10. Boyd, R. W., & Fortune, J. (2021). Design thinking: A framework for diversity and inclusion in healthcare organizations. *Journal of Healthcare Management*, 66(2), 102–110.
11. Brown, T. (2008). Design thinking. *Harvard Business Review*, 86(6), 84–92.
12. Brown, T. (2009). *Change by design: How design thinking transforms organizations and inspires innovation*. Harper Business.
13. Centers for Medicare & Medicaid Services. (2021). *CMS finalizes interoperability and patient access rule to empower patients by giving them access to their health data*. Retrieved from https://www.cms.gov/newsroom/press-releases/cms-finalizes-interoperability-and-patient-access-rule-empower-patients-giving-them-access-their-health
14. Chen, J., & Schulz, P. J. (2016). The effect of information communication technology interventions on reducing social isolation in the elderly: A systematic review. *Journal of Medical Internet Research*, 18(1), e18.
15. Choi, E., Schuetz, A., Stewart, W. F., & Sun, J. (2016). Using recurrent neural network models for early detection of heart failure onset. *Journal of the American Medical Informatics Association*, 24(2), 361–370.
16. Collins, F. S., & Varmus, H. (2015). A new initiative on precision medicine. *New England Journal of Medicine*, 372(9), 793–795.
17. Coughlin, S. S. (2010). The future of medicine—The impact of technology. *Journal of the Medical Association of Georgia*, 99(4), 11–13.

18. Dagdeviren, C., Yang, B. D., Su, Y., Xia, J., & Rogers, J. A. (2017). Flexible piezoelectric devices for gastrointestinal motility sensing. *Advanced Materials Technologies*, 2(5), 1600246.
19. Dixon, M. F. (2018). Ethical considerations in health professions education research. *Journal of Allied Health*, 47(1), 57–64.
20. Dunston, R., Lee, A., & Boud, D. (2009). Interprofessional health education: A literature review. *Nurse Education Today*, 29(6), 549–555.
21. Edmondson, A. C., Bohmer, R. M., & Pisano, G. P. (2011). Disrupted routines: Team learning and new technology implementation in hospitals. *Administrative Science Quarterly*, 46(4), 685–716.
22. Epstein, R. M., & Street, R. L. (2011). The values and value of patient-centered care. *Annals of Family Medicine*, 9(2), 100–103.
23. Esteva, A., Kuprel, B., Novoa, R. A., Ko, J., Swetter, S. M., Blau, H. M., & Thrun, S. (2019). Dermatologist-level classification of skin cancer with deep neural networks. *Nature*, 542(7639), 115–118.
24. Faulkner, W. (2008). Design as a learning process: Insights from engineering design education. *Design Studies*, 29(4), 325–337.
25. Gentry, S., Craig, J., Hutchings, M., & Thwaites, H. (2019). Design thinking in health care. *Quality Management in Health Care*, 28(3), 151–155.
26. Gomes, R., Rosenfeld, L. W., Carneiro, M., & Duff, J. H. (2019). Innovation in health services: Theoretical frameworks and key themes. *Health Research Policy and Systems*, 17(1), 85.
27. Graham, I. D., Tetroe, J., & Pearson, A. (2006). *Turning knowledge into action: practical guidance on how to do integrated knowledge translation research*. Lippincott Williams & Wilkins.
28. Greenhalgh, T., Jackson, C., Shaw, S., & Janamian, T. (2016). Achieving research impact through co-creation in community-based health services: Literature review and case study. *The Milbank Quarterly*, 94(2), 392–429.
29. Halamka, J. D., & Lippman, A. (2018). *Accelerating the adoption of blockchain technology in healthcare: The Stanford medicine experience*. Stanford Medicine White Paper Series.
30. Haque, S., Sze, S. K., Ng, K. C., & Yeo, J. H. (2020). Augmented reality in surgery: The current state and applications in orthopedic surgery. *Journal of Orthopaedic Surgery*, 28(1), 2309499019898984.
31. Hasso Plattner Institute of Design at Stanford (2021). *Design thinking bootleg*. Retrieved from https://dschool.stanford.edu/resources/design-thinking-bootleg
32. Hojat, M., Gonnella, J. S., Nasca, T. J., Mangione, S., Vergare, M., & Magee, M. (2002). Physician empathy: Definition, components, measurement, and relationship to gender and specialty. *American Journal of Psychiatry*, 159(9), 1563–1569.
33. Hojat, M., Louis, D. Z., Markham, F. W., Wender, R., Rabinowitz, C., & Gonnella, J. S. (2011). Physicians' empathy and clinical outcomes for diabetic patients. *Academic Medicine*, 86(3), 359–364.
34. Hojat, M., Vergare, M., Isenberg, G., Cohen, M., Spandorfer, J., & Underwood, K. (2016). Communication skills, empathy, and well-being of medical students: A prospective study. *Academic Medicine*, 91(7), 984–990.

35. Hollander, J. E., & Carr, B. G. (2020). Virtually perfect? Telemedicine for Covid-19. *New England Journal of Medicine*, 382(18), 1679–1681.
36. IDEO. (n.d.). *Redesigning the healthcare experience for patients with chronic illnesses*. Retrieved from https://www.ideo.com/work/redesigning-the-healthcare-experience-for-patients-with-chronic-illnesses
37. IDEO.org (2021). The Field Guide to Human-Centered Design. Retrieved from https://www.designkit.org/resources/1
38. Jameson, J. L., & Longo, D. L. (2015). Precision medicine—Personalized, problematic, and promising. *New England Journal of Medicine*, 372(23), 2229–2234.
39. Jovanov, E., Milenkovic, A., Otto, C., & De Groen, P. C. (2015). A wireless body area network of intelligent motion sensors for computer assisted physical rehabilitation. *Journal of NeuroEngineering and Rehabilitation*, 2(1), 6.
40. Jünger, S., Payne, S. A., Brine, J., Radbruch, L., & Brearley, S. G. (2017). Guidance on conducting and REporting DElphi Studies (CREDES) in palliative care: Recommendations based on a methodological systematic review. *Palliative Medicine*, 31(8), 684–706.
41. Kaplan, B., & Dretler, S. (2020). Telehealth and telemedicine: Strategies for effective implementation. *Journal of Healthcare Information Management*, 34(4), 39–45.
42. Karppinen, P. (2012). A study of the concept of iterative design and its implications for the development of educational systems. *Procedia - Social and Behavioral Sciences*, 45, 266–275.
43. Kelley, D., & Kelley, T. (2013). *Creative confidence: Unleashing the creative potential within us all*. Crown Business.
44. Kelley, K., & Kelley, D. (2016). *Creative confidence: Unleashing the creative potential within us all*. Currency.
45. Kelm, Z., Womer, J., Walter, J. K., Feudtner, C., & Lantos, J. D. (2014). Interventions to cultivate physician empathy: A systematic review. *BMC Medical Education*, 14(1), 219.
46. Kim, B., Park, K., Kim, K. K., Kim, S., Park, J., & Lee, H. (2018). Deep learning in medical imaging. *Neuroimaging Clinics of North America*, 28(1), 11–24.
47. Kim, S. S., Kaplowitz, S., & Johnston, M. V. (2004). The effects of physician empathy on patient satisfaction and compliance. *Evaluation & the Health Professions*, 27(3), 237–251.
48. Kim, Y. E., & Kim, Y. (2018). Design thinking for wearable devices: Case study of a wearable fitness tracker. *International Journal of Design*, 12(1), 1–18.
49. Kuo, T. T., Kim, H. E., & Ohno-Machado, L. (2017). Blockchain distributed ledger technologies for biomedical and health care applications. *Journal of the American Medical Informatics Association*, 24(6), 1211–1220.
50. Lyu, Y., Zhang, Y., Hu, X., & Su, Y. (2019). Exploring the potential of deep learning and its applications in oncology. *IEEE Access*, 7, 73020–73034.
51. Ma, M., Fallavollita, P., & Seelbach, I. (2020). Virtual reality and augmented reality in surgery: Challenges and opportunities. *Medical & Biological Engineering & Computing*, 58(5), 1073–1080.

52. Meng, Q. (2020). Applying design thinking in telemedicine service design. *International Journal of Design*, 14(2), 109–124.
53. Mettler, M. (2016). *Blockchain technology in healthcare: The revolution starts here*. Proceedings of the 2016 IEEE 18th International Conference on e-Health Networking, Applications and Services (Healthcom), pp. 1–3. IEEE.
54. Muller, M. J. (2009). Participatory design: The third space in HCI. In J. A. Jacko & A. Sears (Eds.), *The human-computer interaction handbook: Fundamentals, evolving technologies and emerging applications* (pp. 1051–1068). CRC Press.
55. Nie, X., Zhang, A., Chen, J., Qu, Y., & Yu, S. (2022). Blockchain-empowered secure and privacy-preserving health data sharing in edge-based IoMT. *Security and Communication Networks*. https://doi.org/10.1155/2022/8293716.
56. Nishi, F. K., Khan, M. M., Alsufyani, A., Bourouis, S., Gupta, P., & Saini, D. K. (2022). Electronic healthcare data record security using blockchain and smart contract. *Journal of Sensors*. https://doi.org/10.1155/2022/7299185.
57. Obermeyer, Z., & Emanuel, E. J. (2016). Predicting the future—Big data, machine learning, and clinical medicine. *New England Journal of Medicine*, 375(13), 1216–1219.
58. Obermeyer, Z., Powers, B., Vogeli, C., & Mullainathan, S. (2019). Dissecting racial bias in an algorithm used to manage the health of populations. *Science*, 366(6464), 447–453.
59. Palmiero, A. J., Bien, Z., Tkacz, N., & Norrie, J. (2019). The role of blockchain technology in medical imaging. *Journal of Digital Imaging*, 32(1), 18–26.
60. Plattner, H., Meinel, C., & Leifer, L. (2010). *Design thinking: Understand – improve – apply*. Springer.
61. Rahmani, M. K. I., Shuaib, M., Alam, S., Siddiqui, S. T., Ahmad, S., & Bhatia, S. (2022). Blockchain-based trust management framework for cloud computing-based internet of medical things (IoMT): A systematic review. *Computational Intelligence and Neuroscience*. https://doi.org/10.1155/2022/9766844.
62. Rajasekaran, A. S., & Azees, M. (2022). An anonymous blockchain-based authentication scheme for secure healthcare applications. *Security and Communication Networks*. https://doi.org/10.1155/2022/2793116.
63. Rajkomar, A., Oren, E., Chen, K., Dai, A. M., Hajaj, N., Hardt, M., ... Dean, J. (2018). Scalable and accurate deep learning with electronic health records. *NPJ Digital Medicine*, 1(1), 1–10.
64. Ries, E. (2011). *The lean startup: How today's entrepreneurs use continuous innovation to create radically successful businesses*. Crown Business.
65. Saeed, H., Malik, H., Bashir, U., Ahmad, A., Riaz, S., Ilyas, M., & Khan, M. I. A. (2022). Blockchain technology in healthcare: A systematic review. *PLoS One*, 17(4). https://doi.org/10.1371/journal.pone.0265207.
66. Sankar, S. V., Subramanian, R., & Ramkumar, P. (2019). *IoT in healthcare: Design thinking framework for healthcare 4.0*. Proceedings of the International Conference on Computing Methodologies and Communication, pp. 182–185. IEEE.

67. Saria, S., & Subbaswamy, A. (2019). *Tutorial: Safe and reliable machine learning in healthcare*. Proceedings of the 25th ACM SIGKDD International Conference on Knowledge Discovery & Data Mining, pp. 441–442. IEEE.
68. Shanafelt, T. D., Bradley, K. A., Wipf, J. E., & Back, A. L. (2005). Burnout and self-reported patient care in an internal medicine residency program. *Annals of Internal Medicine*, 142(4), 10.7326/0003-4819-142-4-200502150-00009.
69. Sharma, V., Gupta, A., Hasan, N. U., Shabaz, M., & Ofori, I. (2022). *Blockchain in secure healthcare systems: State of the art, limitations, and future directions*. Security and Communication Networks. https://doi.org/10.1155/2022/9697545.
70. Singh, K., & Gans, N. (2017). *AI-based predictive analytics holds the promise of revolutionizing patient flow*. NEJM Catalyst. Retrieved from https://catalyst.nejm.org/ai-predictive-analytics-patient-flow/
71. Srivastava, P., Hopkinson, G. C., & Chen, M. A. (2015). Design thinking: a human-centered approach to innovation. *International Journal of Engineering Pedagogy*, 5(3), 1–22.
72. Stanford Medicine X. (n.d.). *Medicine X | CHANGE*. Retrieved from https://medicinex.stanford.edu/
73. Thompson, C. (2009). Interdisciplinary research: Where to from here? *Journal of Interprofessional Care*, 23(3), 219–221.
74. Topol, E. J. (2019). High-performance medicine: The convergence of human and artificial intelligence. *Nature Medicine*, 25(1), 44–56.
75. Ulrike, H. (2018). Retrieved from https://globalwa.org/2018/04/how-ideos-design-thinking-methodology-supports-innovative-solutions-to-global-challenges
76. Van Gogh, C. D., Yassine, A., & Braziotis, C. (2018). An integrative framework of design thinking and agile for innovative information systems development. *International Journal of Information Management*, 38(1), 184–196.
77. Vermeulen, J., Verweij, M., & Dechesne, F. (2018). Ethical issues in personalized medicine: A systematic literature review. *Personalized Medicine*, 15(5), 457–467.
78. Wang, H., Song, S., Zhai, E., & Zheng, L. (2020). Blockchain-based data preservation system for electronic medical records. *Journal of Medical Systems*, 44(6), 115.
79. Wong, C. A., & Osterwalder, J. J. (2020). Ethical implications of design thinking in healthcare innovation. *Nursing Ethics*, 27(5), 1123–1133.
80. Wootton, R. (2020). Telemedicine from the arctic. *Journal of Telemedicine and Telecare*, 26(1–2), 3–5.
81. World Health Organization. (2020). *Digital health*. Retrieved from https://www.who.int/westernpacific/health-topics/digital-health
82. World Health Organization. (2021). *Telemedicine: Opportunities and developments in Member States: Report on the second global survey on eHealth*. Retrieved from https://www.who.int/news-room/detail/19-01-2010-telemedicine-opportunities-and-developments-in-member-states.

Chapter 2

# Next-gen health analytics

## Meta-heuristic bi-clustering of gene expression data with k-means

*Biswajit Jana, Bireshwar Dass Mazumdar, Anindya Ghatak, and Ram Gopal Gupta*

### 2.1 INTRODUCTION

High throughput technologies are being used to investigate the core mechanism of complex diseases and the identification of disease associations. It helps to improve the treatment of patients. DNA is the most vital component of the biological unit as it transfers genetic knowledge to the next generations. Thus, understanding DNA functions will provide a deeper knowledge of the mechanism of biological units. Protein-coded segments of DNA are referred to as genes. Genes consist of many unknown or complicated biological functions. Microarray technology [1, 2] can generate a massive volume of highly spatial expression values of genes. The fundamental rule behind DNA microarray is to bind integral sequences. Figure 2.1 represents the structure of DNA, and Figure 2.2 is the representation of a microarray.

To identify the gene functions and to recognize the backend mechanism of diseases, microarrays play a vital role. An in-depth utility was also provided by microarray technology in medication or drug finding research. Drugs are the combinations of some chemical substance applied for remedy, therapy or to prevent biological disorders. Microarrays help in drug discovery through monitoring adjustments in gene expression in response to drug treatment. Integration of genomic data in yeast and humans is helping in defining gene-related diseases.

In human genetics, the number of human disease-related gene variants is increasing due to advancements in next-generation sequencing technologies. Identifying precise genes that are the main cause of a disease is a significant challenge. Growing evidence suggests that model organisms are extremely important for addressing this issue. *Saccharomyces cerevisiae* (yeast) is very helpful in achieving the objectives of genomic studies. *S. cerevisiae* is a valuable model organism for understanding human genetic variability because of its genetic tractability. In the current work, we demonstrate how yeast has been used to study variants of various genes, highlighting the multifaceted capability of this model organism. By analyzing the gene expression data, similar genes and their functions can be discovered by recognizing the relationship between the nature of the condition

 DOI: 10.1201/9781003634089-2

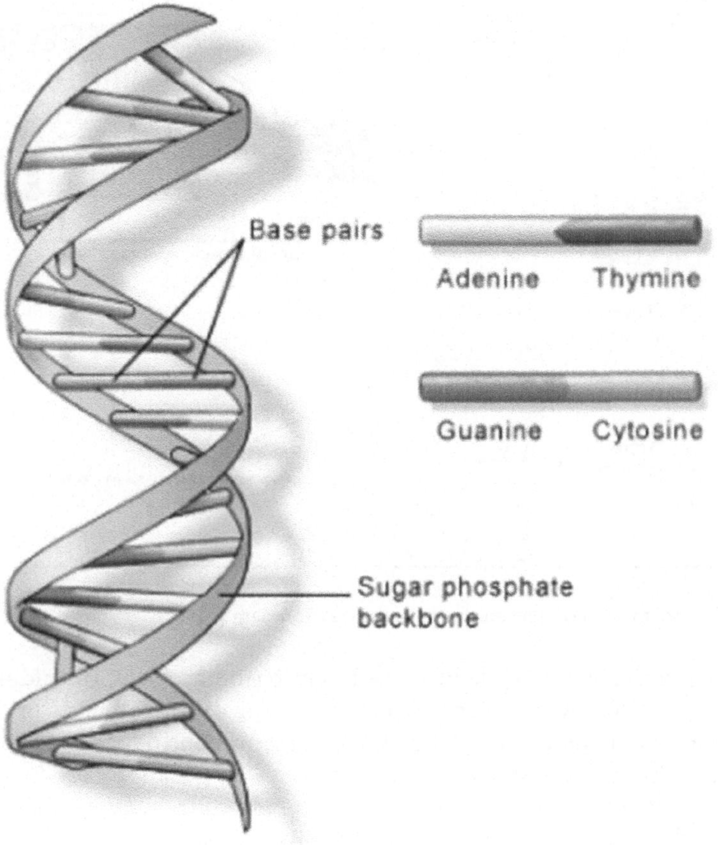


*Figure 2.1* Representation of DNA structure.

and the genes. However, to gain accurate biological understanding is a very challenging task by conventional single gene-based investigation of gene microarray expression data because of the diversity in disease samples and patients. To bring solutions to these challenges, mining techniques like bi-clustering have been introduced. Bi-clustering allows clustering of rows and columns simultaneously in a matrix format dataset. Bi-clustering in microarray data is described as the subset of expression values of genes that consist of a coherent pattern over some subsets of experimental time stamp or conditions. This technique is used to discover homogeneous submatrices in a bigger data matrix. Bi-clustering was first introduced by Hartigan [1] in the year 1970, although it was first applied to bi-cluster the gene data by Cheng and Church in the year 2000 [2]. Over the last two decades, the bi-clustering technique has generated large interest among researchers to analyze gene data and other big data.

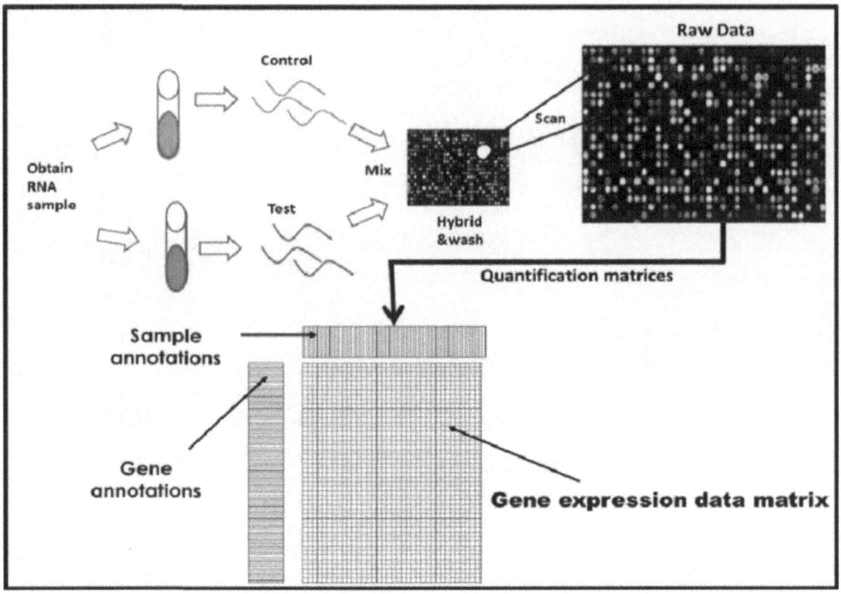


*Figure 2.2* Formation of microarray gene expression data [3].

Cheng and Church [2] defined the bi-clustering problem, or finding the biggest bi-cluster within gene expression data, as an NP-hard problem. Therefore, many new and modified techniques are introduced to solve the bi-clustering problem based on meta-heuristic methods to produce estimated results in a reasonable amount of time. Each technique is associated with single or multiple objective functions, which define the quality of the discovered bi-clusters. Like many different bi-clustering algorithms, there are also a variety of combinations of algorithms and objective functions to address the problem of bi-clustering in gene expression data. Cheng and Church first applied the mean square ratio (MSR) as the objective function in their greedy algorithm to solve the bi-clustering problem [2], then Chakraborty and Maka used a ratio-based objective function on genetic algorithms [4], and other methods are also available. However, there a considerable gap can be found among bi-clustering techniques due to lack of knowledge of the selection of the most relevant bi-clustering technique and corresponding objective functions for the specific data. Selection of a most relevant technique is a challenging and complicated task for sure, but it is also very important to find the most relevant and accurate bi-clusters considered to be connected to a disease mechanism because if the bi-clustering algorithm cannot determine the bi-clusters connected to diseases accurately, then the treatment cannot be applied perfectly or sometimes the treatment will be totally wrong. And, it is important to understand gene functions accurately.

In this work, a hybrid method of k-means clustering algorithm and a meta-heuristic approach called binary particle swarm optimization (BPSO) has been implemented to get bi-clusters from expression data. Analysis is conducted on the cell cycle expression dataset of yeast. This yeast expression data matrix consists of 2884 varieties of genes and 17 experimental situations with two rows of missing values. A portion of this dataset is represented in Figure 2.3. First, the k-means algorithm is applied to generate the gene/row and condition/column clusters separately, then a bi-cluster is generated from the gene and condition clusters. In the next step, the MSR of all bi-clusters is calculated and the bi-clusters selected have MSR value less than the threshold MSR. These seeds or swarms are selected for BPSO to generate larger bi-clusters within the threshold MSR value. And, a comparison has been provided among the objective functions to understand how the objective function works in BPSO.

The chapter is organized as follows. The related work on bi-cluster algorithms is described in Section 2.2. The process of bi-clustering is described in Section 2.3. Section 2.4 provides an overview of meta-heuristics and discusses the importance of meta-heuristic methods in bi-clustering of gene data. A brief overview of different objective functions that are used for comparison in this report is provided in Section 2.5. Section 2.6 elaborates the methods applied to solve the bi-clustering problem of gene expression data. Section 2.7 describes the details of the dataset and the hardware–software setup used for the experiment. The experiment's results are described in Section 2.8. The conclusion of this report and the future direction of this work are presented in Section 2.9.

| | sample1 | sample2 | sample3 | sample4 | sample5 |
|---|---|---|---|---|---|
| YAL001C | 161 | 110 | 139 | 139 | 161 |
| YAL002W | 208 | 139 | 69 | 110 | 139 |
| YAL003W | 425 | 429 | 451 | 423 | 465 |
| YAL004W | 289 | 248 | 220 | 161 | 161 |
| YAL005C | 366 | 364 | 340 | 256 | 283 |
| YAL007C | 271 | 300 | 347 | 300 | 304 |
| YAL009W | 179 | 69 | 139 | 110 | 161 |
| YAL010C | 240 | 179 | 139 | 161 | 179 |
| YAL011W | 179 | 161 | 139 | 139 | 208 |
| YAL012W | 337 | 326 | 322 | 330 | 397 |

*Figure 2.3* Example of a real-life microarray gene expression data (yeast data).

## 2.2 LITERATURE REVIEW

After the first application of bi-clustering in gene expression data in 2000 [2], researchers introduced many other methods to improve the result or to discover the best results considering time and efficiency. In this review, methods published in previous years are introduced.

To bi-cluster the gene matrix, the Cheng and Church (C&C) algorithm was the first of its kind [2]. This algorithm used the deterministic greedy approach to find bi-clusters of coherent patterns from the gene data matrix. The greedy method of this algorithm is to minimize the MSR values of the converged submatrix. MSR is a technique to measure bi-cluster homogeneity. This algorithm is able to discover a predefined number of bi-clusters by users within a permissible MSR score by applying a heuristic approach. The iterative signature algorithm (ISA) by Bergmann et al. in 2003 [5] was able to discover bi-clusters from noisy datasets using a non-deterministic approach. It describes the bi-clusters as transcription modules (TM), which are some coregulated genes with significant experimental conditions. This algorithm selects random genes at first, then it starts to refine the genes and conditions continuously until selected genes and conditions are matched to the TM. ISA was also evaluated as a non-heuristic based approach by Pontes et al. [6]. Although, because of its iterative greedy characteristic, Prelic et al. in 2006 [7] and Eren et al. in 2012 [8] evaluated it as a heuristic-based search approach.

BenDor et al. introduced the order-preserving submatrices algorithm (OPSM) in 2003 [9] and with a deterministic approach, order-preserving submatrices were discovered. In the order-preserved submatrix, expression values of a set of genes are increased or ordered in a similar fashion with respect to some set of experimental conditions. Numerous, possibly overlapped bi-clusters can be efficiently found by the OPSM algorithm. A stochastic iterative-based approach used by Yang et al. in 2005 [10] to explore the bi-clusters was named the flexible overlapped bi-clustering algorithm. And this algorithm used a probabilistic model to explore overlapping bi-clusters in particular. The MSR function is used to access the detected bi-cluster's quality in this evaluation-based scheme. The method is divided into two steps. The first step is to build "crude" bi-clusters initially on a probabilistic basis. Improving of these bi-clusters is done in the second step iteratively. This process reduces the MSR score of bi-clusters by applying a greedy approach of row and column removal. Chakraborty and Maka proposed two genetic algorithms that embed the greedy search algorithm as a local search procedure and found the best bi-clusters without being reliant on the threshold score, i.e., MSR score [11]. By these algorithms, they were able to discover larger bi-clusters, which means bi-clusters accommodate more genes and conditions with a smaller residue score. A generative multiplicative model was introduced by Hochreiter et al. in 2010 [12] and named the FABIA or factor analysis for bi-cluster acquisition to find bi-clusters from the genome matrix. The bi-clusters are shaped as the outer product of two infrequent vectors in FABIA. The "probability of memberships" is returned by this "fuzzy" based bi-clustering approach. Users can define the threshold parameters of this algorithm to find "crisp" bi-clusters by this approach. The Bayesian framework was used by Chekouo and Murua in 2015 for the PPM or penalized plaid model of bi-clustering [13]. This technique is an altered extension of the Bayesian plaid model. The PPM algorithm can find general overlapped bi-clusters and this feature differed it from other algorithms like the Bayesian bi-clustering model by Gu and Liu in 2008 [14], which can only discover one-dimensional overlapping. Unlike the sequential algorithm defined by Zhang in 2010 [15], all parameters of PPM are discovered at once with the help of a devoted Markov chain Monte Carlo sampler. This is a meta-heuristic approach. The BicPAMS algorithm by Henriques et al. in 2017 [16] is a combination of state-of-the-art pattern discovery approaches to the bi-clustering task. BicPAMS is one of the recently introduced pattern discovery algorithms. This algorithm is an enhanced variant of previous pattern mining bi-clustering algorithms since the first publication of BicPAM by Henriques and Madeira [17]. This is not a heuristic algorithm.

Like many different bi-clustering algorithms, there are also different types of objective functions applied to answer the bi-clustering problem in gene expression data. Cheng and Church first applied MSR as the objective function in their greedy algorithm to solve the bi-clustering problem [2], then Chakraborty and Maka used a ratio-based objective function on the genetic algorithm [4] to find the bi-cluster from gene expression data. They used the same MSR [2] to measure the correlation of a subset of genes co-regulated by a subset of conditions. The ratio-based objective function is the ratio of a bi-cluster's residue (MSR) over its size or volume. Divina and Aguilar-Ruiz [18] presented the SEBI algorithm, a sequential evolutionary bi-clustering approach. In this research, they used an objective function called row variance to determine the quality bi-clusters within an MSR threshold value. Then Mukhopadhyay et al. [19] introduced a new coherence function called scaling mean squared residue (SMSR) that can detect bi-clusters with scaling patterns.

## 2.3 BI-CLUSTERING USING META-HEURISTIC APPROACHES

In genetics, the main challenge or problem is to find the set of coherently expressed genes in some different set of conditions, bi-clustering has been applied vastly to address the challenge. The main goal of bi-clustering is to find a subset of genes based on the condition from the gene expression matrix. For example, an expression matrix G of dimension M×N (M genes and N conditions); now find bi-cluster B of dimension I×J (I rows and J

$$G = \begin{bmatrix} a_{11} & a_{12} & \cdots & a_{1N} \\ a_{21} & a_{22} & \cdots & a_{2N} \\ \vdots & \vdots & \ddots & \vdots \\ a_{M1} & a_{M2} & \cdots & a_{MN} \end{bmatrix} \Longrightarrow B = \begin{bmatrix} b_{11} & b_{12} & \cdots & b_{1J} \\ b_{21} & b_{22} & \cdots & b_{2J} \\ \vdots & \vdots & \ddots & \vdots \\ b_{I1} & b_{I2} & \cdots & b_{IJ} \end{bmatrix}$$

*Figure 2.4* A generalized representation of expression matrix G and its bi-cluster B.

columns are the subsets of M and N, respectively). Figure 2.4 represents a generalized structure of a matrix G and its bi-cluster B.

Bi-clusters are the submatrices that reveal some logical understanding or tendency. And a bi-cluster is a matrix I×J, denoted as (I, J), where I and J are the set of genes (or rows) and conditions (or columns), respectively, and $|I| \leq |M|$ and $|J| \leq |N|$. $|I|.|J|$ denotes the size or volume of a bi-cluster.

Let's elaborate the bi-clustering problem with a simple example. Suppose the expression matrix G consists of ten genes or rows and six conditions or columns shown in Table 2.1.

Now say a condition or logic to get a bi-cluster from this expression matrix, the values in the submatrix are all odd numbers.

All odd numbers of the expression matrix are marked with an underline. Rows and columns of odd numbers only will form bi-clusters. A single expression matrix may contain multiple numbers of bi-clusters of different sizes. Some of the submatrix of the main expression matrix that satisfy the condition means the bi-cluster of the G matrix is expressed in the following tables.

In Table 2.2 and 2.3, only two bi-clusters are shown, but the expression matrix G contains many more bi-clusters of different size. A real-life gene expression data may contain thousands of genes and conditions, and that makes it complicated to discover all bi-clusters in the expression matrix for

*Table 2.1* An example of expression matrix G of size 10 × 6

| | *N1* | *N2* | *N3* | *N4* | *N5* | *N6* |
|---|---|---|---|---|---|---|
| M1 | 1 | 5 | 2 | 6 | 9 | 0 |
| M2 | 2 | 8 | 8 | 1 | 5 | 4 |
| M3 | 7 | 3 | 6 | 1 | 1 | 9 |
| M4 | 4 | 6 | 8 | 8 | 2 | 3 |
| M5 | 5 | 5 | 4 | 3 | 2 | 7 |
| M6 | 6 | 6 | 6 | 6 | 6 | 6 |
| M7 | 8 | 9 | 7 | 7 | 7 | 0 |
| M8 | 0 | 0 | 0 | 0 | 0 | 0 |
| M9 | 3 | 5 | 7 | 1 | 9 | 0 |
| M10 | 5 | 1 | 4 | 4 | 7 | 3 |

*Table 2.2* Bi-cluster of G

| | *N1* | *N2* |
|---|---|---|
| M1 | 1 | 5 |
| M3 | 7 | 3 |
| M5 | 5 | 5 |
| M9 | 3 | 5 |
| M10 | 5 | 1 |

a certain condition. In real-life data, the conditions to discover bi-clusters are usually the objective functions.

In big datasets like gene datasets, it is possible to discover different types of bi-clusters. Figures 2.5 and 2.6 represent some structures, and the main types of bi-clusters can be discovered in a dataset. A dataset may also consist of only a single structure or multiple bi-cluster structures at the same time, and the next one is more common in big datasets.

### 2.3.1 Meta-heuristics

The fields of engineering, operation research, and bioinformatics are generating a huge amount of information day by day. This vast number of data leads to the optimization problem. But unfortunately, most of them are unsolvable in polynomial time, and for that, these are determined as the NP-hard problems [20]. Thus, very few of these types of problems can be answered by the usual exact mathematical or numerical techniques. But without giving up, the researchers think of a possible approximation technique that can find a quality solution in an equitable time. These approximation techniques are categorized as heuristic and meta-heuristic. The main difference between these two methods is that meta-heuristics are more problem independent than heuristic techniques. It can also be said that the meta-heuristics can be applied to almost all types of optimization problems, unlike heuristics, which can be applied to a specific problem only.

In simple words, meta-heuristics can be defined as an efficient guide to the searching process in order to find (near-)optimal solution. The term meta-heuristics was first introduced by Glover in 1986 [21] to explain the heuristic technique but without the problem-specific nature. Precisely it can

*Table 2.3* Bi-cluster of G

| | *N2* | *N3* | *N4* | *N5* |
|---|---|---|---|---|
| M7 | 9 | 7 | 7 | 7 |
| M9 | 5 | 7 | 1 | 9 |

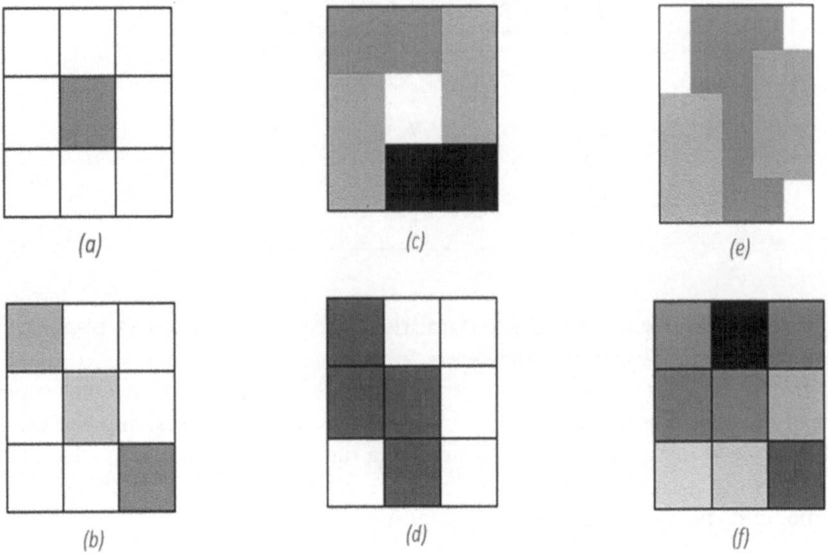


*Figure 2.5* Different structured bi-clusters: (a) single bi-cluster, (b) exclusive row–column bi-clusters, (c) non overlapping nonexclusive bi-clusters, (d) exclusive rows bi-clusters, (e) overlapped arbitrarily positioned bi-clusters, (f) checkerboard structure.

be said that meta-heuristics are the high-level, heuristic-based soft-computing algorithms that can be applied to different types of optimization problems by detecting the general structure of a specific problem with few desired modifications. In meta-heuristics, it is not guaranteed that optimal solutions can be found by the algorithm, but in a reasonable amount of time, a quality solution of a difficult optimization problem can be found. In meta-heuristics, it is assumed that the algorithms will work as desired most of the time but not every time.

Basically, meta-heuristics are an algorithmic architecture that can be applied to heterogeneous optimization problems with few modifications to solve the given problem. Some fundamental characteristics of metaheuristics are [20]:

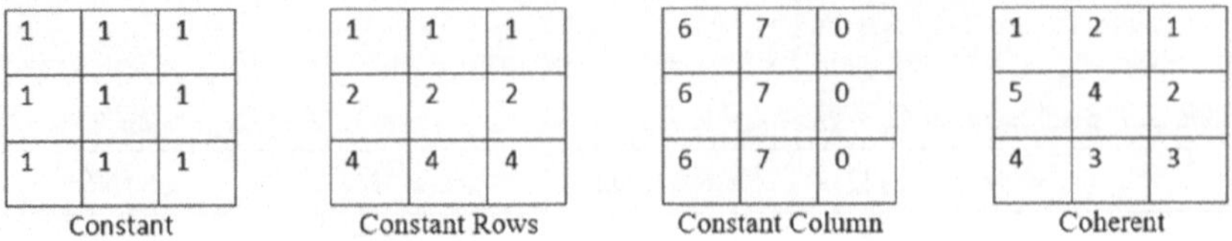


*Figure 2.6* Main types of bi-clusters.

- Meta-heuristics are not only for one or a particular problem.
- It is not precise but more approximate.
- Meta-heuristics are used to find "good enough" or quality solutions.
- Meta-heuristics can be extended to the advanced learning technique from basic local search.

Getting the bi-cluster from a gene data matrix is NP-hard. For that reason, normal or conventional mathematical ways are ineffective on the bi-clustering problem. But now many metaheuristics are available to address this problem. However, metaheuristics will not guarantee to provide accurate or perfectly desired results, but within a sensible amount of time, an efficient result can be discovered.

### 2.3.2 Objective functions

The main goal of bi-clustering is to find the submatrices from a big gene expression matrix. Objective functions are mainly a filtering condition to select a particular type of bi-cluster or select only bi-clusters within desired conditions. Many researchers used objective functions for selection of bi-clusters in bi-clustering algorithms. Some objective functions like MSR, ratio, row variance, size of the bi-cluster, and scaling MSR objective functions are mainly considered in the study of bi-clustering of gene expression data. The objective functions are described next.

#### 2.3.2.1 *MSR*

Mean square ratio (MSR) is to evaluate the degree of coherence in a bi-cluster. It is the sum of squared residue score divided by the size of the bi-cluster [2]. In this third step, MSR has been calculated for each bi-cluster. If RS is the residue score of an element Bij in a bi-cluster B, then it can be defined by Equation 2.1:

$$RS(Bij)=Bij-BIj-BiJ+BIJ \tag{2.1}$$

Here, Bij is an element of bi-cluster B, BIj is the *j*th column mean of bi-cluster B, BiJ is the *i*th row mean of bi-cluster B, and BIJ is the mean of whole bi-cluster B. So, the mean square ratio (MSR) score for the bi-cluster B can be defined by Equation (2.2):

$$MSR(B)=\frac{1}{|I||J|}\Sigma i\in I,j\in J\left(Bij-BIj-BiJ+BIJ\right)^2 \tag{2.2}$$

Here, I is the total number of rows and J is the total number of columns in bi-cluster B, hence $|I|.|J|$ is the size of the bi-cluster.

Cheng and Church [2] used a threshold value of MSR in their algorithm, meaning they choose or discover only those bi-clusters that are within a threshold MSR value. Algorithm 1 defines the pseudocode of the MSR function.

**Algorithm 1. msr_fun()**

```
Output: MSR value of the bicluster B
Compute size, |I|.|J| of the bicluster
Calculate mean, BIJ of the bi – cluster
For row number i = 1 to I do
   Calculate ith row mean, BiJ
   For column number j = 1 to J do
      Calculate jth column mean, BIj
      Compute ith row and jth column value, Bij
      Compute residue score(RS)
      RS = Bij - BIj - BiJ + BIJ
   End for
End for
Compute mean square ratio(MSR)
```

$$MSR\ (B) = \frac{1}{|I||J|} \sum (RS)^2$$

#### 2.3.2.2 Ratio

Chakraborty and Maka used a ratio-based objective function on genetic algorithm [4] to find the bi-cluster from the gene expression data. They used the same MSR [2] to measure the correlation of a subset of genes co-regulated by a subset of conditions. The ratio-based objective function is the ratio of a bi-cluster's residue (MSR) over its size or volume, i.e., residue/ volume, provided in Equation 2.3. This objective function determines that the smaller the residue and/or the larger the volume, the better the quality of the discovered bi-cluster.

$$Fitness\left(Bi-cluster\right) = \frac{MSR}{|I|.|J|} \tag{2.3}$$

Here, $|I|.|J|$ is the size of the bi-cluster.

#### 2.3.2.3 Size of bi-cluster

It is a general objective function that determines the large bi-cluster within a threshold MSR value is the better quality bi-cluster. The higher the value of $|I|.|J|$ of a bi-cluster within a threshold MSR value is the better bi-cluster to choose. $|I|.|J|$ is the size of the bi-cluster.

#### 2.3.2.4 Row variance

Divina and Aguilar-Ruiz [18] presented the SEBI algorithm. In this research, they used an objective function called row variance to determine the quality bi-clusters within an MSR threshold value.

Row variance of a bi-cluster B (I, J) is defined as in Equation 2.4:

$$VAR(B) = \frac{1}{|I||J|} \Sigma i \in I, j \in J \left(Bij - BiJ\right)^2 \tag{2.4}$$

Here, Bij is an element of bi-cluster B, BiJ is the *i*th row mean of bi-cluster B and $|I|.|J|$ is the size of the bi-cluster.

**Algorithm 2. OF_rowvariance()**

***Input: bicluster B of size I × J***
***Output: MSR value of the bicluster B***
***Compute size, |I|. |J| of the bicluster***
***For row number i = 1 to I do***
  ***Calculate ith row mean, BiJ***
  ***For column number j = 1 to J do***
    ***Compute ith row and jth column value, Bij***
    ***Compute variance,***
    ***variance = Bij - BiJ***
  ***End for***
***End for***
***Compute row variance(RV),***

$$RV(B) = \frac{1}{|I||J|} \sum (variance)^2$$

The row variance score is used to determine how well a bi-cluster captures genes exhibiting a fluctuating yet consistent tendency under some set of conditions. So, the high row variance score indicates the quality bi-clusters in terms of fluctuating characteristics of a bi-cluster within a threshold MSR value. Algorithm 2 represents the row variance objective function, and the output of the algorithm is the result of Equation 2.4.

#### 2.3.2.5 Scaling mean squared residue

Mukhopadhyay et al. [19] introduced a new coherence function called SMSR that is able to detect bi-clusters with scaling patterns.

The SMSR of a bi-cluster B (I, J) is defined in Equation 2.5:

$$SMSR(B) = \frac{1}{|I||J|} \Sigma i \in I, j \in J \frac{1}{BiJ^2.BIj^2} (BiJ.BIj - Bij.BIJ)^2 \tag{2.5}$$

Here, Bij is an element of bi-cluster B, BIj is the *j*th column mean of bi-cluster B, BiJ is the *i*th row mean of bi-cluster B, BIJ is the mean of whole bi-cluster B, and $|I|.|J|$ is the size of the bi-cluster.

Like the MSR value, the lower SMSR value indicates the bi-cluster has more coherent values. This objective function was introduced to detect bi-clusters with scaling patterns [19] as the MSR function is able to detect bi-clusters with shifting patterns and constant bi-clusters only, but it cannot discover scaling patterned bi-clusters.

Algorithm 3 defines the SMSR objective function and the result of Equation 2.5 is the output of this algorithm.

---

***Algorithm 3. OF_smsr()***

---

***Input: bicluster B of size I × J***
***Output: MSR value of the bicluster B***
***Compute size, |I|.|J| of the bicluster***
***Calculate mean, BIJ of the bi – cluster***
***For row number i = 1 to I do***
  ***Calculate ith row mean, BiJ***
  ***For column number j = 1 to J do***
    ***Calculate jth column mean, BIj***
    ***Compute ith row and jth column value, Bij***
    ***Compute,***
    $a = BiJ.BIj - Bij.BIJ$
    $b = BiJ.BIj$
  ***End for***
***End for***
***Compute scaling mean square ratio(SMSR)***

$$SMSR\,(B) = \frac{1}{|I||J|} \sum \frac{a^2}{b^2}$$

---

A comparative result is provided in this report among ratio, bi-cluster size, row variance, and SMSR objective function. This result comparison was made to get the idea of the working process of these objective functions.

## 2.4 METHODOLOGIES

It is found that the conventional single gene-based analysis is not very effective to find reliable and accurate biological understanding from the huge datasets like gene expression matrices. In this study, a meta-heuristic approach has been applied to find bi-clusters from gene expression data, and different types of objective functions have been implemented to compare the objective functions. The methodologies of bi-clustering using k-means clustering and binary PSO hybridization are discussed in detail in the following steps.

### 2.4.1 Step 1: K-means clustering

In the first step to get bi-clusters from gene expression data, the k-means clustering algorithm is applied to make row clusters and column clusters separately.

First, understand the concept of clustering. The basic concept of the clustering can be defined as "the process of organizing objects into groups whose members are similar in some way" [22].

Clustering is an important method to analyze gene expression data; it aims to identify the group of genes that have similar expression value over several gene conditions. A pictorial representation of clustering is provided in Figure 2.7.

> K-means clustering is the most famous and uncomplicated "unsupervised" machine learning algorithm [30].

The pseudocode of the k-means clustering algorithm is provided in Algorithm 4 and explained with an example of expression matrix G of dimension $10 \times 5$ in Table 2.4.

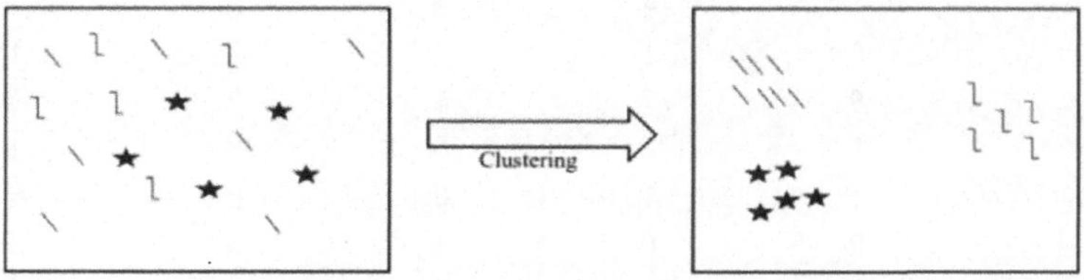


*Figure 2.7* A pictorial representation of clustering.

***Algorithm 4. k-means ()***

*Input: k i.e, the number of clusters*
*and the set of points (x_1, x_2, ...., x_n)*
*Output: k number of clusters*
*1. Choose the number of clusters(K)*
*and obtain the data points*
*2. Place the centroids c_1, c_2, ..... c_k randomly*
*3. Repeat steps 4 and 5 until convergence*
*4. for each data point x_i:*
*find the nearest centroid* $(c_1, c_2 .. c_k)$
*assign the point to that cluster*
*5. for each cluster j = 1..k*
*new centroid = mean of*
*all points assigned*
*to that cluster*
*6. End*

Row clustering:

I. Select the number of row cluster RC will generate, RC = 3.
II. Calculate each row's average GM.

| *GM1* | *GM2* | *GM3* | *GM4* | *GM5* | *GM6* | *GM7* | *GM8* | *GM9* | *GM10* |
|---|---|---|---|---|---|---|---|---|---|
| 3 | 5.4 | 3.4 | 1 | 5.4 | 3 | 2.2 | 3.4 | 2.2 | 2.6 |

III. Generate three (RC = 3) random numbers between the minimum and maximum value of GM (1 and 5.4) for initial cluster centroid. RC1 = 1, RC2 = 5.4, RC3 = 3.

*Table 2.4* G matrix

| | *C1* | *C2* | *C3* | *C4* | *C5* |
|---|---|---|---|---|---|
| G1 | 4 | 2 | 8 | 0 | 1 |
| G2 | 7 | 1 | 9 | 5 | 5 |
| G3 | 1 | 4 | 3 | 8 | 1 |
| G4 | 0 | 1 | 2 | 1 | 1 |
| G5 | 9 | 7 | 6 | 2 | 3 |
| G6 | 5 | 1 | 0 | 8 | 1 |
| G7 | 1 | 1 | 0 | 0 | 9 |
| G8 | 2 | 0 | 7 | 3 | 5 |
| G9 | 3 | 2 | 5 | 1 | 0 |
| G10 | 1 | 2 | 2 | 0 | 8 |

IV. Find which GM is nearest to which RC, |GM-RC|.

| | *GM1* | *GM2* | *GM3* | *GM4* | *GM5* | *GM6* | *GM7* | *GM8* | *GM9* | *GM10* |
|---|---|---|---|---|---|---|---|---|---|---|
| RC1(1) | 2 | 4.4 | 2.4 | **0** | 4.4 | 2 | 1.2 | 2.4 | 1.2 | 1.6 |
| RC2(5.4) | 2.4 | **0** | 2 | 4.4 | **0** | 2.4 | 3.2 | 2 | 3.2 | 2.8 |
| RC3(3) | **0** | 2.4 | **0.4** | 2 | 2.4 | **0** | **0.8** | **0.4** | **0.8** | **0.4** |

V. The nearest GMs to each row cluster RC will form clusters with corresponding rows to GMs in matrix G. RC1 contains one row {G4}, RC2 contains two rows {G2, G5} and RC3 contains seven rows {G1, G3, G6, G7, G8, G9, G10}.
VI. Update RC by finding the average value of GMs in a cluster RC. RC1 = 1, RC2 = 5.4, RC3 = 2.8.

Repeat steps IV, V and VI until there is no change in the value of RCs or the defined number of iterations is achieved.

Column clustering:

I. Select the number of column clusters CC will generate, CC = 2.
II. Calculate each column's average CM.

| *CM1* | *CM2* | *CM3* | *CM4* | *CM5* |
|---|---|---|---|---|
| 3.3 | 2.1 | 4.2 | 2.8 | 3.4 |

III. Generate two (CC = 3) random numbers between the minimum and maximum value of CM (2.1 and 4.2) for the initial cluster centroid. CC1 = 2.1, CC2 = 4.2.
IV. Find which CM is nearest to which CC, |CM–CC|.

| | *CM1* | *CM2* | *CM3* | *CM4* | *CM5* |
|---|---|---|---|---|---|
| CC1(2.1) | 1.2 | **0** | 2.1 | **0.7** | 1.3 |
| CC2(4.2) | **0.9** | 2.1 | **0** | 1.4 | **0.8** |

V. The nearest CMs to each column cluster CC will form clusters with corresponding columns to CMs in matrix G. CC1 contains two columns {C2, C4}, CC2 contains three columns {C1, C3, C5}.
VI. Update CC by finding the average value of CMs in cluster CC. CC1 = 2.4, CC2 = 3.6.

Repeat steps IV, V and VI until there is no change in the value of RCs or the defined number of iterations is achieved.

### 2.4.2 Step 2: Bi-clustering

In the second step, initial bi-clusters are generated by applying the Cartesian product among row clusters RC (RC1, RC2 and RC3) and column clusters CC (CC1 and CC2). Algorithm 5 describes the initial bi-cluster generation process.

***Algorithm 5. initial_biclust()***

```
Input: row set of m number row clusters and column set of n number column cluster
Output: Bi_cluster set of m × n umber bi − clusters
Initialization: bic_Count = 0
For i = 1 to m do
  For j = 1 to n do
    bic_Count = bic_Count + 1
    Bi_cluster(bic_Count) = {row[i].column[j]}
  End for
End for
```

$\{RC1, RC2, RC3\} \times \{CC1, CC2\}$

B1 = {RC1, CC1}, B2 = {RC1, CC2}, B3 = {RC2, CC1}, B4 = {RC2, CC2}, B5 = {RC3, CC1}, B6 = {RC3, CC2}

For example, six bi-clusters are generated, labelled as B1 to B6 in Figure 2.8.

### 2.4.3 Step 3: Calculating MSR

The MSR score, or Hscore, was introduced by Cheng and Church [2] to evaluate the degree of coherence in a bi-cluster. It is the sum of the squared residue score divided by the size of the bi-cluster. In this third step, the MSR is calculated for each bi-cluster.

The MSR was calculated by Equations 2.1 and 2.2.

Let's calculate the residue score (RS) for bi-cluster B3:

$BIJ = 3.7$

| | C2 | C4 |
|---|---|---|
| G4 | 1 | 1 |

Bi-cluster B1

| | C1 | C3 | C5 |
|---|---|---|---|
| G4 | 0 | 2 | 5 |

Bi-cluster B2

| | C2 | C4 |
|---|---|---|
| G2 | 1 | 5 |
| G5 | 7 | 2 |

Bi-cluster B3

| | C1 | C3 | C5 |
|---|---|---|---|
| G2 | 7 | 9 | 5 |
| G5 | 9 | 6 | 3 |

Bi-cluster B4

| | C2 | C4 |
|---|---|---|
| G1 | 2 | 0 |
| G3 | 4 | 8 |
| G6 | 1 | 8 |
| G7 | 1 | 0 |
| G8 | 0 | 3 |
| G9 | 2 | 1 |
| G10 | 2 | 0 |

Bi-cluster B5

| | C1 | C3 | C5 |
|---|---|---|---|
| G1 | 4 | 8 | 1 |
| G3 | 1 | 3 | 1 |
| G6 | 5 | 0 | 1 |
| G7 | 1 | 0 | 9 |
| G8 | 2 | 7 | 5 |
| G9 | 3 | 5 | 0 |
| G10 | 1 | 2 | 8 |

Bi-cluster B6

*Figure 2.8* Generated bi-clusters.

$$RS(1) = (1 - 4 - 3 + 3.7) = -2.3[Bij = 1, BIj = 4, BiJ = 3, BIJ = 3.7]$$

$$RS(5) = (5 - 3.5 - 3 + 3.7) = 2.2$$

$$RS(7) = (7 - 4 - 4.5 + 3.7) = 2.2$$

$$RS(2) = (2 - 3.5 - 4.5 + 3.7) = -2.3$$

Now the MSR value for bi-cluster B3 is

$$MSR(B3) = \frac{(-2.3)^2 + (2.2)^2 + (2.2)^2 + (-2.3)^2}{2 \times 2} = 5.06$$

Therefore, MSR (B1) = 0, MSR (B2) = 0, MSR (B4) = 1.16, MSR (B5) = 3.18.

### 2.4.4 Step 4: Bi-cluster selection

In this fourth step, bi-clusters within the given threshold of MSR with non-zero values are selected for initial particles of BPSO. The MSR value is different for the distinct dataset. The MSR value for the yeast dataset is 300, but the MSR value for the human lymphoma dataset is 1200. The pseudo-code for particle selection is given in Algorithm 6.

```
Algorithm 6. particle_selection()
Input: MSR threshold value, all initial bi
                - clusters and their MSR values
Output: bi - clusters within given MSR threshold value
Initialization: count = 0
For i = 1 to number of bi - clusters do
  If MSR value <= MSR threshold value
    count = count + 1
    Selected_BIC(count) = initial bi - cluster(i)
  End if
End for
```

Say, for example, the MSR threshold is 4, then only bi-clusters B4 and B5 will be selected for initial particles of BPSO.

### 2.4.5 Step 5: Bi-cluster encoding

The fifth step is to encode the selected bi-clusters in binary bits (0, 1) in a single string [23] for BPSO. The length of the binary bit is the number of rows plus the number of columns of the initial expression matrix G of size M × N, i.e., M + N, where M is the total number of rows and N is the total number of columns. Each of the first M bits of the binary string is related to the rows, in the order in which the bits appear in the string. In the same way, the remaining N bits are related to columns. If a bit is set to 1, it means that the relative row or column belongs to the encoded bi-cluster; otherwise it does not [24]. In Algorithm 7, the process of encoding is explained as pseudocode.

Figure 2.9 represents a generalized array of encoded bi-cluster of length M+N.

```
Algorithm 7. encode()
Determine the number of row(M) and number of column(N) of gene matrix(G)
Compute, a = M + N
For each bicluster B do
   Make an array, E of size (M + N) containing all zeros
   Fetch row indices and column indices of selected bicluster
   Change values of zeros(0) to ones(1) in E at the positions of row indices and
              + (column indices) positions for column indices
End for
```

It will be encoded as:

| | | | | | | | | | | | | | | |
|---|---|---|---|---|---|---|---|---|---|---|---|---|---|---|
| 0 | 1 | 0 | 0 | 1 | 0 | 0 | 0 | 0 | 0 | 1 | 0 | 1 | 0 | 1 |

As the sum of the row and column of the matrix G was 10 + 5 = 15, the string length is 15. For B4 row 2 and 5 are in the bi-cluster, so the second and fifth bit is 1, and the 11th, 13th and 15th bit is 1 for the column. Bi-cluster B5 will be encoded as:

| | | | | | | | | | | | | | | |
|---|---|---|---|---|---|---|---|---|---|---|---|---|---|---|
| 1 | 0 | 1 | 0 | 0 | 1 | 1 | 1 | 1 | 1 | 0 | 1 | 0 | 1 | 0 |

### 2.4.6 Step 6: Initial population for BPSO

In this step, the previously selected and encoded bi-clusters are given as the initial particles of the BPSO to generate high-quality bi-clusters. B4 and B5 have been selected for the initial population.

| | | | | | | | | | | |
|---|---|---|---|---|---|---|---|---|---|---|
| $P_1$ | $P_2$ | $P_3$ | ... | $P_{M-1}$ | $P_M$ | $P_{1+M}$ | $P_{2+M}$ | ... | $P_{N-1}$ | $P_N$ |

*Figure 2.9* Representation of encoded bi-cluster of length M + N.

### 2.4.7 Step 7: Optimization functions

As BPSO is an optimization problem, there must be an objective function to evaluate the quality of the bi-clusters and or to optimize the result based on the objective function. In this study, the main objective is to find maximum-sized bi-clusters with low MSR value or at least within the given MSR value threshold. The quality of each bi-cluster B can be assessed by the following fitness function, $G(B) = |I|.|J|$ for the MSR value within the threshold, and $MSR > 0$. $I \times J$ is the size of the bi-cluster.

And for comparison among optimization functions, the ratio used as cost function, row variance used as fitness function and scaling MSR used as cost function can optimize the problem.

### 2.4.8 Step 8: BPSO-based bi-clustering

In this study, the binary version of the PSO is implemented as the meta-heuristic, so it is needed to introduce the sigmoid function to force the real values to stay between 1 and 0 [25]. Binary particle swarm optimization or BPSO is the binary version of the normal PSO algorithm, and it was introduced by Kennedy and Eberhart in 1997 [26]. This version allows the PSO algorithm to operate in a binary problem space. The normal version of the PSO uses two update functions: one is the velocity and the other is the position of the particle. In the original version of PSO, the position of the particle is updated by combining its current position and velocity. But in case of BPSO, the current position is only updated based on the velocity. Generally, a function named sigmoid updates the position of the particle in BPSO.

The general steps of BPSO with a numerical example can be defined as:

- Initialize BPSO with a particle (p1, p2, p3, ...) string containing 0 or 1.
  - B4 and B5 are selected as the initial particles, p1 and p2.

| | | | | | | | | | | | | | | | |
|---|---|---|---|---|---|---|---|---|---|---|---|---|---|---|---|
| p1(t) | 0 | 1 | 0 | 0 | 1 | 0 | 0 | 0 | 0 | 0 | 1 | 0 | 1 | 0 | 1 |
| p2(t) | 1 | 0 | 1 | 0 | 0 | 1 | 1 | 1 | 1 | 1 | 0 | 1 | 0 | 1 | 0 |

- Define the cost or fitness function.
  - Let's take the size of the bi-cluster as fitness function, fp = Number of rows · Number of columns:
  - fp(p1) = 6 and fp(p2) = 14.

- Generate the initial velocity for particles; it is the array of random numbers. It is the same as the size of the particle, as the velocity is generated for each vector of the particle.

| | | | | | | | | | | | | | | | |
|---|---|---|---|---|---|---|---|---|---|---|---|---|---|---|---|
| v1(t) | 0.8 | 1 | 1.2 | 0.7 | 0.2 | 0.9 | 0.6 | 2 | 0.5 | 0.4 | 0 | 0.1 | 0.4 | 0.8 | 0.9 |
| v2(t) | 2 | 0 | 1.5 | 1.1 | 1 | 0.3 | 0.8 | 1 | 0.5 | 1.1 | 1.2 | 1 | 1.6 | 1.7 | 0.6 |

- Calculate the velocity for updating the position of the particle using Equation 2.6:

$$vij(t+1) = w.vij(t) + c1.r1(pbest(i,j) - xij(t))$$

$$+ \; c2.r2(gbest(i,j) - xij(t)) \tag{2.6}$$

where i is the index of a particle in the swarm (i = 1, …, n), j is the position index of vectors in the particle (j = 1, …, m), t represents the iteration number, $v_{ij}(t)$ is the velocity of the *i*th particle and $x_{ij}(t)$ is the position. r1 and r2 are random numbers uniformly distributed between 0 and 1, c1 and c2 are the acceleration coefficients, and w is the positive inertia weight. And pbest is the initial particle itself in the first step, and gbest is the particle with the best fitness.

Here, gbest is p2, and initially pbest is p1, p2. To get a new velocity, Equation 2.6 is applied for each particle. The parameters are taken as w = 1, c1 = c2 = 2, and r1 and r2 are two uniform random numbers between 0 and 1.

Now apply Equation 2.6 for p1(1,1) position, pbest(1, 1) = 0, gbest(1, 1) = 1, v1(1, 1) = 0.8, x(1, 1) = 0, r1 = 0.1 and r2 = 0.2.

Therefore, $v1(1,1)(t+1) = 1*0.8 + 2*0.1(0-0) + 2*0.2(1-0) = 1.2$.

The other velocities are determined and represented below.

| | | | | | | | | | | | | | | | |
|---|---|---|---|---|---|---|---|---|---|---|---|---|---|---|---|
| v1(t+1) | 1.2 | 0.4 | 1.4 | 0.7 | −0.8 | 1.7 | 1.4 | 3.6 | 0.7 | 1.4 | −1.8 | 0.9 | −0.6 | 1.4 | 0.7 |
| v2(t+1) | 2 | 0 | 1.5 | 1.1 | 1 | 0.3 | 0.8 | 1 | 0.5 | 1.1 | 1.2 | 1 | 1.6 | 1.7 | 0.6 |

- Now update the position of the particle using Equation 2.7:

$$x_{ij}(t+1) = \begin{cases} 1 & \text{if } rand() < S(v_{ij}(t+1)) \\ 0 & \text{if } rand() \geq S(v_{ij}(t+1)) \end{cases} \tag{2.7}$$

where rand () is the random number selected from a uniform distribution over [0.0, 1.0] and S(.) is the sigmoid function for transforming the velocity to the probability (Equation 2.8):

$$S\left(v_{ij}\left(t+1\right)\right)=\frac{1}{1+e^{-v_{ij}(t+1)}} \tag{2.8}$$

The sigmoid function value will be determined for each velocity of each particle.

$$S\left(v1\left(1,1\right)\right)=\frac{1}{1+e^{-v1(1,1)}}=\frac{1}{1+e^{-1.2}}=0.77$$

Other sigmoid function values are calculated as:

| | | | | | | | | | | | | | | | |
|---|---|---|---|---|---|---|---|---|---|---|---|---|---|---|---|
| S(v1) | 0.77 | 0.6 | 0.8 | 0.67 | 0.31 | 0.85 | 0.8 | 0.97 | 0.67 | 0.8 | 0.14 | 0.71 | 0.35 | 0.8 | 0.67 |
| S(v2) | 0.88 | 0.5 | 0.82 | 0.75 | 0.73 | 0.57 | 0.69 | 0.73 | 0.62 | 0.75 | 0.77 | 0.73 | 0.83 | 0.85 | 0.65 |

Now to update the position, a random number between 0 and 1 will be generated for each sigmoid value, compare to each sigmoid value and update the position of the particle with the help of Equation 2.7. After applying Equation 2.7, the updated particles are generated:

| | | | | | | | | | | | | | | | |
|---|---|---|---|---|---|---|---|---|---|---|---|---|---|---|---|
| p1(t+1) | 1 | 0 | 1 | 1 | 1 | 1 | 0 | 0 | 0 | 0 | 0 | 0 | 1 | 0 | 1 |
| p2(t+1) | 1 | 0 | 1 | 0 | 1 | 1 | 0 | 1 | 1 | 1 | 0 | 1 | 1 | 1 | 0 |

New bi-clusters are generated from these encoded particles (see Figure 2.10):

| | C3 | C5 |
|---|---|---|
| G1 | 8 | 1 |
| G3 | 3 | 1 |
| G4 | 2 | 1 |
| G5 | 6 | 3 |
| G6 | 0 | 1 |

| | C2 | C3 | C4 |
|---|---|---|---|
| G1 | 2 | 8 | 0 |
| G3 | 4 | 3 | 8 |
| G5 | 7 | 6 | 2 |
| G6 | 1 | 0 | 8 |
| G8 | 0 | 7 | 3 |
| G9 | 2 | 5 | 1 |
| G10 | 2 | 2 | 0 |

*Figure 2.10* Bi-cluster from particle p1(t + 1).

**Algorithm 8. km_Bpso()**

```
Input: gene expression matrix, G;
Initialization: max_Run, max_iteration, positive constant(c1, c2), inertia weight(iw)
Output: best bi − cluster as global_best
For mr = 1 to max_run do
  k_means(G, row) /* generates row cluster, algorithm 8 */
  k_means(G, column) /* generates column cluster, algorithm 8 */
  initial_biclust()/* generates initial bi − clusters, algorithm 9 */
  msr_fun()/* calculate MSR value of bi − cluster, algoritm 5 */
  particle_selection()/
              * select particles which are within threshold MSR, algorithm 10 */
  encode()/* encode selected bi − clusters, algorithm 11 */
  initial global_best = particle with lowest MSR
  initial personal_best = current value
  randomly initialize particle's velocities for particle dimension N
  for it = 1 to max_iteration do
    for each particle i = 1 to n do
      for each dimension j = 1 to N do
        v_ij(it + 1) = iw.v_ij(it) + c1.r1(pbest.ij - x_ij(it)) + c2.r2(gbest.ij - x_ij(it))
        s(v_ij(it + 1)) = 1 / (1 + e^(-v_ij(it+1)))
        x_ij(it + 1) = { 1   if rand() < s(v_ij(it + 1))
                       { 0   if rand() ≥ s(v_ij(it + 1))
      end for
    end for
    generate bi − clusters
    calculate MSR of new bi − clusters
    if MSR <= threshold MSR then
      calculate objective function, of()
      if of(i) better than personal_best(i) then
        personal_best = of(i)
      end if
      if of(i) better than global_best(i) then
        global_best = of(i)
      end if
    end if
  end for
end for
```

- Calculate the MSR value to check if the solution is within the given threshold value, and if it is, then calculate the cost function or fitness function to update global best($g_{best}$) and personal best($p_{best}$).

Now the MSR of the particles are $MSR\left(p1(t+1)\right)=1.76$ and $MSR\left(p2(t+1)\right)=41.34$. This value is greater than the MSR threshold value, i.e., 4.

So, p1(t+1) will save as pbest and gbest in place of p(t) as it has a better fitness value (i.e., 10) within the MSR threshold value, and p2(t) will remain the same as no better solution was found than the previous one for p2(t).

- Particle updating will continue for n iterations or until a stopping criterion.

From the preceding steps of methodologies, it becomes clear how the process of finding bi-clusters from a gene expression data matrix works with the help of meta-heuristics. It is also observable that the main structure of the program is the same, but it is possible to change between different objective functions to optimize the result in a different way. By keeping this in mind, the comparison between different objective functions is done in this work. The methodology of this technique is summed up in the Algorithm 8.

## 2.5 EXPERIMENTAL RESULTS AND DISCUSSION

The *Saccharomyces cerevisiae* (yeast) cell cycle expression dataset has been used as the benchmark dataset to compare the objective functions because of its availability, and it is widely used among various techniques. The dataset includes 2884 genes, 17 conditions and 0.07% missing data. If the rows containing missing data are deleted, we are left with 2882 genes and 17 conditions. The dataset is available at http://arep.med.harvard.edu /biclustering/.

Each of the datasets has a threshold MSR value for the discovered bi-clusters. This MSR value is an important measure to determine how good a bi-cluster is. A low MSR value indicates a bi-cluster contains much coherent expression value and it will indicate a good quality bi-cluster. In the study of Cheng and Church [2], the threshold value for the yeast dataset was set to 300; this value is the standard threshold for this dataset.

The source code is written in MATLAB, version 2015a, of 64-bit architecture. The program was run on an Intel i5 4th generation machine with 8GB of RAM. Parameters for the k-means algorithm were k = 50 (number of clusters) for rows and k = 5 (number of clusters) for the columns. For BPSO, the iteration number was 100, inertia weight (W) was taken 0.9 initially, and it varied from 0.9 to 0.4 decreasing uniformly, two random numbers (r1 and r2) generated between 0 and 1 were taken, and acceleration coefficient (c1 and c2) was set to 2. A total of five numbers of the run were taken of the whole program.

This study shows the results based on the yeast cell cycle data. The first part of this study was to apply a k-means and use a meta-heuristic-based hybrid algorithm to find the largest bi-cluster within the yeast data matrix.

In Table 2.5, the average, median and standard deviation of the output results of multiple runs are provided. From the table, it can be said that the size of the discovered bi-clusters is more spread, but the ratio (MSR/size) values are nearly the same or very near to each other as the standard deviation values are high and low significantly. This signifies that the larger bi-cluster size also indicates a higher MSR value. Also, the MSR and row variance signify that the bi-clusters are without much variation in data.

*Table 2.5* Average, median and mean values of the experiment results

| | *Average* | *Median* | *Standard deviation* |
|---|---|---|---|
| MSR value | 279.42 | 286.52 | 15.66 |
| Size of bi-clusters | 2791.6 | 2792 | 97.71 |
| Ratio | 0.1002 | 0.103 | 0.0075 |
| Row variance | 288.12 | 294.41 | 21.05 |

By this experiment, it has been observed that the result varies by iteration number, which means the higher iteration number of BPSO will find much bigger bi-clusters, but it will also take much time to run the program. Figure 2.10 provides the convergence graph of BPSO iteration number versus bi-cluster size. Also, it can be said that the starting iterations are able to converge more results than the later ones. Hence, initial iterations take less time to improve the result than later iterations.

As can be seen in Figure 2.11, within iteration 1 to nearly iteration 30, bi-clusters sized nearly 2500 are discovered, but after that, the remaining iterations are not able to find better results than the previous one.

For the second part of this study, the yeast cell cycle dataset was used in the same algorithm for four times with four objective functions for comparison study. All four objective functions are used in a common MSR threshold value (i.e., 300).

The following figures and tables are achieved by comparing objective functions. Figure 2.12 is the representation of the graphs of the bi-clusters generated by the objective functions followed by tables of numerical representation of the results of the experiment.

From Figure 2.12, it is clear that different objective functions are able to discover bi-clusters consisting of different characteristics. It is observable

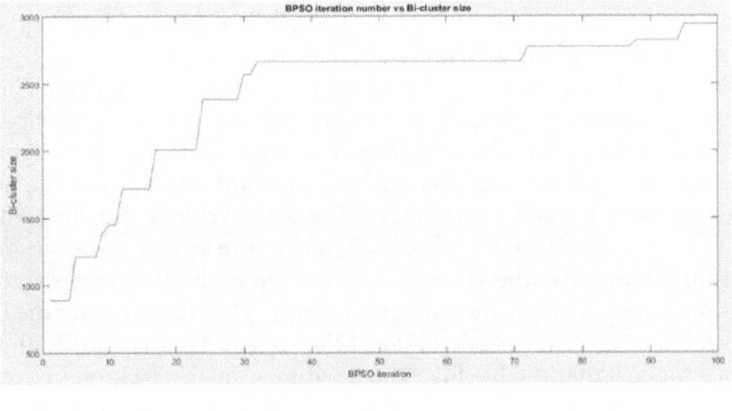


*Figure 2.11* Convergence graph of BPSO iteration versus bi-cluster size.

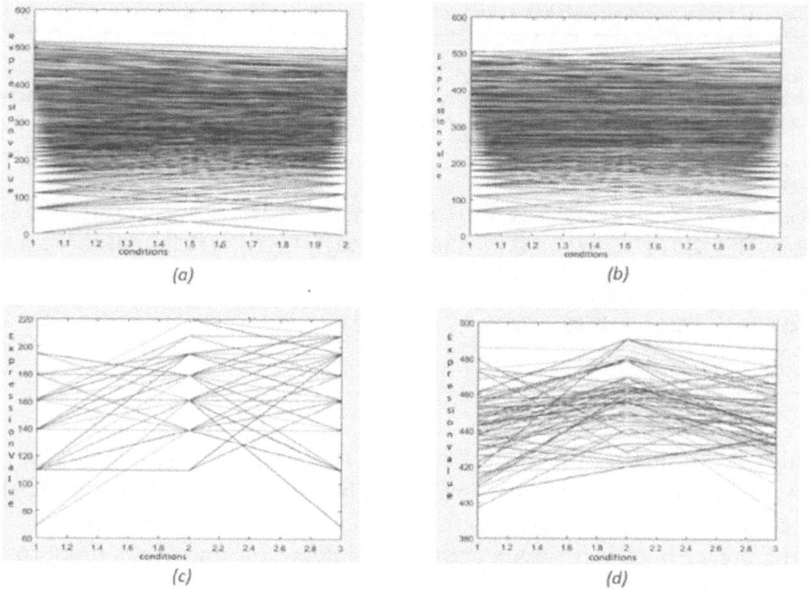


*Figure 2.12* The graphical representation of objective functions: (a) size objective function, (b) ratio function, (c) RowVariance function and (d) sMSR function.

that the bi-cluster generated by the size and ratio objective function does not show a clear pattern, but the bi-cluster of the SMSR function is showing some upregulation and downregulation of gene expression values respective to conditions, and for the bi-cluster of the row variance objective function, a clear upregulation and downregulation of expression level is visible.

Table 2.6 shows the comparative result for yeast cell cycle bi-clustering data among four objective functions with the best results of three parameters: MSR, size and row variance.

Table 2.7 shows the comparative result for yeast cell cycle bi-clustering data among objective functions with mean, median and standard deviation values of three parameters.

From the tables, it is visible that the objective function SMSR was able to achieve the lowest MSR value among the objective functions, but it also

*Table 2.6* Bi-clustering result for yeast dataset

| *Objective function (OF)* | *Best result of each OF value* | *MSR (low is best)* | *Size (high is best)* | *Row variance (high is best)* |
|---|---|---|---|---|
| Size of bi-cluster | Biggest size 2894 | 227.17 | 2894 | 276.57 |
| Ratio | Lowest ratio 0.046 | 124.37 | 2888 | 218.18 |
| Row variance | Highest RV 1268.85 | 136.31 | 411 | 1268.85 |
| Scaling MSR (SMSR) | Lowest SMSR 0.00048 | 119.55 | 213 | 989.84 |

*Table 2.7* Mean, median and the standard deviation values of comparison result

| *Measures Objective function* | *MSR* | | | *Bi-cluster size* | | | *Row variance* | | |
|---|---|---|---|---|---|---|---|---|---|
| | *Mean* | *Median* | *Standard deviation* | *Mean* | *Median* | *Standard deviation* | *Mean* | *Median* | *Standard deviation* |
| i. Size of bi-cluster | 241 | 240.19 | 11.25 | 2784 | 2788 | 76.48 | 258.37 | 254.43 | 15.26 |
| ii. Ratio | 163 | 176.79 | 35.32 | 2798 | 2812 | 67.21 | 170.65 | 177.15 | 43.08 |
| iii. Row variance (RV) | 220.68 | 247.69 | 57.14 | 164.6 | 100 | 141.41 | 712.52 | 525.72 | 378.30 |
| iv. Scaling MSR (SMSR) | 172.64 | 134.80 | 72.70 | 111.6 | 92 | 66.74 | 571.21 | 609.19 | 314.98 |

achieved the smallest bi-cluster. The size function achieved the largest bi-cluster, but it also achieved a significantly higher MSR value among the objective functions. But also, in the size objective function, it is possible to find a bigger bi-cluster within some initial iterations and then no improvement in the upcoming iterations. In the case of the ratio objective function, it was able to discover a significantly large bi-cluster with a significantly low MSR value, and this is a desirable characteristic among bi-clustering methods. For the row variance, it is observable that this function achieved a bi-cluster with a higher row variance, meaning the bi-cluster has values with significant fluctuation but not constant. However, it fails to achieve a very large bi-cluster or very low MSR value. It can also be said that it is not obvious that only bigger bi-clusters will have high variance or higher MSR values, but it is also possible to have small-sized bi-clusters with high row variance in data and not with a very low MSR value.

It is also observable from the table that the bi-clusters generated by the row variance and SMSR functions have much more fluctuating expression value, but the size and ratio functions achieved bi-clusters with more constant values.

## 2.6 CONCLUSION AND FUTURE SCOPE

Identification of the most significant bi-clusters causing disorder from a biological dataset is a challenging task. It is observed that a gene expression dataset normally consists of many bi-clusters of smaller size. The significance of those bi-clusters may be questionable in the context of understanding their biological functions properly. In this work, a k-means meta- heuristic-based hybrid algorithm is used to find bi-clusters from the yeast dataset. The performance of the algorithm used in this work can be measured by the size of a bi-cluster within the permissible or threshold MSR value, and a bigger bi-cluster means better performance. But it also should be kept in mind that a good or relevant bi-cluster cannot be defined only by the size of a bi-cluster. To understand this aspect, a comparison has been provided among different objective functions.

In the comparison of objective functions, differences in the performance are observed among them. By this study, it is observed that each objective function has its own characteristics, and advantages and disadvantages. The objective function "size of bi-cluster" helps to discover much bigger bi-clusters and the objective function "row variance" helps discover bi-clusters of fluctuating patterns. It cannot be strongly stated that a particular objective function is best in every aspect than other available functions in the bi-clustering algorithms. It can be concluded that it is not a good choice to compare objective functions with each other to find which one is superior. Also, comparing them on every parameter to determine which one is the best for all tasks is a very complicated task.

So, this approach will help in various research areas of healthcare. Some of the prominent health sectors are as follows:

**Complex diseases analysis:** Using this technique, researchers can identify specific gene expression patterns for some complex diseases. For example, for autoimmune disorders, there are so many diseases in which multiple genes have complex involvement. Bi-clustering helps to identify the co-regulated gene sets associated with disease pathways.

**Genomic medicine development:** Using this technique, researcher can identify specific gene expression patterns and understand the genetic variations and their impact on human health. This will be helpful for developing targeted genomic medicine.

**Personalized medicine development:** Bi-clustering can help to identify candidate genes of individual patients or specific conditions of individuals. Based on these identifications, researchers can develop or tailor personalized medicine.

**Identify neurodegenerative diseases:** Alzheimer's, Parkinson's, and autism are characterized by genetic disorders. Using this technique, researchers can identify related genetic factors.

Overall bi-clustering, especially when combined with meta-heuristic optimization techniques, can help in various health-related sectors. This technique could be helpful for biomarker discovery, cancer research, and aging and longevity-related issues. *Saccharomyces cerevisiae* for studying gene variants associated with human diseases has wide-ranging implications across various research areas within healthcare. Therefore, multiple objective functions may be used at the same time for better optimization of the results. In the future, it will be observed how this algorithm will behave or improve itself with the help of multiple optimization functions at the same time. Also, it will be tested if the improvement of the algorithm is possible with parameter modifications.

## REFERENCES


1. Hartigan, John A. "Direct clustering of a data matrix." *Journal of the American Statistical Association* 67, no. 337 (1972): 123–129.
2. Cheng, Yizong, and George M. Church. "Biclustering of expression data." *ISMB* 8 (2000): 93–103.
3. Aziz, Rabia, C. K. Verma, and Namita Srivastava. "Dimension reduction methods for microarray data: A review." *AIMS Bioeng* 4, no. 1 (2017): 179–197.
4. Chakraborty, Anupam, and Hitashyam Maka. "Biclustering of gene expression data using genetic algorithm." 2005 IEEE Symposium on Computational Intelligence in Bioinformatics and Computational Biology, pp. 1–8. IEEE, 2005.
5. Bergmann, Sven, Jan Ihmels, and Naama Barkai. "Iterative signature algorithm for the analysis of large-scale gene expression data." *Physical review E* 67, no. 3 (2003): 031902.
6. Pontes, Beatriz, Raúl Giráldez, and Jesús S. Aguilar-Ruiz. "Biclustering on expression data: A review." *Journal of Biomedical Informatics* 57 (2015): 163–180.
7. Prelić, Amela, Stefan Bleuler, Philip Zimmermann, Anja Wille, Peter Bühlmann, Wilhelm Gruissem, Lars Hennig, Lothar Thiele, and Eckart Zitzler. "A systematic comparison and evaluation of biclustering methods for gene expression data." *Bioinformatics* 22, no. 9 (2006): 1122–1129.
8. Eren, K., M. Deveci, O. Küçüktunç, and U. V. Çatalyürek. "A comparative analysis of biclustering algorithms for gene expression data." *Briefings in Bioinformatics* 14, no. 3 (2012): 279–292.
9. Ben-Dor, Amir, Benny Chor, Richard Karp, and Zohar Yakhini. "Discovering local structure in gene expression data: the order-preserving submatrix problem." Proceedings of the Sixth Annual International Conference on Computational Biology, pp. 49–57. IEEE, 2002.
10. Yang, Jiong, Haixun Wang, Wei Wang, and Philip S. Yu. "An improved biclustering method for analyzing gene expression profiles." *International Journal on Artificial Intelligence Tools* 14, no. 05 (2005): 771–789.
11. Chakraborty, Anupam, and Hitashyam Maka. "Biclustering of gene expression data using genetic algorithm." 2005 IEEE Symposium on Computational Intelligence in Bioinformatics and Computational Biology, pp. 1–8. IEEE, 2005.
12. Hochreiter, Sepp, Ulrich Bodenhofer, Martin Heusel, Andreas Mayr, Andreas Mitterecker, Adetayo Kasim, Tatsiana Khamiakova et al. "FABIA: factor analysis for bicluster acquisition." *Bioinformatics* 26, no. 12 (2010): 1520–1527.
13. Chekouo, Thierry, and Alejandro Murua. "The penalized biclustering model and related algorithms." *Journal of Applied Statistics* 42, no. 6 (2015): 1255–1277.
14. Gu, Jiajun, and Jun S. Liu. "Bayesian biclustering of gene expression data." *BMC Genomics* 9 (2008): 1–10.
15. Zhang, Jian. "A Bayesian model for biclustering with applications." *Journal of the Royal Statistical Society Series C: Applied Statistics* 59, no. 4 (2010): 635–656.

16. Henriques, Rui, Francisco L. Ferreira, and Sara C. Madeira. "BicPAMS: software for biological data analysis with pattern-based biclustering." *BMC Bioinformatics* 18 (2017): 1–16.
17. Henriques, Rui, and Sara C. Madeira. "BicPAM: Pattern-based biclustering for biomedical data analysis." *Algorithms for Molecular Biology* 9 (2014): 1–30.
18. Divina, Federico, and Jesus S. Aguilar-Ruiz. "Biclustering of expression data with evolutionary computation." *IEEE Transactions on Knowledge and Data Engineering* 18, no. 5 (2006): 590–602.
19. Mukhopadhyay, Anirban, Ujjwal Maulik, and Sanghamitra Bandyopadhyay. "A novel coherence measure for discovering scaling biclusters from gene expression data." *Journal of Bioinformatics and Computational Biology* 7, no. 05 (2009): 853–868.
20. Abdel-Basset, Mohamed, Laila Abdel-Fatah, and Arun Kumar Sangaiah. "Metaheuristic algorithms: A comprehensive review." *Computational Intelligence for Multimedia Big Data on the Cloud with Engineering Applications* (2018): 185–231.
21. Glover, Fred. "Future paths for integer programming and links to artificial intelligence." *Computers & Operations Research* 13, no. 5 (1986): 533–549.
22. Bashir, Muhammad Adnan, Tabasam Rashid, and Muhammad Salman Bashir. "Generalized ordered intuitionistic fuzzy C-means clustering algorithm based on PROMETHEE and intuitionistic fuzzy C-means." *International Journal of Intelligent Systems* 2023, no. 1 (2023): 6686446.
23. Mitra, Sushmita, and Haider Banka. "Multi-objective evolutionary biclustering of gene expression data." *Pattern Recognition* 39, no. 12 (2006): 2464–2477.
24. Rathipriya, R., K. Thangavel, and J. Bagyamani. "Binary particle swarm optimization based biclustering of web usage data." *arXiv preprint arXiv:1108.0748* (2011).
25. Taşgetiren, M. Fatih, and Yun-Chia Liang. "A binary particle swarm optimization algorithm for lot sizing problem." *Journal of Economic and Social Research* 5, no. 2 (2003): 1–20.
26. Kennedy, James, and Russell C. Eberhart. "A discrete binary version of the particle swarm algorithm." 1997 IEEE International Conference on Systems, Man, and Cybernetics. Computational Cybernetics and Simulation, vol. 5, pp. 4104–4108. IEEE, 1997.

Chapter 3

# Uncovering methods for early Alzheimer diagnosis using machine learning and deep learning

*Rohit Kumar, Ankush Jain, and Surendra Nagar*

## 3.1 INTRODUCTION

Alzheimer's disease (AD) is a type of neurodegenerative impairment in which cells of the cerebral organ stop working over time and eventually die [1]. As per the "2023 Alzheimer's Disease Facts and Figures" report, AD has been found to be the fifth leading factor of fatality among Americans age 65 and over [2]. It's a progressive disease in which the central nervous system of a human deteriorates with time, affecting their thinking skills and daily life activities. It starts with mild memory loss, which is the most general form of dementia, for which one of the main causes is AD. Its symptoms are depicted in Figure 3.1 [3].

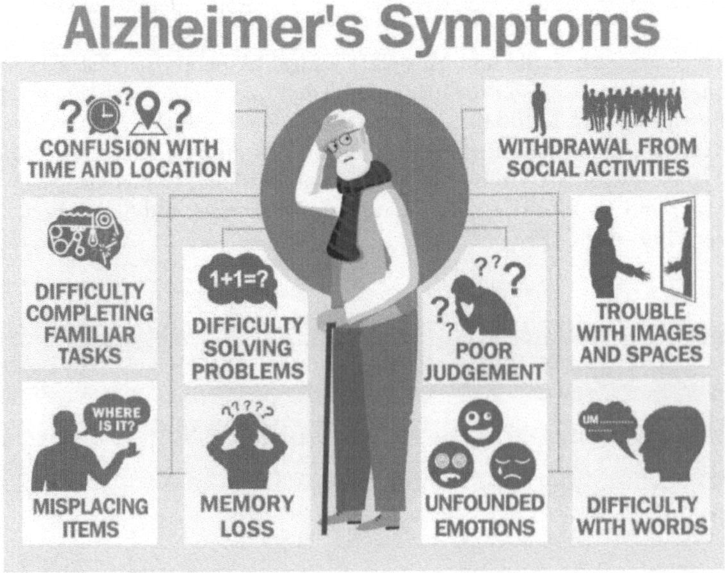


*Figure 3.1* Signs of Alzheimer's disease.


DOI: 10.1201/9781003634089-3

Irregular protein buildup accumulates in the brain, forming amyloid deposits and tau neurofibrillary tangles. The accumulation of beta-amyloid in the brain is considered to have a substantial contribution in the onset and advancement of Alzheimer's disease [4]. Beta-amyloid peptides have a tendency to clump together, forming insoluble aggregates known as amyloid plaques. These plaques accumulate between nerve cells (neurons) in the brain, disrupting communication between neurons and interfering with normal brain function. Beta-amyloid aggregates can become toxic to neurons, leading to their dysfunction and eventual death.

This neuronal toxicity contributes to the progressive cognitive decline seen in AD. Beta-amyloid can initiate a neuroinflammatory response, causing further damage to neurons and contributing to the neurodegenerative process characteristic of AD. Beta-amyloid can interfere with the function of synapses, the connections between neurons where communication occurs. This disruption of synaptic function impairs memory and cognitive processes [5]. The buildup of beta-amyloid is linked to the abnormal phosphorylation of tau protein, which is another characteristic feature of AD. Tau protein aggregates create neurofibrillary tangles inside neurons, which further impair neuronal function and contribute to cell death. The healthy brain and Alzheimer's brain are visualized in Figure 3.2 [6]. Overall, while the precise mechanisms by which beta-amyloid contributes to AD are still being researched, its accumulation and associated effects on neuronal

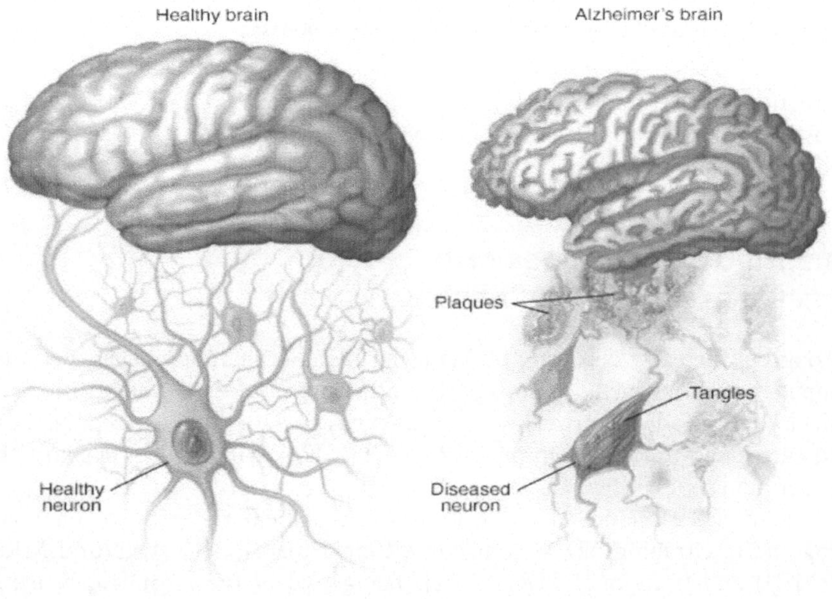


*Figure 3.2* Healthy brain versus Alzheimer's brain (source: Mayo Foundation).

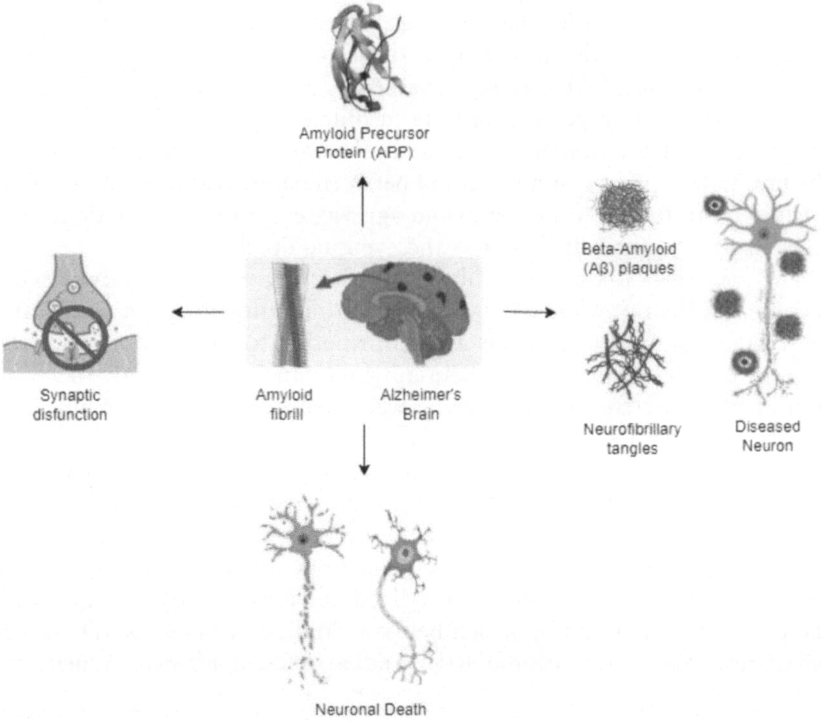


*Figure 3.3* Neuropathological features of Alzheimer's disease.

function and structure are widely recognized as a core factor in the disease's pathogenesis [7]. These neuropathological features of Alzheimer's disease are shown in Figure 3.3.

## 3.2 INPUT MODALITIES AND RELEVANT BIOMARKERS

To aid in the early detection of AD using ML and DL approaches, various input modalities including image and other types of data can be utilized. Each input modality provides different types of data that can be analyzed to detect and predict the progression of AD. Following are some common input modalities.

Magnetic resonance imaging (MRI) is a critical resource in diagnosing and researching AD. It comes in different forms, with structural MRI (sMRI) and functional MRI (fMRI) being two of the most widely used types in this context. sMRI focuses on the anatomy and structure of the brain. It provides high-resolution images that are used to detect changes in brain volume and morphology, which are important indicators of AD [8]. fMRI monitors brain activity by observing variations in blood flow, referred to as the hemodynamic response, which is linked to neuronal activity. It depends upon the blood-oxygen-level-dependent (BOLD) signal to analyze brain regions with accelerated oxygen consumption, indicating increased neuronal activity [9]. AD is often associated with reduced BOLD signals in certain regions, reflecting impaired neural activity. Unlike sMRI, which provides static images, fMRI captures dynamic processes within the brain.

There exist various sorts of fMRI that we generally use in the detection of AD. In AD diagnosis research, resting-state fMRI (rs-fMRI) is widely engaged to monitor the functional connectivity among diverse areas of the brain while the patient is at rest [10]. Alterations in these networks, such as the default mode network (DMN), are often observed in Alzheimer's patients [11]. Then, task-based fMRI involves having patients perform specific cognitive tasks during the scan, which can help to identify those areas of the brain where activity is reduced or abnormal, such as in memory or attention-related regions [12]. Positron emission tomography (PET) is adapted for identifying amyloid deposits and tau tangles, which are key indicators of AD, using radiotracers such as 18F-fluorodeoxyglucose (FDG) [13].

Diffusion tensor imaging (DTI) is also a neuroimaging modality that has been utilized in various studies [14]. It uses MRI-based techniques to measure water molecule diffusion in brain tissue. It primarily targets the brain's white matter tracts, which are the pathways that connect different regions. DTI provides key metrics like fractional anisotropy, radial diffusivity, mean diffusivity, and axial diffusivity to assess the integrity of these white matter fibers [15]. This helps in detecting microstructural changes in white matter, which are often associated with AD. DTI is often used alongside other imaging techniques, such as sMRI, fMRI, and PET, in multimodal research studies. This integration helps to correlate white matter integrity with gray matter atrophy, brain activity, and amyloid/tau deposition.

Electroencephalography (EEG) and magnetoencephalography (MEG) are non-intrusive methods utilized to record and analyze brain activity in the context of diverse cognitive, sensory, and motor activities to understand how the human brain processes information [16]. EEG records electrical activity in the brain. It monitors the electrical activity produced by neurons, mainly from the cerebral gray matter, using electrodes positioned on the scalp. It is useful for detecting abnormal brain waves and patterns associated with Alzheimer's [17]. MEG is similar to EEG but monitors magnetic flux produced by neural activity inside the brain, providing another layer of functional data [18]. These magnetic fields are produced by the electrical currents that occur naturally when neurons communicate with each other. Medical professionals utilize this examination to study brain activity and pinpoint the precise source region of epilepsy-induced seizures. MEG employs highly sensitive detectors known as SQUIDs (superconducting quantum interference devices) to diagnose the magnetic flux outside the head [19]. The data collected by MEG is often combined with MRI to produce detailed maps of brain activity, showing how different brain regions interact over time.

APOE e4 (Apolipoprotein e4) is an allele is considered to be the main genetic predisposition for late-onset AD [20]. Individuals with one APOE e4 allele copy have a higher chance of developing AD, while those having two copies are at a significantly higher risk. However, not everyone with the APOE e4 variant develops the disease, and not all AD patients have the APOE e4 allele [21].

ABCA7 (ATP-binding cassette transporter A7) has a significant involvement in lipid metabolism, the immune response, and phagocytosis [22]. Emerging research has also linked it to AD, primarily through its role in lipid processing and amyloid beta clearance [23]. Genome-wide association studies (GWAS) have identified genetic variations in ABCA7 that increase the chances of late-onset AD. Mutations or loss-of-function variants in this gene can reduce its protective effects, leading to increased susceptibility to AD [24]. Individuals with certain ABCA7 variants have been found to have a higher amyloid burden and more severe neurodegeneration.

Several genes beyond APOE4 and ABCA7 play crucial roles in AD. PSEN1 (presenilin 1) and PSEN2 (presenilin 2) are involved in amyloid-beta production, with mutations leading to early-onset familial Alzheimer's due to increased toxic amyloid-beta fragments [25]. Amyloid precursor protein (APP) mutations similarly contribute by increasing amyloid-beta aggregation. Immune system genes like TREM2 (triggering receptor expressed on myeloid cells 2) affect microglial function, impairing amyloid clearance [26], while CLU (clusterin), CR1 (complement Receptor 1), and PICALM (phosphatidylinositol binding clathrin assembly protein) are linked to disrupted amyloid-beta clearance and neuroinflammation [27]. SORL1 (sortilin-related receptor 1) regulates APP trafficking, and its dysfunction leads to amyloid accumulation [28]. Additionally, BIN1 (bridging integrator 1) and CASS4 (Cas scaffolding protein family member 4) are implicated in synaptic function and neuroinflammation, further contributing to AD risk [29]. These genetic variants collectively influence amyloid metabolism, neuroinflammation, and neuronal signaling, key processes in Alzheimer's pathology.

(Blood-based biomarkers) Plasma amyloid-beta: The Aβ42/40 ratio measures amyloid-beta in the blood and correlates with amyloid plaque accumulation in the brain [30], providing a less intrusive alternative to PET imaging or cerebrospinal fluid (CSF).

Plasma phosphorylated tau (p-tau181, p-tau217, p-tau231): Elevated levels of phosphorylated tau in the blood are indicative of tau pathology and have been observed to predict cognitive loss and brain atrophy [31].

The neurofilament light chain (NfL) marker indicates neural degeneration and neuronal damage. Amplified plasma NfL levels are linked to disease progression in Alzheimer's and other neurodegenerative conditions [32].

## 3.3 ROLE OF MACHINE LEARNING (ML) AND DEEP LEARNING (DL) IN DIAGNOSIS OF ALZHEIMER'S DISEASE

Machine learning (ML) algorithms can process extensive datasets of structural biomolecules and bioassays to find possible drug candidates that may target beta-amyloid. These algorithms can estimate the binding affinity of molecules to beta-amyloid, helping researchers narrow the pool of compounds to be tested experimentally [33]. ML models can process complex datasets, such as imaging, genetic, and clinical data, to detect patterns and biomarkers linked to beta-amyloid accumulation. This can help in the early diagnosis of AD and facilitate the monitoring of disease progression [34].

ML algorithms can analyze neuroimaging data, like PET scans and MRI, to detect and quantify beta-amyloid deposits in the human brain. These algorithms can analyze patient data to predict individual responses to potential treatments targeting beta-amyloid [35]. By identifying biomarkers and patient characteristics associated with treatment response, these models can help optimize therapeutic strategies and improve patient outcomes. These algorithms can improve the accuracy and efficiency of image analysis, providing valuable information for both research and clinical applications. Machine learning models can also integrate multimodal data, including imaging, clinical, and biomarker data, to predict the progression of AD and the accumulation of beta-amyloid over time [36]. These predictive models can assist in identifying individuals who have more chances to develop AD and guide personalized treatment strategies.

Deep learning (DL) also plays an integral role in analyzing complex data related to AD. Convolutional neural networks (CNNs), particularly 3D CNNs, have been broadly applied for processing MRI and PET scan data to identify early signs of AD. They help in extracting spatial features and detecting structural brain changes. They can be used to segment brain regions and identify atrophy patterns associated with AD progression [37]. When working with small datasets, transfer learning has proven beneficial. A study demonstrated how pretrained networks, adapted for AD diagnosis, improved classification accuracy [38]. Generative adversarial networks (GANs) have been used to augment training data by creating synthetic images, enabling CNNs to become more robust and capable of better generalization. This approach tackles the challenge of limited datasets often encountered in medical research [39].

Variational autoencoders (VAEs) have been employed for the dimensionality reduction of proteomic data, helping researchers detect relevant protein interactions [40]. VAEs can be employed to find novel biomarkers that could be linked to AD, providing pathways for potential therapeutic targets. Some studies discussed how deep learning models applied to whole-genome sequencing data could reveal polymorphisms linked with a higher risk of AD. This research highlighted the effectiveness of deep neural networks in identifying complex genetic interactions that contribute to AD [41].

Recurrent neural networks (RNNs), especially long short-term memory (LSTM) networks, are mostly adapted to process sequential cognitive data [42]. LSTM networks are capable of predicting the conversion from mild cognitive impairment (MCI) to AD by assessing clinical test results over time. Integrating attention mechanisms with LSTM models has improved the focus on critical time periods within patient data, enhancing prediction accuracy. Deep reinforcement learning (DRL) models have been applied to optimize treatment plans, suggesting personalized interventions aimed at slowing cognitive decline [43].

Various input modalities of AD research with related different ML and DL approaches are depicted in Figure 3.4. Full forms of some abbreviations used in Figure 3.4 can be found in the footnote of Table 3.1. Multimodal deep learning approaches have also become more prevalent, combining MRI, genetic, and cognitive data for comprehensive AD analysis [44]. CNNs and attention-based models to integrate imaging data with genetic profiles, resulted in improved diagnostic accuracy in AD studies. Transformer-based models have shown potential for assigning weights to various data sources and capturing complex relationships, enhancing both interpretability and performance.

EEG data, combined with clinical and neuroimaging data, has been processed using deep learning for early detection and classification of AD. This approach leverages multimodal data to provide a more detailed and accurate diagnostic process. A review emphasized the need for explainable AI (XAI) to make models more transparent and understandable for clinicians [45]. Techniques such as SHAP (SHapley Additive exPlanations) and LRP (layer-wise relevance propagation) have been adopted to provide insights into which features most influence predictions. Federated learning is also being highlighted as a future direction to train models across multiple institutions without sharing patient data, promoting data privacy while improving generalizability. The future of AD research includes integrating continuous data streams from wearable devices and EHRs to create predictive models capable of real-time monitoring and personalized treatment adaptations.

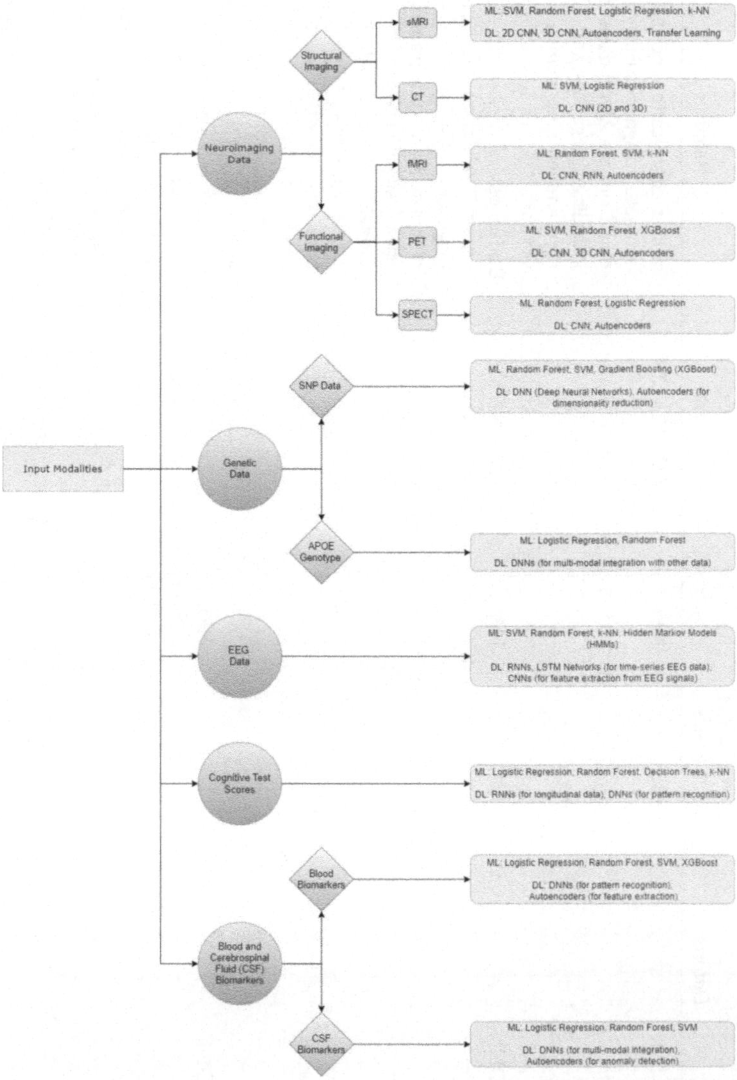


*Figure 3.4* Input modalities of AD research with different ML and DL approaches.

## 3.4 STUDY OF RELATED WORK

Numerous studies have been conducted using both single-modality and multimodality biomarkers, which can be split into two major groups: machine learning and deep learning approaches. ML shows promise in identifying dementia risk from neuroimaging but remains limited in accuracy. A review of studies (2006–2016) found the highest accuracy in identifying AD versus

*Table 3.1* An overview of the papers applying different ML and DL models

| *Reference* | *Model* | *Dataset* | *Number of subjects* | *Input modality* | *Prediction type* | *Remarks* |
|---|---|---|---|---|---|---|
| [55] | LR, KNN, SVM, GNB, DT, RF | ADNI | 485 | MRI | AD-MCI-CN | Various classification models estimated diagnosis using data from the ADNI dataset, including age, gender, and right and left hippocampal volume. |
| [56] | SVM, CNN | ADNI | 1715 | MRI | AD-CN-MCIc-MCInc | Both cross-validation and external validation for diagnosing AD-CN demonstrated comparable effectiveness between DL models and traditional classifiers, with notable improvement when using modulated GM maps compared with raw T1w scans. |
| [57] | XGBoost | ADNI | 12741 | MRI, PET- FDG, and AV45 | AD-CN-EMCI-LMCI-SMC | The XGBoost algorithm outperforms other classifiers in distinguishing between various neurodegenerative diagnoses, demonstrating greater reliability and accuracy. |

(*Continued*)

*Table 3.1* (Continued)

| *Reference* | *Model* | *Dataset* | *Number of subjects* | *Input modality* | *Prediction type* | *Remarks* |
|---|---|---|---|---|---|---|
| [58] | LR | Patients were recruited from hospitals (Mazloum, Dar al-Ajaza, and Vita Nova Polyclinic in Tripoli, Lebanon), while healthy individuals were gathered from local populace. | 41 | EEG | AD-HC | Several classification algorithms were tested, with logistic regression yielding the best results. Hyperparameter combinations were optimized using GridSearchCV, and classifiers have been validated using StratifiedKFold cross-validation with k = 5. |
| [59] | RF, SVM, NB, KNN | Training on NACC dataset Testing on ADNI dataset | 26722 | Categorical and numerical features | AD-MCI-NC | Among 4 models tested—NB, KNN, RF and SVM—RF and SVM reliably achieved the highest accuracy, precision, and recall among all tasks, successfully differentiating between NC and AD, NC and MCI, and MCI and AD individuals. Whereas NB and KNN had also showed notable accuracy, their overall performance was typically inferior to that of RF and SVM. |

*(Continued)*

*Table 3.1* (Continued)

| *Reference* | *Model* | *Dataset* | *Number of subjects* | *Input modality* | *Prediction type* | *Remarks* |
|---|---|---|---|---|---|---|
| [60] | SVM, DT, KNN, RNN, CNN | Data collected over a decade from 5 different hospitals | 668 | EEG | ADA-ADM-CN | CNN approach outperformed other methods, gaining 97.45% classification accuracy for ADM and 97.03% for ADA. |
| [61] | GAN, MLP, GNN | ADNI | 332 (Paired Dataset-MRI-T1WI and FDG-PET) and 760 (Extended Dataset-MRI-T1WI only) | MRI, FDG-PET | AD-MCI-NC | A GAN model was proposed to create synthetic images to address the absence of PET images, followed by MLP and GNN for Alzheimer's disease classification. |
| [62] | DeepCurvMRI model | Kaggle | 6400 | MRI | ND-VMD-MID-MOD | A curvelet transform-based CNN (DeepCurvMRI) model was used to enhance the accuracy of early onset of AD diagnosis from MRI scans. |

(*Continued*)

*Table 3.1* (Continued)

| *Reference* | *Model* | *Dataset* | *Number of subjects* | *Input modality* | *Prediction type* | *Remarks* |
|---|---|---|---|---|---|---|
| [63] | CNN, SDAE, DNN | ADNI | 300 | MRI, SNPs | AD-MCI | 3D ResNet architecture, a CNN model, is used along with stacked denoising autoencoders (SDAE) to extract feature from high-dimensional, sparse SNP data. DNN is then employed to represent the structure of clinical data. |
| [64] | CNN, RNN | ADNI | 830 | MRI | AD- NC- sMCI-pMCI | Separate 3D CNNs were implemented to each point of time, with their resulting feature maps passed into 3-stacked bidirectional GRUs. The outputs were then merged into a dense layer, with Softmax activation applied afterward. |

ADNI: Alzheimer's Disease Neuroimaging Initiative, NACC: National Alzheimer's Coordinating Center, SNPs: single nucleotide polymorphisms, LR: logistic regression, NB: naive Bayes, KNN: k-nearest neighbor, DT: decision tree, SVM: support vector machine, GNB: Gaussian naive Bayes, RF: random forest, XGBoost: eXtreme Gradient Boosting, CNN: convolutional neural network, GAN: generative adversarial network, RNN: recurrent neural network, MLP: multilayer perceptron, GNN: graph neural network, SDAE: stacked denoising autoencoder, DNN: deep neural network, GRUs: gated recurrent units, sMRI: structural magnetic resonance imaging, CT: computed tomography, fMRI: functional magnetic resonance imaging, PET: positron emission tomography, SPECT: single photon emission computed tomography, FDG: fluorodeoxyglucose, AV45: Amyvid (Florbetapir F18), MRI-T1WI: magnetic resonance imaging–T1-weighted imaging, AD: Alzheimer's disease, MCI: mild cognitive impairment, CN: cognitively normal, MCIc: MCI converters, MCInc: MCI non-converters, EMCI: early mild cognitive impairment, LMCI: late mild cognitive impairment, SMC: significant memory concern, HC: healthy controls, NC: normal control, sMCI: stable mild cognitive impairment, pMCI: progressive mild cognitive impairment, ND: neurodegenerative disease, VMD: very mild dementia, MID: mild dementia, MOD: moderate dementia, ADA: advanced Alzheimer's dementia, ADM: moderate Alzheimer's dementia

healthy controls (HC), while differentiation between other groups, like MCI, was less effective [46]. Combining data types improved results, suggesting the need for more diverse datasets and closer clinical integration to advance the field. Neuroimaging now enables in vivo measurement of AD-related brain changes, providing resources for individualized diagnostic and prognostic evaluation through classification frameworks. A review of studies (1985–2016) explored AD and MCI classification using different neuroimaging modalities: sMRI, fMRI, DTI, FDG-PET, and amyloid-PET [47]. These classification frameworks, based on specific extracted features, hold potential in diagnosing and predicting disease progression.

DL, especially through CNNs and the Xception architecture, is advancing AD diagnostics via MRI analysis. Li et. al. used deep learning models to classify MRI images by AD stage, achieving 99.6% accuracy, highlighting its potential in early and precise diagnosis [48]. Automatic diagnosis is critical due to limited expert availability and the demand for precise analysis of MRI brain scans. Traditional machine learning has limitations in feature extraction and accuracy, while deep learning offers automatic feature extraction and improved training. Using an imbalanced MRI dataset of Alzheimer's stages, Mujahid et al. employed synthetic oversampling to balance class distributions and applied an ensemble model of VGG16 and EfficientNet-B2 [49]. This approach gained 97.35% accuracy and 99.64% AUC for multiclass, and 97.09% accuracy and 99.59% AUC for binary class datasets, outperforming previous methods.

Ju et al. [50] developed a deep learning approach that combines brain network data with clinical information (age, gender, ApoE gene) for early Alzheimer's diagnosis. Using R-fMRI data, an autoencoder network distinguished normal aging from mild cognitive impairment, achieving ~31.21% higher accuracy and 51.23% lower standard deviation than traditional methods. Liu et al. [51] introduced a hippocampus analysis procedure for AD diagnosis that combines global and local features using 3D densely connected convolutional networks and shape analysis. Unlike other methods, it doesn't require tissue segmentation or nonlinear registration. Tested on T1-weighted MRIs from 811 subjects, this approach achieved 92.29% accuracy and a 96.95% AUC, outperforming existing methods. Fabietti et al. [52] introduced an explainable ensemble machine learning model (EXML) to detect early markers of AD by analyzing cortical and hippocampal local field potential signals (LFPs). Obtained from healthy and two AD animal models, LFPs were validated with ECG and respiration signals. The model generated features from LFPs in temporal, spatial, and spectral domains, and achieved an impressive 99.4% accuracy using late fusion. It revealed observations of amyloid deposits as early as three months post-onset and demonstrated robustness against artifacts by masking channels during evaluation.

Rogeau et al. [53] designed a 3D convolutional neural network model to classify [18F]-FDG PET scans for AD, frontotemporal dementia (FTD), and cognitively normal (CN) subjects by analyzing glucose metabolism in the brain. After categorizing the dataset into training and test groups (90%–10%), this model employed data augmentation and cross-validation, achieving an overall accuracy of 89.8% on test scans. The area under the ROC curve was 93.3% for AD, 95.3% for FTD, and 99.9% for CN. In comparison, physician consensus achieved 69.5% accuracy, indicating considerable consensus (kappa = 0.61, 95% CI: 0.49–0.73). Neuronal cell segmentation plays a vital role in understanding neuron structure and function, essential for treating neurological disorders. Hasan et al. [54] used a method that combines CNNs and graph attention networks (GATs) to segment medical diagnostic images. Their architecture captures context through a contracting path, then applies GATs to calculate attention coefficients between nodes for precise segmentation. Evaluated on a dataset of 606 microscopic images from different cell types, the U-GAT algorithm achieved 86.5% accuracy and an F1 score of 0.719, outperforming models like CNN and U-Net. This approach could enhance drug development by improving segmentation of complex neuronal images. A review of some AD research papers is presented in Table 3.1.

## 3.5 CONCLUSION AND FUTURE DIRECTIONS

Alzheimer's disease (AD), a chronic neurological disorder, benefits from early detection to alleviate symptoms. This report presents the different machine learning and deep learning approaches utilized for the early diagnosis of AD. These approaches have been targeted on relevant different aspects related to AD. A literature review of some of these approaches is included to represent their significant targets. Here we observed that for such complex tasks like medical image processing, deep learning approaches are more effective than machine learning solutions since they are better at identifying abnormal conditions. The integration of multimodal data, such as neuroimaging and genetic information, holds promise for more accurate early diagnosis of AD. Future developments in explainable AI and transfer learning may enhance diagnostic transparency and efficiency. Additionally, real-time AI support could transform clinical workflows, enabling better monitoring of disease progression and treatment outcomes.

## REFERENCES

1. Khojaste-Sarakhsi, M., Haghighi, S. S., Ghomi, S. M. T. F., & Marchiori, E. (2022). Deep learning for Alzheimer's disease diagnosis: A survey. *Artificial Intelligence in Medicine*, *130*. Elsevier B.V. https://doi.org/10.1016/j.artmed.2022.102332

2. 2023 Alzheimer's disease facts and figures (2023). *Alzheimer's & Dementia, 19*, 1598–1695.
3. Alzheimer's Diagnosis and Treatment, Alzheimer's Research and Prevention Foundation™, a 501(c)(3) charitable organization. https://alzheimersprevention.org/alzheimers-info/diagnosis-and-treatment/
4. Duchateau, L., Wawrzyniak, N., & Sleegers, K. (2024). The ABC's of Alzheimer risk gene ABCA7. *Alzheimer's and Dementia, 20*(5), 3629–3648. John Wiley and Sons Inc. https://doi.org/10.1002/alz.13805
5. Sadigh-Eteghad, S., Sabermarouf, B., Majdi, A., Talebi, M., Farhoudi, M., & Mahmoudi, J. (2015). Amyloid-beta: A crucial factor in Alzheimer's disease. *Medical Principles and Practice, 24*(1), 1–10. S. Karger AG. https://doi.org/10.1159/000369101
6. Healthy brain and brain with Alzheimer's disease, Mayo Foundation for Medical Education and Research. https://www.mayoclinic.org/diseases-conditions/alzheimers-disease/multimedia/img-20543517
7. Rajmohan, R., & Reddy, P. H. (2017). Amyloid-beta and phosphorylated Tau accumulations cause abnormalities at synapses of Alzheimer's disease neurons. *Journal of Alzheimer's Disease, 57*(4), 975–999). IOS Press. https://doi.org/10.3233/JAD-160612
8. Zhang, F., Pan, B., Shao, P., Liu, P., Shen, S., Yao, P., & Xu, R. X. (2022). A single model deep learning approach for Alzheimer's disease diagnosis. *Neuroscience, 491*, 200–214. https://doi.org/10.1016/J.NEUROSCIENCE.2022.03.026
9. Ahmadi, H., Fatemizadeh, E., & Motie-Nasrabadi, A. (2021). Deep sparse graph functional connectivity analysis in AD patients using fMRI data. *Computer Methods and Programs in Biomedicine, 201*, 105954. https://doi.org/10.1016/J.CMPB.2021.105954
10. Dai, P., Xiong, T., Zhou, X., Ou, Y., Li, Y., Kui, X., Chen, Z., Zou, B., Li, W., Huang, Z., & The REST-meta-MDD Consortium. (2022). The alterations of brain functional connectivity networks in major depressive disorder detected by machine learning through multisite rs-fMRI data. *Behavioural Brain Research, 435*, 114058. https://doi.org/10.1016/J.BBR.2022.114058
11. Hao, S., Yang, C., Li, Z., & Ren, J. (2022). Distinguishing patients with temporal lobe epilepsy from normal controls with the directed graph measures of resting-state fMRI. *Seizure, 96*, 25–33. https://doi.org/10.1016/J.SEIZURE.2022.01.007
12. König, P., Zwiky, E., Küttner, A., Uhlig, M., & Redlich, R. (2025). Brain functional effects of cognitive behavioral therapy for depression: A systematic review of task-based fMRI studies. *Journal of Affective Disorders, 368*, 872–887. https://doi.org/10.1016/J.JAD.2024.09.084
13. Rowley, P. A., Samsonov, A. A., Betthauser, T. J., Pirasteh, A., Johnson, S. C., & Eisenmenger, L. B. (2020). Amyloid and Tau PET imaging of Alzheimer disease and other neurodegenerative conditions. *Seminars in Ultrasound, CT and MRI, 41*(6), 572–583. https://doi.org/10.1053/J.SULT.2020.08.011
14. Qu, Y., Wang, P., Liu, B., Song, C., Wang, D., Yang, H., Zhang, Z., Chen, P., Kang, X., Du, K., Yao, H., Zhou, B., Han, T., Zuo, N., Han, Y., Lu, J., Yu, C., Zhang, X., Jiang, T., Liu, Y. (2021). AI4AD: Artificial intelligence analysis for Alzheimer's disease classification based on a multisite DTI database. *Brain Disorders, 1*, 100005. https://doi.org/10.1016/J.DSCB.2021.100005

15. Alexander, A. L., Lee, J. E., Lazar, M., & Field, A. S. (2007). Diffusion tensor imaging of the brain. *Neurotherapeutics*, *4*(3), 316–329. https://doi.org/10.1016/J.NURT.2007.05.011
16. Beppi, C., Ribeiro Violante, I., Scott, G., & Sandrone, S. (2021). EEG, MEG and neuromodulatory approaches to explore cognition: Current status and future directions. *Brain and Cognition*, *148*, 105677. https://doi.org/10.1016/J.BANDC.2020.105677
17. Safi, M. S., & Safi, S. M. M. (2021). Early detection of Alzheimer's disease from EEG signals using Hjorth parameters. *Biomedical Signal Processing and Control*, *65*, 102338. https://doi.org/10.1016/J.BSPC.2020.102338
18. Mandal, P. K., Banerjee, A., Tripathi, M., & Sharma, A. (2018). A comprehensive review of magnetoencephalography (MEG) studies for brain functionality in healthy aging and Alzheimer's disease (AD). *Frontiers in Computational Neuroscience*, *12*. Frontiers Media S.A. https://doi.org/10.3389/fncom.2018.00060
19. Ellenbogen, J. R., & Ashkan, K. (2018). Neurosurgery of epilepsy, movement disorders and pain. *Surgery (United Kingdom)*, *36*(11), 655–663. https://doi.org/10.1016/j.mpsur.2018.09.002
20. Troutwine, B. R., Hamid, L., Lysaker, C. R., Strope, T. A., & Wilkins, H. M. (2022). Apolipoprotein E and Alzheimer's disease. *Acta Pharmaceutica Sinica B*, *12*(2), 496–510. https://doi.org/10.1016/J.APSB.2021.10.002
21. Husain, M. A., Laurent, B., & Plourde, M. (2021). APOE and Alzheimer's disease: From lipid transport to physiopathology and therapeutics. *Frontiers in Neuroscience*, *15*. Frontiers Media S.A. https://doi.org/10.3389/fnins.2021.630502
22. de Roeck, A., van Broeckhoven, C., & Sleegers, K. (2019). The role of ABCA7 in Alzheimer's disease: evidence from genomics, transcriptomics and methylomics. *Acta Neuropathologica*, *138*(2), 201–220. Springer Verlag. https://doi.org/10.1007/s00401-019-01994-1
23. Aikawa, T., Holm, M. L., & Kanekiyo, T. (2018). ABCA7 and pathogenic pathways of Alzheimer's disease. *Brain Sciences*, *8*(2). MDPI AG. https://doi.org/10.3390/brainsci8020027
24. Zhang, J., Wang, Y., Zhang, Y., & Yao, J. (2023). Genome-wide association study in Alzheimer's disease: A bibliometric and visualization analysis. *Frontiers in Aging Neuroscience*, *15*. https://doi.org/10.3389/fnagi.2023.1290657
25. Petit, D., Fernández, S. G., Zoltowska, K. M., Enzlein, T., Ryan, N. S., O'Connor, A., Szaruga, M., Hill, E., Vandenberghe, R., Fox, N. C., & Chávez-Gutiérrez, L. (2022). Aβ profiles generated by Alzheimer's disease causing PSEN1 variants determine the pathogenicity of the mutation and predict age at disease onset. *Molecular Psychiatry*, *27*(6), 2821–2832. https://doi.org/10.1038/s41380-022-01518-6
26. Li, Y., Xu, H., Wang, H., Yang, K., Luan, J., & Wang, S. (2023). TREM2: Potential therapeutic targeting of microglia for Alzheimer's disease. *Biomedicine & Pharmacotherapy*, *165*, 115218. https://doi.org/10.1016/J.BIOPHA.2023.115218
27. Khan, T. K. (2016). Genetic biomarkers in Alzheimer's disease. In *Biomarkers in Alzheimer's Disease* (pp. 103–135). Elsevier. https://doi.org/10.1016/B978-0-12-804832-0.00004-3

28. Hung, C., Tuck, E., Stubbs, V., van der Lee, S. J., Aalfs, C., van Spaendonk, R., Scheltens, P., Hardy, J., Holstege, H., & Livesey, F. J. (2021). SORL1 deficiency in human excitatory neurons causes APP-dependent defects in the endolysosome-autophagy network. *Cell Reports*, *35*(11), 109259. https://doi.org/10.1016/J.CELREP.2021.109259
29. Karch, C. M., & Goate, A. M. (2015). Alzheimer's disease risk genes and mechanisms of disease pathogenesis. *Biological Psychiatry*, *77*(1), 43–51. https://doi.org/10.1016/J.BIOPSYCH.2014.05.006
30. Fandos, N., Pérez-Grijalba, V., Pesini, P., Olmos, S., Bossa, M., Villemagne, V. L., Doecke, J., Fowler, C., Masters, C. L., & Sarasa, M. (2017). Plasma amyloid β 42/40 ratios as biomarkers for amyloid β cerebral deposition in cognitively normal individuals. *Alzheimer's & Dementia: Diagnosis, Assessment & Disease Monitoring*, *8*, 179–187. https://doi.org/10.1016/J.DADM.2017.07.004
31. Ashton, N. J., Janelidze, S., Mattsson-Carlgren, N., Binette, A. P., Strandberg, O., Brum, W. S., Karikari, T. K., González-Ortiz, F., di Molfetta, G., Meda, F. J., Jonaitis, E. M., Koscik, R. L., Cody, K., Betthauser, T. J., Li, Y., Vanmechelen, E., Palmqvist, S., Stomrud, E., Bateman, R. J., Hansson, O. (2022). Differential roles of Aβ42/40, p-tau231 and p-tau217 for Alzheimer's trial selection and disease monitoring. *Nature Medicine*, *28*(12), 2555–2562. https://doi.org/10.1038/s41591-022-02074-w
32. Xiong, Y. L., Meng, T., Luo, J., & Zhang, H. (2021). The potential of neurofilament light as a biomarker in Alzheimer's disease. *European Neurology*, *84*(1), 6–15. S. Karger AG. https://doi.org/10.1159/000513008
33. Rehman, A. U., Li, M., Wu, B., Ali, Y., Rasheed, S., Shaheen, S., Liu, X., Luo, R., & Zhang, J. (2024). Role of artificial intelligence in revolutionizing drug discovery. *Fundamental Research*. https://doi.org/10.1016/J.FMRE.2024.04.021
34. Gao, S., & Lima, D. (2022). A review of the application of deep learning in the detection of Alzheimer's disease. *International Journal of Cognitive Computing in Engineering*, *3*, 1–8.
35. Angelucci, F., Ai, A. R., Piendel, L., Cerman, J., & Hort, J. (2024). Integrating AI in fighting advancing Alzheimer: diagnosis, prevention, treatment, monitoring, mechanisms, and clinical trials. *Current Opinion in Structural Biology*, *87*, 102857. https://doi.org/10.1016/J.SBI.2024.102857
36. Li, Z., Jiang, X., Wang, Y., & Kim, Y. (2021). Applied machine learning in Alzheimer's disease research: Omics, imaging, and clinical data. *Emerging Topics in Life Sciences*, *5*(6), 765–777. Portland Press Ltd. https://doi.org/10.1042/ETLS20210249
37. Zhang, J., Zheng, B., Gao, A., Feng, X., Liang, D., & Long, X. (2021). A 3D densely connected convolution neural network with connection-wise attention mechanism for Alzheimer's disease classification. *Magnetic Resonance Imaging*, *78*, 119–126. https://doi.org/10.1016/j.mri.2021.02.001
38. Shanmugam, J., Duraisamy, B., Simon, B., & Bhaskaran, P. (2022). Alzheimer's disease classification using pre-trained deep networks. *Biomedical Signal Processing and Control*, *71*, 103217. https://doi.org/10.1016/j.bspc.2021.103217

39. Islam, S., Aziz, M. T., Nabil, H. R., Jim, J. R., Mridha, M. F., Kabir, M. M., Asai, N., & Shin, J. (2024). Generative Adversarial Networks (GANs) in medical imaging: Advancements, applications, and challenges. *IEEE Access, 12*, 35728–35753. https://doi.org/10.1109/ACCESS.2024.3370848
40. Mansoor, S., Baek, M., Park, H., Lee, G. R., & Baker, D. (2024). Protein ensemble generation through variational autoencoder latent space sampling. *Journal of Chemical Theory and Computation, 20*(7), 2689–2695. https://doi.org/10.1021/acs.jctc.3c01057
41. Park, C., Ha, J., & Park, S. (2020). Prediction of Alzheimer's disease based on deep neural network by integrating gene expression and DNA methylation dataset. *Expert Systems with Applications, 140*, 112873. https://doi.org/10.1016/J.ESWA.2019.112873
42. Alessandrini, M., Biagetti, G., Crippa, P., Falaschetti, L., & Luzzi, S. (2022). EEG-based Alzheimer's disease recognition using robust-PCA and LSTM recurrent neural network. *Sensors, 22*, 3696. https://doi.org/10.3390/s22103696
43. El-Dosuky, M. A. (2024). Optimization of treatment plans using deep reinforcement learning with the human-in-the-loop. *International Journal of Computer Applications, 186*(4).
44. Venugopalan, J., Tong, L., Hassanzadeh, H. R., & Wang, M. D. (2021). Multimodal deep learning models for early detection of Alzheimer's disease stage. *Scientific Reports, 11*(1). https://doi.org/10.1038/s41598-020-74399-w
45. Sadeghi, Z., Alizadehsani, R., CIFCI, M. A., Kausar, S., Rehman, R., Mahanta, P., Bora, P. K., Almasri, A., Alkhawaldeh, R. S., Hussain, S., Alatas, B., Shoeibi, A., Moosaei, H., Hladík, M., Nahavandi, S., & Pardalos, P. M. (2024). A review of explainable artificial intelligence in healthcare. *Computers and Electrical Engineering, 118*, 109370. https://doi.org/10.1016/J.COMPELECENG.2024.109370
46. Pellegrini, E., Ballerini, L., Hernandez, M. del C. V., Chappell, F. M., González-Castro, V., Anblagan, D., Danso, S., Muñoz-Maniega, S., Job, D., Pernet, C., Mair, G., MacGillivray, T. J., Trucco, E., & Wardlaw, J. M. (2018). Machine learning of neuroimaging for assisted diagnosis of cognitive impairment and dementia: A systematic review. *Alzheimer's & Dementia: Diagnosis, Assessment & Disease Monitoring, 10*, 519–535. https://doi.org/10.1016/J.DADM.2018.07.004
47. Rathore, S., Habes, M., Iftikhar, M. A., Shacklett, A., & Davatzikos, C. (2017). A review on neuroimaging-based classification studies and associated feature extraction methods for Alzheimer's disease and its prodromal stages. *NeuroImage, 155*, 530–548. https://doi.org/10.1016/J.NEUROIMAGE.2017.03.057
48. Li, S., Qu, H., Dong, X., Dang, B., Zang, H., & Gong, Y. (2024). *Leveraging deep learning and xception architecture for high-accuracy MRI classification in Alzheimer diagnosis.* http://arxiv.org/abs/2403.16212
49. Carlsen, J. F., Ladefoged, C. N., Mujahid, M., Rehman, A., Alam, T., Alamri, F. S., Fati, S. M., & Saba, T. (2023). *An efficient ensemble approach for Alzheimer's disease detection using an adaptive synthetic technique and deep learning.* https://doi.org/10.3390/diagnostics

50. Ju, R., Hu, C., Zhou, P., & Li, Q. (2019). Early diagnosis of alzheimer's disease based on resting-state brain networks and deep learning. *IEEE/ACM Transactions on Computational Biology and Bioinformatics*, *16*(1), 244–257. https://doi.org/10.1109/TCBB.2017.2776910
51. Cui, R., & Liu, M. (2019). Hippocampus analysis by combination of 3-D DenseNet and shapes for Alzheimer's disease diagnosis. *IEEE Journal of Biomedical and Health Informatics*, *23*(5), 2099–2107. https://doi.org/10.1109/JBHI.2018.2882392
52. Fabietti, M., Mahmud, M., Lotfi, A., Leparulo, A., Fontana, R., Vassanelli, S., & Fasolato, C. (2023). Early detection of Alzheimer's disease from cortical and hippocampal local field potentials using an ensembled machine learning model. *IEEE Transactions on Neural Systems and Rehabilitation Engineering*, *31*, 2839–2848. https://doi.org/10.1109/TNSRE.2023.3288835
53. Rogeau, A., Hives, F., Bordier, C., Lahousse, H., Roca, V., Lebouvier, T., Pasquier, F., Huglo, D., Semah, F., & Lopes, R. (2024). A 3D convolutional neural network to classify subjects as Alzheimer's disease, frontotemporal dementia or healthy controls using brain 18F-FDG PET. *NeuroImage*, *288*, 120530. https://doi.org/10.1016/J.NEUROIMAGE.2024.120530
54. Hasan, M. E., & Wagler, A. (2024). A novel deep learning graph attention network for Alzheimer's disease image segmentation. *Healthcare Analytics*, *5*, 100310. https://doi.org/10.1016/J.HEALTH.2024.100310
55. Uysal, G., & Ozturk, M. (2020). Hippocampal atrophy based Alzheimer's disease diagnosis via machine learning methods. *Journal of Neuroscience Methods*, *337*, 108669. https://doi.org/10.1016/J.JNEUMETH.2020.108669
56. Bron, E. E., Klein, S., Papma, J. M., Jiskoot, L. C., Venkatraghavan, V., Linders, J., Aalten, P., de Deyn, P. P., Biessels, G. J., Claassen, J. A. H. R., Middelkoop, H. A. M., Smits, M., Niessen, W. J., van Swieten, J. C., van der Flier, W. M., Ramakers, I. H. G. B., & van der Lugt, A. (2021). Cross-cohort generalizability of deep and conventional machine learning for MRI-based diagnosis and prediction of Alzheimer's disease. *NeuroImage: Clinical*, *31*, 102712. https://doi.org/10.1016/J.NICL.2021.102712
57. Bogdanovic, B., Eftimov, T., & Simjanoska, M. (2022). In-depth insights into Alzheimer's disease by using explainable machine learning approach. *Scientific Reports*, *12*(1). https://doi.org/10.1038/s41598-022-10202-2
58. Chedid, N., Tabbal, J., Kabbara, A., Allouch, S., & Hassan, M. (2022). The development of an automated machine learning pipeline for the detection of Alzheimer's Disease. *Scientific Reports*, *12*(1). https://doi.org/10.1038/s41598-022-22979-3
59. Alatrany, A. S., Khan, W., Hussain, A., Kolivand, H., & Al-Jumeily, D. (2024). An explainable machine learning approach for Alzheimer's disease classification. *Scientific Reports*, *14*(1). https://doi.org/10.1038/s41598-024-51985-w
60. Roncero-Parra, C., Parreño-Torres, A., Sánchez-Reolid, R., Mateo-Sotos, J., & Borja, A. L. (2024). Inter-hospital moderate and advanced Alzheimer's disease detection through convolutional neural networks. *Heliyon*, *10*(4), e26298. https://doi.org/10.1016/J.HELIYON.2024.E26298

61. Chen, K., Weng, Y., Hosseini, A. A., Dening, T., Zuo, G., & Zhang, Y. (2024). A comparative study of GNN and MLP based machine learning for the diagnosis of Alzheimer's disease involving data synthesis. *Neural Networks, 169*, 442–452. https://doi.org/10.1016/J.NEUNET.2023.10.040
62. Chabib, C. M., Hadjileontiadis, L. J., & Shehhi, A. al. (2023). DeepCurvMRI: Deep convolutional curvelet transform-based MRI approach for early detection of Alzheimer's disease. *IEEE Access, 11*, 44650–44659. https://doi.org/10.1109/ACCESS.2023.3272482
63. Lu, P., Hu, L., Mitelpunkt, A., Bhatnagar, S., Lu, L., & Liang, H. (2024). A hierarchical attention-based multimodal fusion framework for predicting the progression of Alzheimer's disease. *Biomedical Signal Processing and Control, 88*, 105669. https://doi.org/10.1016/J.BSPC.2023.105669
64. Cui, R., & Liu, M. (2019). RNN-based longitudinal analysis for diagnosis of Alzheimer's disease. *Computerized Medical Imaging and Graphics, 73*. https://doi.org/10.1016/j.compmedimag.2019.01.005

Chapter 4

# Comparative analysis of transfer learning models versus ensemble transfer learning models for multiclass cutaneous carcinoma classification

*Rashmi Nair, Rohit Agrawal, and Sudheesh Sudhakaran*

## 4.1 INTRODUCTION

One of the major types of cancers is cutaneous carcinoma (Barata et al., 2021; Liu et al., 2021), which leads to a high number of deaths. Screening methods include biopsy; asymmetry of lesion, border irregularity, color variation, diameter and evolving (ABCDE) rule (Bandic et al., 2020); seven-point checklist (Argenziano et al., 1998); dermoscopy; and microscopic images (Singh et al., 2019). The seven-point criteria relies on seven dermatoscopic characteristics: unusual melanin pattern, bluish-white overlay, abnormal vascular arrangement, disordered stripes, uneven pigmentation, uneven spots/clusters and receding structures.

Diagnosis requires expert dermatologists. It requires lots of attention and is considered extremely time-intensive, subjective and prone to errors. Table 4.1 shows the statistics of the cutaneous carcinoma patients globally as per World Cancer Research Fund International (www.wcrf.org). Developing an effective strategy for preliminary identification of cutaneous carcinoma patients is increasingly critical, aiming to mitigate mortality rates through accurate diagnosis.

*Table 4.1* Statistics of cutaneous carcinoma patients globally as per World Cancer Research Fund International

| *Cutaneous carcinoma type* | *Total number of people affected all over the world* | *Total number of men affected* | *Total number of women affected* | *Number of cancer deaths all over the world* | *Number of cancer deaths in men* | *Number of cancer deaths in women* |
|---|---|---|---|---|---|---|
| Melanoma | 324,635 | 173,844 | 150,791 | 57,043 | 32,385 | 24,658 |
| Non-melanoma | 1,198,073 | 722,348 | 475,725 | 63,731 | 37,596 | 26,135 |


DOI: 10.1201/9781003634089-4

Several works have been carried out for binary categorization of dermal layer abnormalities. Works related to dermal layer lesion categorization require feature extraction followed by detection. Computer-aided diagnostics (CAD) are less time-consuming and provide accurate diagnosis (Kassem et al., 2019; Szaleniec et al., 2014). The overall accuracy of CAD is constrained by manual intervention, which requires preprocessing and hand-crafted feature extraction followed by classification. This chapter compares various transfer learning models and ensembles of transfer learning models based on their accuracy of classification. The purpose of this investigation is to develop a proficient model for classifying cutaneous carcinoma images across multiple categories, ensuring accurate identification of dermal layer lesions.

The remaining sections of the chapter are organized as follows: Section 4.2 provides a review of prior research, and Section 4.3 outlines the dataset, data augmentation methods, various transfer learning models and ensembles of transfer learning models. Section 4.4 presents the investigative findings and discussions. Lastly, Section 4.5 offers conclusions.

## 4.2 RELATED WORKS

Categorizing images of dermal layer lesions can streamline the process of identifying multiple varieties of cutaneous carcinoma. Dermal layer lesion images can be broadly categorized as malignant and benign. These images can be further classified as basal cell carcinoma, actinic keratosis, squamous cell carcinoma, seborrheic keratosis, dermatofibroma, nevi, melanoma and vascular lesions. This section delves into both conventional and cutting-edge classification techniques.

Conventional classification algorithms encompass either picture element-based or region-based methodologies. Jamil and Khalid (2014) proposed an instance-based classifier that includes the k-nearest neighbor algorithm and kernel machines. However, it is time-consuming and becomes computationally complex and insensitive.

Alquran (2017) proposed a binary classification supervised learning model called support vector machines (SVM). It helps to optimize the cost function. The disadvantage of this learning model is that it cannot process uncertain information and produces biased results for unavailable class membership probability.

Khan et al. (2019) proposed a decision tree that makes use of the parent node to create decision rules for image classification. The outcomes of this method can be affected by noise and may lack predictive capability beyond the training data scope. Xception deep learning architecture (Lu et al., 2022) employs depth-wise separable convolution. It is considered to be computationally expensive as it employs cardinality to understand abstract characteristics.

Cutting-edge convolutional neural network (CNN) frameworks are investigated for cutaneous carcinoma visualization categorization. Simonyan and Zisserman (2016) proposed VGG, which makes use of algorithmically exorbitant fully connected layers. Szegedy et al. (2015) proposed GoogleNet that utilizes multiscale filters embedded within its layers and incorporates a split, transform, and merge process. The performance is affected by the presence of a representational bottleneck.

Szegedy et al. (2016) proposed the Inception deep learning architecture, which makes use of asymmetric filters and a bottleneck layer. Wu et al. (2018) proposed ResNet, which utilizes an identity-driven residual-based framework.

Tschandl et al. (2019) proposed a technique that makes use of ResNet34 layers for dermal layer lesion segmentation and a fully CNN for classification of segmented images. Mahbod et al. (2020) explored the impact of image scaling and cropping on pretrained CNN models for categorization of dermal layer lesions. The CNN architectures used in this study include SeReNeXt-50, EfficientNetB0 and EfficientNetB1.

Al-masni et al. (2020) presented a hybrid model that makes use of a full-resolution convolutional network (FrCN) for segmentation of lesions segments followed by deep CNN architecture for multiclass cutaneous carcinoma classification. Mahbod et al. (2019) proposed a method that employed the extracted features from multiple pretrained CNNs to train different SVM classifiers for cutaneous carcinoma classification.

The aforementioned methods propose image segmentation followed by classification networks to augment the exactness of the CNN models for dermal layer lesion categorization. The proposed study tries to maximally utilize the features of available CNN models that have been extensively trained on large datasets for the performance of ensembles of transfer learning models. To keep the system simple and to build an automated system free from human intervention, preprocessing steps such as segmentation are avoided. The performance of four transfer learning models (VGGNet, Xception, ResNet and Inception) along with the different combinations of ensembles of transfer learning models are compared.

## 4.3 MATERIALS AND METHODOLOGY

This section delves into the dataset utilized in the study, data augmentation techniques for increasing the image dataset size, different transfer learning models used and different ensembles of transfer learning frameworks utilized for multiclass dermal layer lesion classification.

### 4.3.1 Standard dermal layer lesion image databases

Table 4.2 lists the different dermal layer lesion image databases available for evaluation of traditional and deep learning models. The proposed study

*Table 4.2* Dermal layer lesion image databases available for assessment of the model

| *Database name* | *Number of images available* | *Remarks* |
|---|---|---|
| DERMOFIT | 1300 | Ten various categories of cutaneous carcinoma images are available. It is owned by the University Edinburgh. |
| PH2 | 200 | Medical annotation available. Three different types of cutaneous carcinoma images are available. |
| ISIC2018 | 2594 | Has corresponding ground truth. |
| ISIC2019 | 25,331 | Contains metadata of patients like age, gender and overall anatomical location. |
| HAM10000 | 10,000 | Publicly available in ISIC archive. |

considers only one dataset (HAM10000), which is publicly available and consists of different types of cutaneous carcinoma images to perform multiclass image categorization.

The HAM10000 dataset (Tschandl et al., 2018) consists of seven classes of cutaneous carcinoma images: basal cell carcinoma (BCC), squamous cell carcinoma (SCC), melanoma (MEL), benign keratosis (BKL), melanocytic nevi (NV), vascular lesion (VASC) and actinic keratosis (AKIEC). BCC, if untreated, grows invasively. BKL is often mistaken for melanoma. AKIEC can be managed locally without the need for surgery. NV are mild malformations of melanocytes. When MEL is identified in its preliminary stages, surgical excision can lead to a cure. HAM10000 is a publicly accessible archive of anonymous dermoscopic images taken from different camera systems. Figure 4.1 shows some of the sample images from the dataset under study. Duplicate images were removed by lesion ID. Each category consists of 350 samples, out of which 200 of each sample were used for multiclass classification training, 100 of each sample were used for validation and the remaining for testing. HAM10000 is among the top intricate visualization databases accessible for multiclass dermal layer lesion classification. To validate the effectiveness of the approach, a small subset of images from the benchmark dataset representing seven distinct types of lesions is utilized.

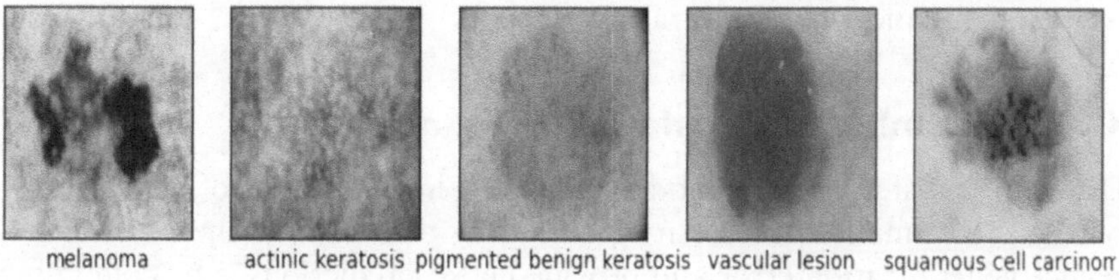


*Figure 4.1* Sample images from HAM10000 dermal layer lesion image dataset.

### 4.3.2 Data augmentation

All input images were resized to 224 × 224 × 3. The pixel intensity values were rescaled to the range [0,1] as part of the image normalization process. For image augmentation, the input images were subjected to shear, zoom, horizontal and vertical flip. These techniques mitigate the adverse impact of significant class imbalances, thereby enhancing the functioning of deep learning frameworks.

### 4.3.3 Transfer learning models

Transfer learning is utilized so as to reduce training time and utilize the knowledge of the network trained on another but similar dataset to provide efficient network performance on a small dataset.

- **Xception architecture**
  Xception is a deep neural network model developed by Francois Chollet (Chollet, 2017). It was inspired by Inception and has 36 depth-wise separable convolutional layers of significant image features.

- **VGGNet architecture**
  Simonyan and Zisserman (2016) introduced the Visual Geometry Group network (VGGNet). It was trained on ImageNet. It provided better feature extraction from images by using 3 × 3 filters. In this study, VGG16 is utilized, as VGG19 has a deeper architecture and is considered to be expensive to train.

- **ResNet architecture**
  He et al. (2016) proposed the deep residual neural network (ResNet). These networks make use of bottleneck features to improve efficiency and recognition accuracy.

- **InceptionV3 architecture**
  Inception V3 (Benedetti et al., 2020) was developed from Keras models pretrained on the ImageNet dataset. Inception V3 uses the convolution kernel splitting method, which splits 3 × 3 convolutions into 3 × 1 and 1 × 3 convolutions. This diminishes the count of parameters and enhances network training speed.

### 4.3.4 Ensemble of transfer learning models

Different transfer learning models can show high variance of performance on the same small dataset. An efficient way to overcome these variances, reduce generalization error and provide better predictions is by combining several transfer learning models. Transfer learning models were combined with top layers frozen and appended by three dense layers to form a new ensemble model.

Figure 4.2 presents the ensemble of the transfer learning models of VGGNet and XceptionNet. Likewise, various combinations of the transfer learning models have been experimented to find the most efficient multi-class classifier for the dermal layer lesion for a minimum of ten epochs.

Figure 4.3 presents the ensemble of the transfer learning models of ResNet and Inception. They were combined with the top layers frozen and appended by three dense layers to form a new ensemble model.

Figure 4.4 presents the ensemble of the transfer learning models of VGG and Inception. They were combined with the top layers frozen and appended by three dense layers to form a new ensemble model.

Figure 4.5 presents the ensemble of the transfer learning models of ResNet, VGG and Inception. They were combined with the top layers frozen and appended by three dense layers to form a new ensemble model.

Figure 4.6 presents the ensemble of the transfer learning models of ResNet, Xception and Inception. They were combined with the top layers frozen and appended by three dense layers to form a new ensemble model.

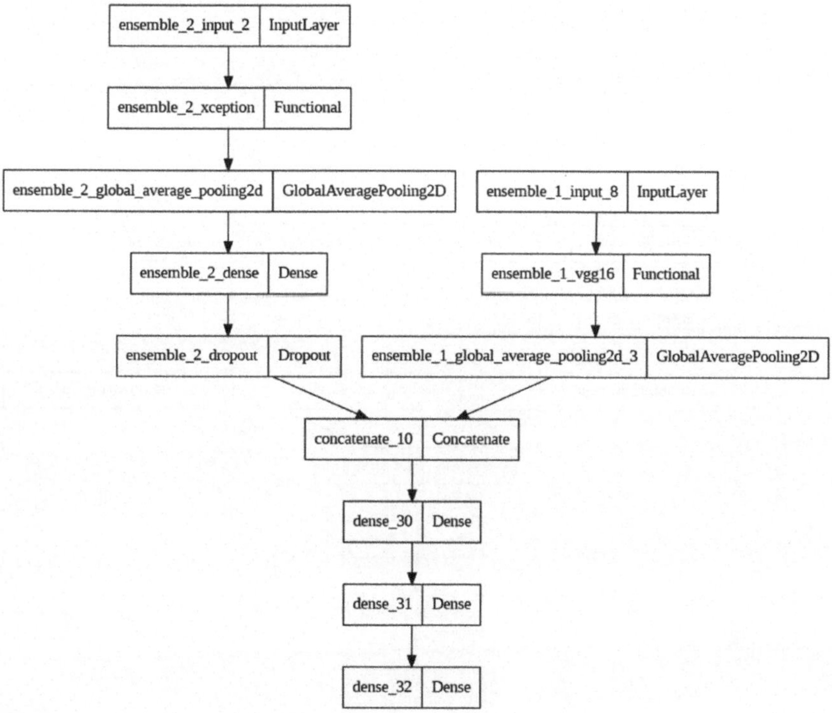


*Figure 4.2* Ensemble of VGGNet and XceptionNet.

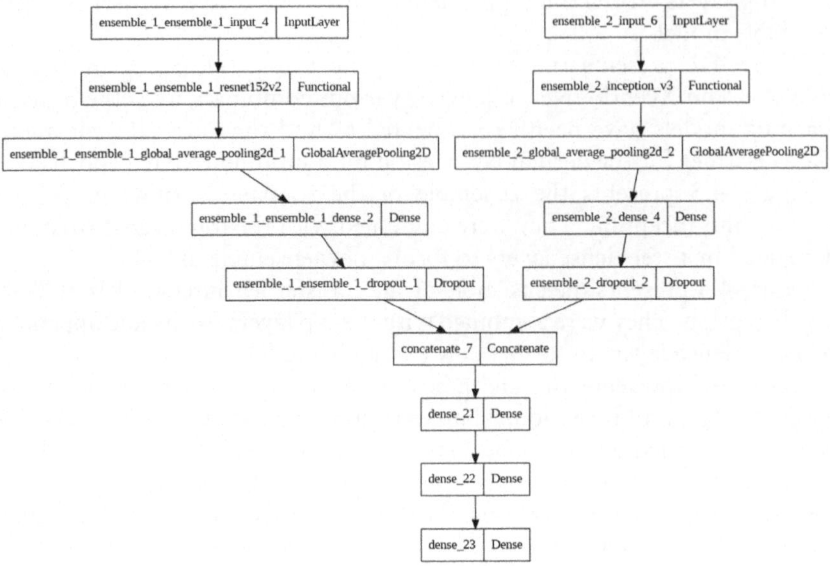


*Figure 4.3* Ensemble of ResNet and Inception.

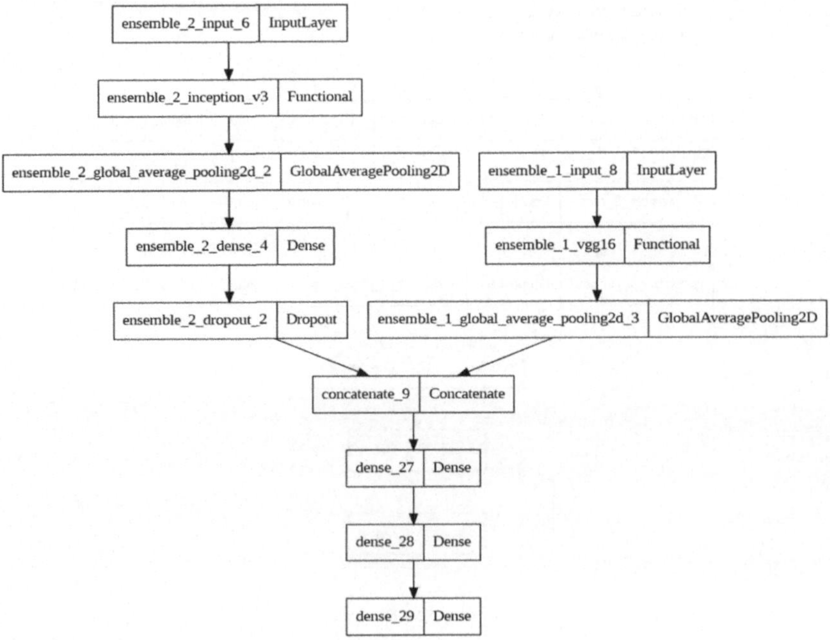


*Figure 4.4* Ensemble of VGG and Inception.

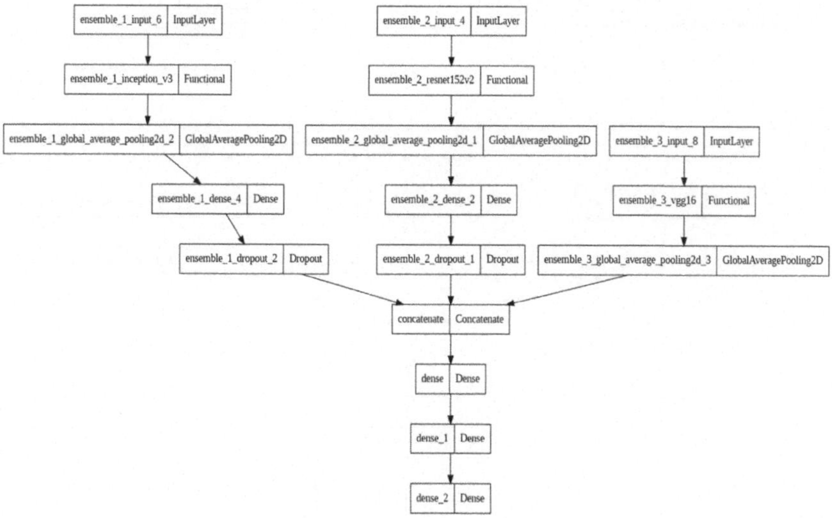


*Figure 4.5* Ensemble of ResNet, VGG and Inception.

Figure 4.7 presents the ensemble of the transfer learning models of VGG, Xception and Inception. They were combined with the top layers frozen and appended by three dense layers to form a new ensemble model.

Figure 4.8 presents the ensemble of the transfer learning models of ResNet, VGG, Xception and Inception. They were combined with the top layers frozen and appended by three dense layers to form a new ensemble model.

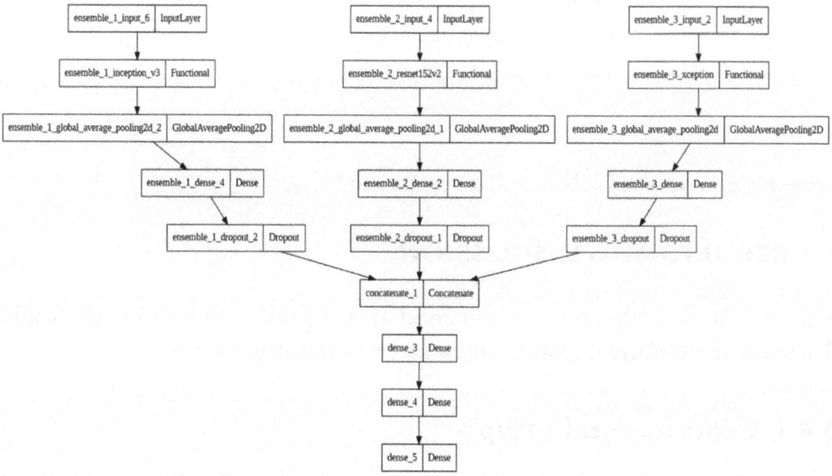


*Figure 4.6* Ensemble of ResNet, Xception and Inception.

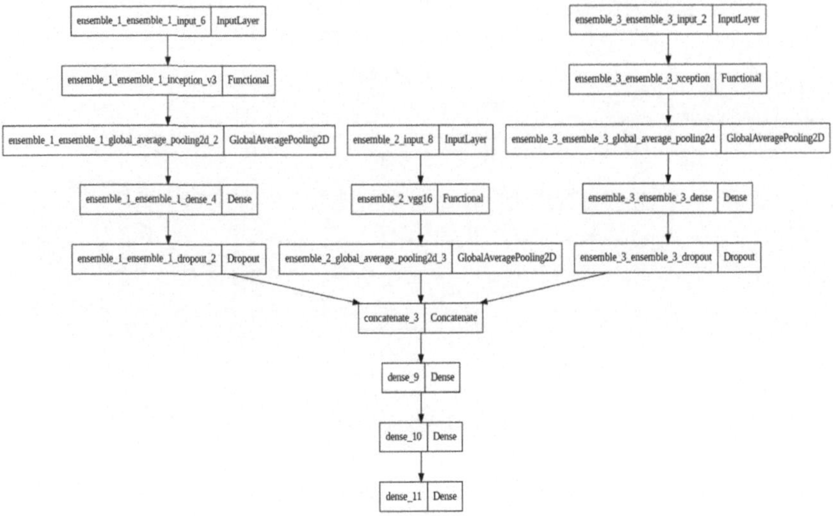


*Figure 4.7* Ensemble of VGG, Xception and Inception.

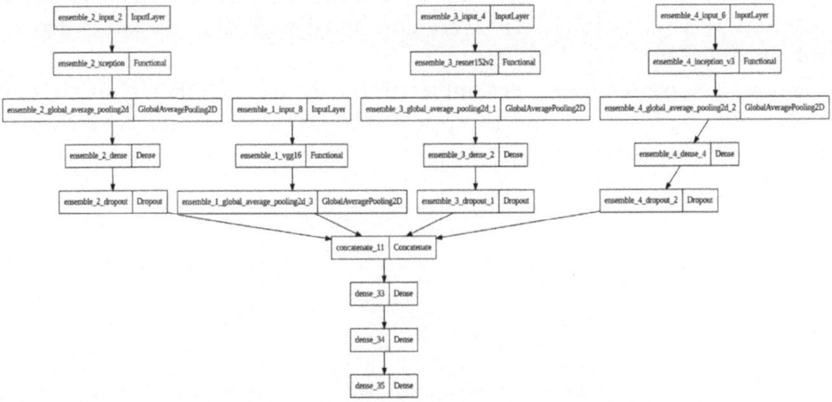


*Figure 4.8* Ensemble of ResNet, VGG, Xception and Inception.

## 4.4 RESULTS AND DISCUSSION

This section describes the experimental arrangement employed in the study, discusses the obtained results and addresses the study's limitations.

### 4.4.1 Experimental setup

All the frameworks were executed in Python using Keras with TensorFlow backend on NVIDIA TESLA T4 GPU of Google Colab.

### 4.4.2 Performance assessment measures

The primary measures employed for assessing the effectiveness of multiclass classification by both transfer learning models and ensembles of transfer learning models were training time, accuracy, recall, precision and F1 score. These metrics are described next:

- Accuracy
  Accuracy, as depicted in Equation 4.1, assesses the ratio of correctly classified dermal layer lesions to the aggregate count of dermal layer lesions:

$$Accuracy = \frac{TP + TN}{TP + TN + FP + FN} \tag{4.1}$$

  where TP (true positive) denotes the count of correctly predicted instances, TN (true negative) indicates the number of occurrences incorrectly predicted, FN (false negative) signifies the instances that are incorrectly predicted and FP (false positive) represents the number of negative instances inaccurately anticipated.

- Precision
  Precision defines the proportion of predicted positives that is truly positive as illustrated in Equation 4.2:

$$Precision = \frac{TP}{TP + FP} \tag{4.2}$$

- Recall
  Recall defines the proportion of actual positives is correctly classified as illustrated in Equation 4.3:

$$Recall = \frac{TP}{TP + FN} \tag{4.3}$$

- F-measure
  The F-measure (F1 score) is characterized as the weighted average of precision and recall, amalgamating both metrics, as depicted in Equation 4.4.

$$F-measure = 2 * \frac{(precision * recall)}{(precision + recall)} \tag{4.4}$$

### 4.4.3 Discussion

The comparison of transfer learning on cutting edge frameworks such as VGG, Inception, ResNet and Xception is carried out. The results also show the performance evaluation of ensembles of the transfer learning models.

Table 4.3 demonstrates that as the complexity of the framework rises, the training time also increases. The ensemble of VGG, Inception, ResNet and Xception gives the highest accuracy at ten epochs when compared to the other ensemble models under study. Had the model been trained for a few more epochs, it would have given results comparable to ResNet.

Table 4.4 compares all the models on three additional parameters: precision, recall, F-measure. It is observable that the ensemble framework of VGG, Inception, ResNet and Xception achieves the highest F1 score, which represents the harmonic mean of precision and recall.

### 4.4.4 Limitations

Enhancing the accuracy and efficiency of transfer learning models and their ensembles can be achieved through cutaneous carcinoma visual preprocessing, visual segmentation and visual extraction procedures.

The presence of noise, such as hair, blood vessels, oils and bubbles, makes the interpretation of dermal layer lesion pixels difficult as shown in Figure 4.9. For this there is a need for a dermal layer image preprocessing step.

Image segmentation is necessary to reduce the input image size and improve lesion classification accuracy. Feature extraction helps in reducing the complexity of the learning framework.

*Table 4.3* Comparative analysis of the performance of transfer learning models and ensembles of transfer learning models

| *Model* | *Epochs* | *Training time* | *Training accuracy* |
|---|---|---|---|
| Inception | 50 | 24 min 46 s | 0.7214 |
| ResNet | 50 | 26 min 23 s | **0.8536** |
| VGG | 50 | 17 min 48 s | 0.4357 |
| Xception | 50 | 17 min 57 s | 0.7893 |
| Xception + VGG | 10 | 1 hr 26 min 28 s | 0.6771 |
| Inception + VGG | 10 | 1 hr 26 min 56 s | 0.6541 |
| Inception + ResNet | 10 | 1 hr 22 min 18 s | 0.7216 |
| Inception + ResNet + Xception | 10 | 2 hr 3 min 50 s | 0.7624 |
| Inception + ResNet + VGG | 10 | 2 hr 2 min 18 s | 0.7637 |
| VGG + ResNet + Xception | 10 | 2 hr 3 min 56 s | 0.7648 |
| Inception + VGG + ResNet + Xception | 10 | 2 hr 46 min 18 s | **0.7863** |

*Table 4.4* Comparison of precision, recall and F-measure for the models under study

| *Model* | *Precision* | *Recall* | *F1 score* |
|---|---|---|---|
| Inception | 0.9643 | 0.2975 | 0.45472 |
| ResNet | 0.9875 | 0.3193 | 0.48256 |
| VGG | 0.2268 | 0.6287 | 0.33334 |
| Xception | 0.9821 | 0.3205 | 0.48328 |
| Xception + VGG | 0.5600 | 0.7875 | 0.65454 |
| Inception + VGG | 0.5568 | 0.7875 | 0.65235 |
| Inception + ResNet | 0.5678 | 0.8123 | 0.66839 |
| Inception + ResNet + Xception | 0.6989 | 0.8486 | 0.76650 |
| Inception + ResNet + VGG | 0.6890 | 0.8318 | 0.75369 |
| VGG + ResNet + Xception | 0.6835 | 0.8265 | 0.74822 |
| Inception + VGG + ResNet + Xception | 0.7286 | 0.8462 | **0.78300** |

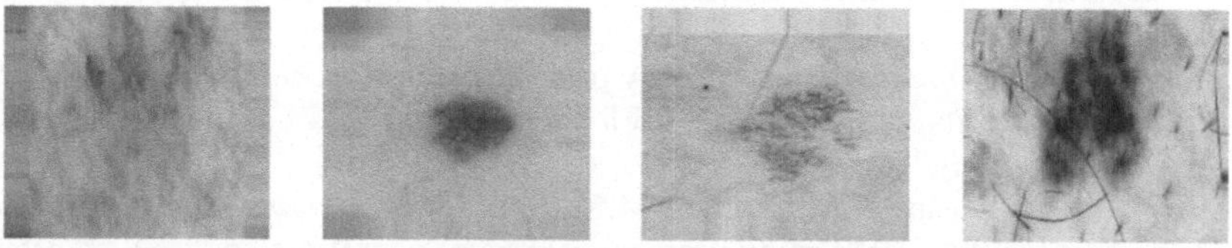

*Figure 4.9* Sample images showing the noise present in the dataset under study.

## 4.5 CONCLUSION

The purpose of this research was to assess the performance of innovative multiclass visual categorization models using transfer learning, both individually and in ensemble configurations. Results indicate that the ensemble comprising VGG, Inception, ResNet and Xception outperforms other model combinations in multiclass classification after ten epochs. Additionally, it demonstrates superior performance compared to individual transfer learning models. These findings warrant careful consideration in future prospective clinical trials.

## REFERENCES

Al-masni, M.A.; Kim, D.-H.; Kim, T.-S. Multiple skin lesions diagnostics via integrated deep convolutional networks for segmentation and classification. *Comput Methods Programs Biomed*. 2020, 190, 105351.

Alquran, H., Qasmieh, I. A., Alqudah, A. M., Alhammouri, S., Alawneh, E., Abughazaleh, A., & Hasayen, F. (2017, October). The melanoma skin cancer detection and classification using support vector machine. In *2017 IEEE Jordan conference on applied electrical engineering and computing technologies (AEECT)* (pp. 1-5). IEEE.

Argenziano, G.; Fabbrocini, G.; Carli, P.; De Giorgi, V.; Sammarco, E.; Delfino, M. Epiluminescence microscopy for the diagnosis of doubtful melanocytic skin lesions. *Arch Dermatol.* 1998, 134, pp. 1563–1570.

Bandic, J.; Kovacevic, S.; Karabeg, R.; Bandic, M.; Lazarov, A.; Opric, D. Teledermoscopy for skin cancer prevention: A comparative study of clinical and teledermoscopic diagnosis. *Acta Inform Med.* 2020, 28, 37.

Barata, C.; Celebi, M.E.; Marques, J.S. Explainable skin lesion diagnosis using taxonomies. *Pattern Recognit.* 2021, 110, 107413.

Benedetti, P., Perri, D., Simonetti, M., Gervasi, O., Reali, G., & Femminella, M. *Skin cancer classification using inception network and transfer learning.* Computational Science and Its Applications–ICCSA 2020: 20th International Conference, Cagliari, Italy, Proceedings, Part I 20, July 1–4, 2020, pp. 536–545. Springer International Publishing.

Chollet, F. *Xception: Deep learning with Depthwise separable convolutions.* Proceedings - 30th IEEE Conference on Computer Vision and Pattern Recognition, CVPR, 2017.

He, K., Zhang, X., Ren, S., Sun, J. *Deep residual learning for image recognition.* 2016 IEEE Conference on Computer Vision and Pattern Recognition (CVPR), 2016.

Jamil, U.; Khalid, S. *Comparative study of classification techniques used in skin lesion detection systems.* 17th IEEE International Multi Topic Conference, 2014, pp. 266–271.

Kassem, M.A.; Hosny, K.M.; Fouad, M.M. Skin lesions classification into eight classes for ISIC 2019 using deep convolutional neural network and transfer learning. *IEEE Access.* 2020, 8, 114822–114832.

Khan, M.Q.; Hussain, A., Rehman, S.U.; Khan, U.; Maqsood, M.; Mehmood, K.; Khan, M.A. Classification of melanoma and nevus in digital images for diagnosis of skin cancer. *IEEE Access.* 2019, 7, 90132–90144.

Lu, X.; Firoozeh Abolhasani Zadeh, Y. A. Deep learning-based classification for melanoma detection using xceptionnet. *Journal of Healthcare Engineering.* 2022, no. 1, 2196096.

Liu, L.; Tsui, Y.Y.; Mandal, M. Skin lesion segmentation using deep learning with auxiliary task. *J Imaging.* 2021, 7, 67.

Mahbod, A.; Schaefer, G.; Ellinger, I.; Ecker, R.; Pitiot, A.; Wang, C. Fusing fine-tuned deep features for skin lesion classification. *Comput Med Imaging Graph.* 2019, 71, 19–29.

Mahbod, A.; Schaefer, G.; Wang, C.; Dorffner, G.; Ecker, R.; Ellinger, I. Transfer learning using a multi-scale and multi-network ensemble for skin lesion classification. *Comput Methods Programs Biomed.* 2020, 193, 105475.

Simonyan, K.; Zisserman, A. Very deep convolutional networks for large-scale image recognition. *arXiv preprint arXiv:1409.1556.* 2016.

Singh, V.K.; Abdel-Nasser, M.; Rashwan, H.A.; Akram, F.; Pandey, N.; Lalande, A.; Presles, B.; Romani, S.; Puig, D. FCA-net: Adversarial learning for skin lesion segmentation based on multi-scale features and factorized channel attention. *IEEE Access.* 2019, 7, 130552–130565.

Szaleniec, J.; Szaleniec, M.; Str˛ek, P.; Boro ´n, A.; Jabło ´nska, K.; Gawlik, J.; Składzie ´n, J. Outcome prediction in endoscopic surgery for chronic rhinosinusitis—A multidimensional model. *Adv Med Sci.* 2014, 59, 13–18.

Szegedy, C.; Liu, W.; Jia, Y.; Sermanet, P.; Reed, S.; Anguelov, D.; Erhan, D.; Vanhoucke, V.; Rabinovich, A. *Going deeper with convolutions*. Proceedings of the IEEE Conference on Computer Vision and Pattern Recognition, 2015, pp. 1–9.

Szegedy, C.; Vanhoucke, V.; Iofe, S.; Shlens, J.; Wojna, Z. *Rethinking the inception architecture for computer vision*. Proceedings of the IEEE Conference on Computer Vision and Pattern Recognition, 2016, pp. 2818–2826.

Tschandl, P., Rosendahl, C., Kittler, H. The HAM10000 dataset, a large collection of multi-source dermatoscopic images of common pigmented skin lesions. *Sci Data*. 2018. 5, 180161.

Tschandl, P.; Sinz, C.; Kittler, H. Domain-specific classification-pretrained fully convolutional network encoders for skin lesion segmentation. *Comput Biol Med*. 2019, 104, 111–116.

World Cancer Research Fund International. n.d. https://www.wcrf.org/cancer-trends/skin-cancer-statistics.

Wu, S.; Zhong, S.; Liu, Y. Deep residual learning for image steganalysis. *Multimed Tools Appl*. 2018, 77(9), 10437–10453.

Chapter 5

# Benefits and drawbacks of using AI technologies in healthcare businesses

## An ethical perspective

*Marwa Abdellateef and R. V. Palanivel*

### 5.1 INTRODUCTION

For several years recently, applications of artificial intelligence (AI) technologies in various businesses have been prominent. The healthcare business is no exception. The traditional procedures of providing services have been replaced with novel AI technological ones that revolutionized the industry. Eventually, this evolution brought in several advantages including preciseness, proficiency, and promptness. These advantages are reflected in diagnoses, treatment, and data analysis. Thus, this leads to better diagnoses and even early ones. Hence, healthcare has turned into a protective industry instead of being a treating one. This package of advantages makes it difficult for decision-makers in the industry to ignore using AI technologies or exclude them. Nevertheless, this package also includes several breaches of healthcare ethics. It's a double-edged weapon.

Healthcare services have been revolutionized due to the ability of AI technologies to analyze massive data efficiently within a few minutes. Evidently, this advantage is necessary for getting the most accurate diagnosis that eventually leads to an accurately tailored treatment plan. When examining medical images, for instance, AI applications have the ability to scan and examine these images faster than human beings. Meanwhile, these applications have a higher level of accuracy. This leads to an early diagnosis of chronic diseases, e.g., cancer (Mazurowski et al., 2019). Another example is when AI applications have the ability to analyze big data in order to decide on the percentage of being prone to specific diseases. This means leaving more space for preventive procedures rather than treatment (Hoppe et al., 2023).

The long list of benefits attached to utilizing AI technologies in the healthcare industry does not negate the existence of another list of ethical issues that contributed to it. Breaching patient's privacy by exposing confidential data to AI systems is the first one on this list. Since AI technology tools necessitate access to massive data of patients, all individuals controlling these technologies also have access to the same massive data. Hence, there is no way to guarantee the privacy of this data (Li et al., 2022). Further

 DOI: 10.1201/9781003634089-5

strict regulations are needed to guarantee the privacy of this data and avoid any misuse. Meanwhile, all sensitive data of patients remain confidential (Nassar & Kamal, 2021).

The second ethical issue on the list is transparency when making decisions using AI tools. Highly complicated algorithms are utilized by AI technologies. These algorithms cannot be easily comprehended by healthcare providers or patients. This leads to transparency blockage. Hence, reliance on AI technologies cannot be trusted as the best option for attaining transparency. Therefore, health providers become reluctant when receiving AI-driven resolutions or recommendations (Kiseleva et al., 2022). When it comes to stakeholders or shareholders, they need transparent information to trust the process. Lack of understanding the AI-driven decisions makes them hesitant when accepting the integration of AI technologies in healthcare systems (Fazakarley et al., 2024).

A third ethical issue related to AI technology applications in healthcare is accountability. It is difficult to hold a specific person responsible for errors when enforcing decisions made based on AI technology applications. Here, three parties can be responsible, i.e., healthcare service providers, developers of AI technologies, or healthcare institutions applying this technology (Rosemann & Zhang, 2022). Therefore, drawing clear lines to decide on who should be held responsible for errors is necessary. As well, all parties sharing in the process must stick to the ethics of using AI technologies in the healthcare industry.

Equity is a major principle of using AI technologies in the healthcare industry. It entails making sure that all personnel involved in the process are unbiased when handling data collected. This leads to unbiased AI-driven decisions. However, when data collectors are biased, the AI-driven decisions become biased, as well. This results in treating specific patients differently based on the biased data collected (Krishnan Ganapathy, 2021). Hence, data should be diversified and representative to guarantee equity among all patients and avoid biased decisions made based on biased data collected (Karimian et al., 2022).

As for beneficence and non-maleficence, they are basic principles of AI technology applications in the healthcare industry. They entail using these technologies ethically in the field. Beneficence, for instance, necessitates enhancing the accuracy of diagnosis and tailoring the remedial process to improve the patient's medical condition (Kasula, 2021). Non-maleficence, however, entails making sure that AI-driven technologies are unbiased, precise, and efficient to guarantee patients' well-being and make sure that they avoid any potential danger (Chikhaoui et al., 2022). The previously mentioned principles play a vital role in reassuring the safety of patients via adhering to ethical practices when providing the service.

Autonomy is a third principle of ethical use of AI technologies in the healthcare realm. Here, patients are granted the right to make decisions based on information presented about their health condition. This includes but is not restricted to, being fully informed about their AI-driven treatment plan (Prakash et al., 2022). This process entails keeping patients informed about all aspects of the process, e.g., the mechanism of AI tools utilized, benefits of AI tools used, risks of AI tools utilized, and signing a consent approving the application of these AI tools to their medical condition.

Ethical principles of AI technology applications in healthcare cannot be explored without addressing justice as a major principle. This entails ensuring all patients have equal access to the advantages of AI technologies without taking any other factors of discrimination into consideration, e.g., social status, origin, and culture (Karimian et al., 2022). Here, all AI-related practices should be monitored closely to make sure that the principle of justice is achieved.

In light of the previously mentioned ethical issues related to AI technology applications in healthcare systems, it becomes evident that some regulations have to be developed to guarantee the applications of AI technologies in healthcare. This is the responsibility of institutions such as the Food and Drug Administration (FDA) in the United States and the European Union's Medical Devices Regulation (MDR). They ensure that all regulations are reinforced to achieve the highest level of accuracy, efficiency, and transparency (Food and Drug Administration, 2019; Floridi, 2021). Thus, patients are fully protected via the fair use of AI technologies in the healthcare system.

## 5.2 LITERATURE REVIEW

### 5.2.1 Ethical issues in AI-driven healthcare

The same concept is supported by recent studies that investigate ethical issues related to the use of AI technologies in healthcare businesses. For instance, Lysaght et al. (2019) referred to the ethical impact of using AI tools for making decisions in healthcare institutions. Meanwhile, using algorithms in making such decisions necessitates a solid application of transparency, accountability, and equity. This is confirmed by Nassar and Kamal (2021) when asserting the drawbacks resulting from applying AI-driven technologies in healthcare businesses that can be avoided by upgrading privacy policies that guarantee patients' rights.

Additionally, machines are not the only party responsible for these ethical concerns. Professionals working for healthcare institutions are also responsible for enforcing the appropriate regulations that guarantee the ethical use of AI tools in the field (Rosemann & Zhang, 2022). When it comes to human interactions and relationships with the healthcare organization, clear policies governing the relationship between the service provider and the patient have to be framed and communicated thoroughly (Kraft, 2020).

Accordingly, the purpose of the current chapter is to shed light on ethical aspects related to using AI technologies in healthcare businesses. This can be achieved by exploring previous literature exploring the issue. Hence, this leads to unraveling various principles governing utilizing AI technologies in healthcare. This may include justice, accountability, and transparency.

AI technologies are investigated based on benefits resulting from using them as well as drawbacks represented in the ethical issues since this is the main concern of the current chapter. Benefits include big data mastery, diagnosis accuracy, and medical proficiency. However, drawbacks related to ethical aspects include areas such as privacy, algorithms, and accountability. This enriches the current debate on using AI technologies in healthcare businesses and may result in getting to more convenient resolutions.

This can be attained by investigating policies and regulations used for managing AI technologies in healthcare businesses. Eventually, this creates a path for better strategies for handling ethical issues and bridging the gap in the current situation. This is beneficial in improving transparency and accountability. This presentation concludes with exploring suggested solutions and recommendations to reinforce using AI technologies ethically in healthcare businesses, which eventually leads to enhancing the benefits of using these technologies as opposed to the drawbacks of using them.

### 5.2.2 Key AI technologies principles in healthcare businesses

As depicted earlier, using AI technologies in healthcare businesses entails considering several ethical aspects. Hence, various key ethics have to be investigated thoroughly to make sure that they are followed by service providers in healthcare institutions. Meanwhile, the enormous growth of AI utilization in the healthcare business led to the pressing need to highlight how ethics are managed and preserved within this context. Here, adopting the key ethical principles guarantees reinforcing accountability, transparency, and justice when providing healthcare services. Unfolding these principles leads to better performance, which consequently leads to developing healthcare businesses altogether. These key ethical principles are as follows.

#### *5.2.2.1 Beneficence*

As a key ethical principle in healthcare, Kasula (2021) asserts that this principle guarantees restricting service providers to present the optimum level of service in a manner that achieves the highest level possible of patient well-being. When applying the same principle to using AI technologies in healthcare businesses, this principle guarantees the utilization of these technologies to the maximum possible level that improves patients' health, advances treatment, and elevates the accuracy of diagnosis. In brief, it ensures that healthcare providers make their maximum efforts to serve patients using the AI technologies available. This may include but is not restricted to using advanced AI diagnostic technology to provide accurate diagnosis, which consequently leads to medical intervention at the appropriate time for the patient before suffering from further complications. Hence, benefits are maximized and risks are minimized as much as possible.

#### *5.2.2.2 Non-maleficence*

Another key principle is non-maleficence, which is presented by Chikhaoui et al. (2022) as the necessity of preventing any potential risk that may result in severe injuries to patients. When using AI technologies in providing healthcare services, the role of the healthcare provider is to diminish the risks related to using AI technologies. These risks may include misdiagnosis due to algorithm biases, which is a major risk threatening patient well-being. Constant testing of AI technologies is mandatory for attaining reliability, accountability, and accuracy when using these technologies in the healthcare sector (Chikhaoui et al., 2022). Meanwhile, healthcare providers have to be alert to any potential risks emerging to take precautions instead of resolving issues later. This helps them preserve non-maleficence as a major principle of ethics in healthcare.

## 5.3 AUTONOMY

While the previous principles focus on healthcare providers' practices for maintaining the reliability of the service provided, the autonomy principle shifts focus to the patient who has the complete right to decide on which medical procedures to follow for approaching their medical condition. Consequently, when using AI technologies in handling patients' health conditions, they have to be granted the absolute right to decide on the manner via which these technologies are used in their conditions. Moreover, they have to be provided with all the necessary information while being fully enlightened based on information presented transparently. This leads to a more effective decision-making process (Prakash et al., 2022). As per the privacy of patients' data when using AI technologies, it must be fully guaranteed by healthcare personnel based on declared policies shared with patients and preferably documented and signed by them.

### 5.3.1 Justice

In practice, all patients must have access to healthcare services equally with no consideration of their gender, ethnicity, religion, belongingness, etc. Integrating AI technologies in healthcare services requires following procedures that guarantee accessibility to AI technologies when receiving healthcare services to avoid injustice practices. This may entail minimizing algorithm biases. Meanwhile, creating reliable databases and directing technologies to have more equity can achieve justice in this sector (Karimian et al., 2022). Maintaining this ethical principle complies with international human rights and enables AI technologies to improve the healthcare services provided.

### 5.3.2 Transparency

Providing healthcare services requires interaction between the service provider (i.e., professionals) and the service receiver (i.e., patients). This includes communication on various levels and for several purposes, which consequently results in exchanging information. This process requires the highest possible level of clarity and openness. Integrating AI technologies in the healthcare system elevates the necessity of transparency when providing information. Patients have the right to gain access to all the required data that enables them to make the right decision. In addition, they need to be informed about the drawbacks of using these technologies to avoid any future misrepresentation or frustrations (Kiseleva et al., 2022). Apart from the benefit of this principle to patients, the healthcare system operators must have transparency to assess the validity and reliability of AI technologies used. This leads to huge improvements and quick fixing of potential issues.

## 5.4 PROPOSED WORK

With the emerging potentials accompanying AI integration in healthcare businesses, optimism increases based on the revolutionized advancement and possibilities in the field. This expands to include almost all aspects of the process, e.g., diagnosis, medication, accessibility, and quality assurance. Nevertheless, this comes along with all the downsides associated with using AI technologies in healthcare services. Several drawbacks and concerns have to be taken into consideration when approaching this issue. Most of these concerns are directly connected with ethical considerations. The goal is to attain and preserve the key principles of using AI technologies in healthcare businesses as mentioned earlier. The benefits and drawbacks associated with using AI technologies in healthcare are elaborated in further detail.

## 5.5 INFERENCES

Undoubtedly, seeking assistance from AI technologies in healthcare procedures brings several benefits to the system. However, improving the accuracy of diagnosis as well as the efficiency of medical treatment remain to be the most significant ones. Big medical data analysis is a task that can be professionally fulfilled using AI applications. This data includes all healthcare documents and information, e.g., patients' records, MRI scans, medical history, injections, and genetic history. Processing this data using AI tools leads to detecting abnormalities and making the right decision with no delay. This process saves both time and effort. Meanwhile, misdiagnosis rates decrease to the minimum when compared to processing diagnoses manually. It's a lifesaving process (Ali et al., 2023).

## 5.6 EXPERIMENTAL FINDINGS

According to Mazurowski et al. (2019), integrating AI-driven tools in checking MRI images led to the detection of abnormalities and identifying cancer as well as diabetes in an early stage. Using AI algorithms has proven to be highly beneficial in these cases.

In addition, data is analyzed collectively. Utilizing AI tools can also assist in individualizing and personalizing the diagnosis process to design a medical treatment for a patient. This exceeds the mere mass processing of data randomly. Algorithms can expect the potential result of the suggested treatment and assume medical interventions accordingly. This increases the effectiveness of treatment and decreases potential risks taken (Le Nguyen & Do, 2019). On an organizational level, using AI-powered technologies enables managers of healthcare institutions to define the needs of their patients and adjust available resources accordingly, which eventually leads to advancement in medical care outcomes (Hoppe et al., 2023). Table 5.1 sheds light on supporting statistics related to applications of AI technologies in healthcare services. Accordingly, the accuracy of predicting the health issue goes up to 85% while the effectiveness of treatment elevates to 25%.

## 5.7 ETHICAL DRAWBACKS OF INTEGRATING AI-POWERED TECHNOLOGIES IN HEALTHCARE

All the benefits mentioned earlier do not nullify the fact that there are ethical concerns resulting from using AI-driven technologies in healthcare

*Table 5.1* Machine learning in healthcare

| *Application* | *Principle* | *Example* | *Supporting statistic* |
|---|---|---|---|
| Predictive analytics | Data-driven Insights | Predictive analytics for patient outcomes | Predictive accuracy: 85% |
| Personalized medicine | Data-driven Insights | Tailoring treatment to patient data | Increase in treatment effectiveness: 25% |

businesses. These concerns need to be tackled to preserve the attained benefits of AI-powered technologies in the realm. Most of these concerns are directly related to the key ethical principles mentioned earlier.

Privacy and confidentiality of patients' data represent a significant concern related to integrating AI technologies in healthcare. This entails gathering highly sensitive health information. Consequently, concerns arise when considering parties authorized to have access to data, privacy policies, and the possibility of hacking or misusing data. Hence, it is highly essential to present procedures for encrypting data and controlling parties that have access to confidential data. Meanwhile, improving governance practices elevates trust in integrating AI technologies into healthcare services (Li et al., 2022). Figure 5.1 highlights the major drawbacks of using AI technologies in healthcare services.

Meeting justice requirements is a basic principle of ethics when using AI-driven technologies, which necessitates avoiding algorithm biases. Usually, AI technologies are fed with patients' history and personal data to be processed using machine learning algorithms. Thus, it is exposed to historical data already existing. This may result in biases and the extension of misrepresentation of equity. Therefore, patients may not have the ability to receive the required medical care equally (Krishnan Ganapathy, 2021). Hence, these AI-powered systems have to be thoroughly tested and inspected to detect potential biases. This is to be followed by suggesting strategies to avoid these biases and preserve the required level of justice and equity with no consideration of any irrelevant factors.

Transparency represents a major concern when applying AI technologies in healthcare businesses. The mechanism based on which these technologies perform is usually incomprehensible to most professionals involved in the process. This makes the decision-making process vague and challenging. Hence, attaining transparency becomes a huge obstacle. It is highly difficult to comprehend how suggestions and conclusions have been drawn. Therefore, professionals and patients find it difficult to trust AI technologies (Fazakarley et al., 2024). This issue can be solved by introducing

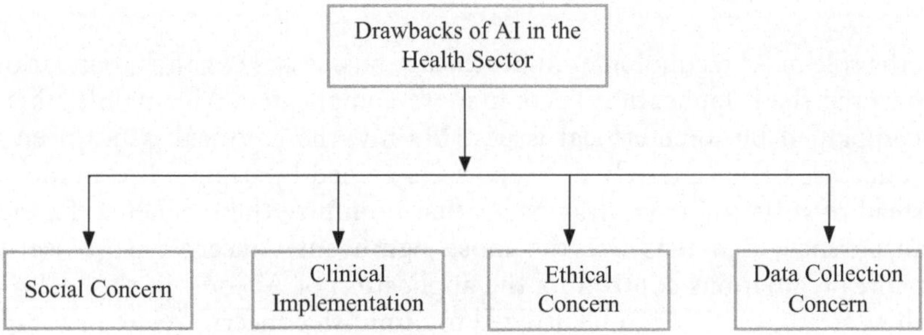


*Figure 5.1* Ethical drawbacks of AI in healthcare.

*Table 5.2* Ethical drawbacks of AI in healthcare

| *Ethical concern* | *Description* | *Supporting statistics* |
|---|---|---|
| Bias and fairness | AI systems can inherit biases from training data, leading to unfair treatment of certain patient groups | 25% of AI systems showed radical bias in healthcare outcomes |
| Privacy and security | AI systems require large datasets, raising concerns about patient data privacy and security breaches | 70% of patients worried about their data privacy |
| Transparency and accountability | Lack of transparency in AI decision-making processes can make it difficult to hold systems accountable | 60% of AI systems lack explainability features |
| Informed consent | Patients may not fully understand how AI technologies are used in their care, impacting their ability to give informed consent | 40% of patients were unaware of AI usage in their care |

professionals and patients to AI-powered technologies and explaining them in a manner that suits their technological capacities. This will make using AI technologies more trustworthy to them. Eventually, this leads to increasing investment in these technologies by stakeholders since they all get the rationale governing AI-powered decisions. As depicted in Table 5.2, the percentage of most drawbacks exceeds 25%, a percentage that should be taken into consideration when using AI technologies in healthcare systems.

Monitoring these concerns closely leads to minimizing their negative impact and amplifies the influence of benefits. To achieve this, healthcare professionals need to consider ethics related to AI applications in the sector. Major principles of AI-powered technologies ethics in the realm answer most drawbacks and suggest resolutions to encounter them. This increases reliability, accountability, and transparency when using these technologies.

## 5.8 THE FRAMEWORK OF REGULATIONS GOVERNING AI TECHNOLOGIES INTEGRATION AND MINIMIZING DRAWBACKS

As the role of AI technologies in healthcare businesses expands, regulations governing their application become more complicated. Meanwhile, this is accompanied by some ethical issues. Mainly, these ethical issues need to be addressed appropriately to keep assets gained by using AI technologies instead of suffering from drawbacks that minimize these benefits. Privacy, transparency, and bias are the most significant concerns. This section explores regulations controlling the application of AI tools in the realm as well as strategies that can be utilized to diminish concerns related to transparency, reliability, and bias resulting from using AI-powered technologies in healthcare businesses.

## 5.9 EXPERIMENTAL RESULTS BASED ON THE REALITY OF AI TECHNOLOGY APPLICATION IN EGYPT

Table 5.3 shows the advancement in statistics collected about using AI technologies in healthcare services presented in Egypt based on a random sample of hospitals and clinics. Meanwhile, based on an official statement released by the Public Authority of Healthcare, the government is investigating possible ways of digitalizing the whole healthcare system with Huawei Technologies Co. This leads to applying AI technologies to all medical services presented to families.

## 5.10 AVAILABLE FRAMEWORK OF REGULATIONS

The regulation framework controlling the application of AI technologies in healthcare businesses varies based on context and legislation. Nevertheless, there is a permanent opportunity to allow advancements to participate in promoting healthcare services. This is accompanied by some drawbacks, though. Food and Drug Administration (FDA) regulates the application of AI-driven tools in the healthcare realm. This includes medical devices and software utilized. To guarantee the reliability, accountability, and trustworthiness of using these technologies in healthcare businesses, the FDA runs a whole system in which these technologies are examined before being presented to the public and after application to ensure quality (Food and Drug Administration, 2019).

The same approach is also followed by the European Union when passing similar regulations, i.e., the Medical Devices Regulation (MDR) and the

*Table 5.3* Experimental results of AI applications in healthcare institutions in Egypt

| *Healthcare service presented* | *Assistance presented by AI technology* | *Quantitative data collected in Egypt* |
|---|---|---|
| Disease diagnosis | Providing various types of scans | 15–20% of accuracy in diagnosis |
| Cancer research | Diagnosing cancer | 30% advancement in early identification of breast cancer |
| Pandemic reaction | Investigating symptoms | 25–30% reduction of hospital visits |
| Organ failure identification | Identifying while staying at ICUs | 15% reduction of mortality |
| Presenting healthcare remotely | Presenting remote consultations | 40% advancement in medical services presented remotely |
| Analysis to predict diseases | Monitoring pandemic outbreaks | 85% accuracy in predicting diseases |
| Cancer research in children | Presenting personalized treatment | 10–15% advancement in treatment |

General Data Protection Regulation (GDPR). Like FDA regulations, the latter monitors various processes of AI-powered technologies in medicine, e.g., development, application, and generating data. Here, AI-driven healthcare technologies are encouraged to be developed. Nevertheless, security, transparency, and accountability are prioritized as main ethical principles. This puts the interests of patients, as service receivers, first (Floridi, 2021).

## 5.11 APPROACH FOR MINIMIZING DRAWBACKS

Several aspects must be considered when approaching the ethical drawbacks of integrating AI technologies into healthcare businesses. These aspects include regulations and the technologies involved. According to Khan et al. (2023), the main concerns can be confronted by highlighting transparency when using AI-powered technologies to make decisions. This elevates the level of trust between healthcare service providers and patients, on the one hand. On the other hand, this eliminates any doubts presented by regulators and makes them aware of all the technicalities. Hence, they can be enlightened when making decisions. Developers of AI systems play a vital role here. They can simplify systems and create an accessible user interface that enables regulators to have an accurate image of how these systems function.

The application of AI technologies leads to another concern, as well. Bias caused by algorithms is a challenging issue that affects justice and equity negatively. Hence, healthcare services can be distributed unevenly. Consequently, this reduces patients' trust in such AI systems. An approach that can be utilized here is the diversification of data feeding these AI-generated systems. In addition, AI-generated analysis has to be revised manually regularly to make sure that data is validated. Some techniques for tackling data biases and asserting justice can also be adopted (Sun & Medaglia, 2019).

As for accountability when applying AI-powered technologies in healthcare businesses, it is necessary to maintain it to elevate patients' well-being and sustain ethical practices among professionals. Issues associated with AI technology applications can be addressed using techniques in which all professionals realize their roles and responsibilities following a specific organizational structure. Hence, it becomes easy to track issues based on the personnel responsible for fulfilling the relevant task (Lopes et al., 2023). It is highly recommended for all professionals to follow a declared guideline or a code of ethics. This helps them comprehend how to tackle AI-relevant issues in the healthcare context.

Presenting successful solutions to ethical concerns related to the application of AI technologies in healthcare requires having mutual understanding and consistent collaboration among several parties, including legislators, service providers, patients, lawmakers, and AI system developers, to generate the best practices that can be adopted. Meanwhile, presenting them to the public leads to building a powerful foundation based on which comprehension of AI applications in the field increases. Eventually, this leads to addressing ethical challenges in a healthier context (He et al., 2021).

## 5.12 THE ROADMAP TO ENHANCED AI-POWERED PRACTICES IN HEALTHCARE BUSINESSES

Based on the previous exploration of ethical principles, benefits, and concerns of integrating AI-driven technologies in healthcare businesses, future guidelines, as well as recommendations, can be presented to help professionals and stakeholders in the industry master these technologies to the extent of amplifying their benefits and minimizing their drawbacks. Meanwhile, these guidelines can be drawn from suggested future studies and research.

## 5.13 SUGGESTED STUDIES

There are several areas suggested for future investigation. Mainly, there are four areas strongly recommended, i.e., developing ethical principles of AI-powered systems, massive cooperation on various interest levels, assessing the effect of using AI technologies, and humanizing AI systems.

As per developing ethical principles of AI-powered systems, more research is highly recommended for generating key principles covering applications of AI-powered technologies in the healthcare realm, in particular. Principles include transparency, justice, accountability, reliability, privacy, and confidentiality. Studies need to be tailored based on the unique characteristics of this field (Char et al., 2018).

Creating a profound foundation for connecting all parties, e.g., professionals, technologists, stakeholders, patients, and lawmakers, has to be another area of research handling the integration of AI technologies in healthcare businesses. This allows all parties involved to collaborate to address ethical challenges resulting from this application. Future studies can stress efforts that can be exerted to highlight this collaboration in practice (Vo et al., 2023).

A few studies investigate the ethical influence of AI technologies in healthcare. Therefore, more studies have to be conducted to shed light on scientific methods that can be used to assess the ethical impact of these technologies on healthcare within the frame of methodological and reliable techniques. The impact can include but is not restricted to treatment outcomes, diagnosis, transparency, and privacy. Meanwhile, using various research designs, e.g., longitudinal design, can lead to more accurate results (Mittelstadt, 2019).

Despite the reliability attributed to AI-generated systems, it is time to design more humanized systems that can help professionals avoid the drawbacks resulting from these technologies. These systems would focus on the values and health condition of patients rather than any other less important considerations. This can be attained by receiving feedback from the service receivers as well as the service providers. The system can be more efficient and reliable than the currently used one (Topol, 2019).

## 5.14 RECOMMENDATIONS

Policies followed can be amended based on the parties involved, as well as the expanding practices when using AI technologies in healthcare businesses. Based on the drawback mentioned earlier, most malpractices result from misconceptions accruing due to lack of information. Hence, sharing declared and written policies with all stakeholders can minimize this misunderstanding. Meanwhile, it serves the principle of transparency as a key ethical principle when using AI technologies in healthcare.

Since policies are to be declared and shared with all parties involved, those same parties can share in making them, as well. This follows the process of clarifying the nature of these technological systems to the non-specialized parties. This fosters collaboration based on the availability of information. Again, this is another occasion through which transparency can be attained on a wider scale.

Providing consistent training to professionals is another recommendation resulting in promoting the level of healthcare services presented to patients. Based on the accountability level, training can be provided to parties involved directly or indirectly in the process. Since integrating AI technologies into the healthcare system is the main reason for some ethical drawbacks, explaining these technologies to the training professionals or parties involved serves two purposes. First, it improves the level of service provided. Second, it enlightens parties and eliminates misunderstandings.

## 5.15 CONCLUSION

To put it in a nutshell, implementations of AI technologies in healthcare systems represent a breakthrough in this realm with all the evident implications it has on patients and professionals. There are several benefits resulting from the application of AI technologies in healthcare systems. They include efficiency, accuracy, and tailored treatment plans (Ali et al., 2023; Le Nguyen & Do, 2019). Nevertheless, this advancement is accompanied by some ethical issues that need to be addressed for better performance in different aspects of the field.

As an ethical challenge, privacy can be difficult to achieve when handling data using AI tools. This arouses worries regarding the confidentiality of sensitive data collected (Li et al., 2022). Encoding data collected and having restricted access to data may seem a profound solution. Nevertheless, this can be difficult to achieve when several parties are able to gain access to data. Furthermore, data has to be diversified regularly to avoid biased processing of data based on the algorithms utilized. This endangers transparency as a basic ethical principle in healthcare systems (Krishnan Ganapathy, 2021; Sun & Medaglia, 2019).

To promote transparency, stakeholders can share in the policymaking process. This helps them understand the mechanism of the process. Thus, trust can be gained as a result (Fazakarley et al., 2024). When patients have the right to gain access to AI tools used in their therapy, they make decisions more efficiently. Meanwhile, this gesture increases transparency. All patients should have access to this right regardless of their background, social status, or origin (Kiseleva et al., 2022).

As a legislative procedure needed for better practices, regulations enacted by the FDA and the EU led to implementing AI-driven technologies in healthcare systems more efficiently (Food and Drug Administration, 2019; Floridi, 2021). Current ethical issues can be addressed based on these regulations that tackle the relevant issues professionally.

In conclusion, despite the challenging nature of ethical issues resulting from the application of AI technologies in healthcare systems, these issues are still solvable. Commitment to specific principles such as equity, transparency, and autonomy, can lead to better applications of AI technologies in the field while controlling the drawbacks of these applications. This makes it possible to achieve the optimal benefits of AI applications promised when starting this revolutionary era of advancement.

## REFERENCES

Ali, O., Abdelbaki, W., Shrestha, A., Elbasi, E., Alryalat, M. A. A., & Dwivedi, Y. K. (2023). A systematic literature review of artificial intelligence in the healthcare sector: Benefits, challenges, methodologies, and functionalities. *Journal of Innovation & Knowledge*, *8*(1), 100333.

Char, D. S., Shah, N. H., & Magnus, D. (2018). Implementing machine learning in health care—addressing ethical challenges. *The New England Journal of Medicine*, *378*(11), 981.

Chikhaoui, E., Alajmi, A., & Larabi-Marie-Sainte, S. (2022). Artificial intelligence applications in healthcare sector: Ethical and legal challenges. *Emerging Science Journal*, *6*(4), 717–738.

Fazakarley, C. A., Breen, M., Thompson, B., Leeson, P., & Williamson, V. (2024). Beliefs, experiences and concerns of using artificial intelligence in healthcare: A qualitative synthesis. *Digital Health*, *10*, 20552076241230075.

Floridi, L. (2021). The European legislation on AI: A brief analysis of its philosophical approach. *Philosophy & Technology*, *34*(2), 215–222.

Food and Drug Administration. (2019). *Proposed regulatory framework for modifications to artificial intelligence/machine learning (AI/ML)-based software as a medical device (SaMD).* U.S. Food and Drug Administration.

He, W., Zhang, Z. J., & Li, W. (2021). Information technology solutions, challenges, and suggestions for tackling the COVID-19 pandemic. *International Journal of Information Management*, *57*, 102287.

Hoppe, N., Härting, R. C., & Rahmel, A. (2023). Potential benefits of artificial intelligence in healthcare. In N. Hoppe, R. C. Härting, & A. Rahmel (Eds.), *Artificial intelligence and machine learning for healthcare* (pp. 225–249). Springer.

Karimian, G., Petelos, E., & Evers, S. M. (2022). The ethical issues of the application of artificial intelligence in healthcare: a systematic scoping review. *AI and Ethics*, *2*(4), 539–551.

Kasula, B. Y. (2021). Ethical and regulatory considerations in AI-driven healthcare solutions. *International Meridian Journal*, *3*(3), 1–8.

Khan, B., Fatima, H., Qureshi, A., Kumar, S., Hanan, A., Hussain, J., & Abdullah, S. (2023). Drawbacks of artificial intelligence and their potential solutions in the healthcare sector. *Biomedical Materials & Devices*, *1*(2), 731–738.

Kiseleva, A., Kotzinos, D., & De Hert, P. (2022). Transparency of AI in healthcare as a multilayered system of accountabilities: Between legal requirements and technical limitations. *Frontiers in Artificial Intelligence*, *5*, 879603.

Kraft, S. A. (2020). Respect and trustworthiness in the patient-provider-machine relationship: Applying a relational lens to machine learning healthcare applications. *The American Journal of Bioethics*, *20*(11), 51–53.

Krishnan Ganapathy, M. N. (2021). Artificial intelligence and healthcare regulatory and legal concerns. *Telehealth and Medicine Today*, *6*(2), 2–4.

Le Nguyen, T., & Do, T. T. H. (2019, August). *Artificial intelligence in healthcare: A new technology benefit for both patients and doctors.* 2019 Portland International Conference on Management of Engineering and Technology (PICMET). IEEE, pp. 1–15.

Li, F., Ruijs, N., & Lu, Y. (2022). Ethics & AI: A systematic review on ethical concerns and related strategies for designing with AI in healthcare. *AI*, *4*(1), 28–53.

Lopes, A. R., Dias, A. S., & Sá-Moura, B. (2023). Application of technology in healthcare: tackling COVID-19 challenge–the integration of blockchain and Internet of Things. Khosrow, M. (Editor-in-Chief), Clarke, S., Jennex, M. E., and Anttiraiko, A. (Associate Eds.) *In Research anthology on convergence of blockchain, internet of things, and security* (pp. 108–131). IGI Global.

Lysaght, T., Lim, H. Y., Xafis, V., & Ngiam, K. Y. (2019). AI-assisted decision-making in healthcare: the application of an ethics framework for big data in health and research. *Asian Bioethics Review, 11*, 299–314.

Mazurowski, M. A., Buda, M., Saha, A., & Bashir, M. R. (2019). Deep learning in radiology: An overview of the concepts and a survey of the state of the art with focus on MRI. *Journal of Magnetic Resonance Imaging*, *49*(4), 939–954.

Mittelstadt, B. (2019). Principles alone cannot guarantee ethical AI. *Nature Machine Intelligence*, *1*(11), 501–507.

Nassar, A., & Kamal, M. (2021). Ethical dilemmas in AI-powered decision-making: A deep dive into big data-driven ethical considerations. *International Journal of Responsible Artificial Intelligence*, *11*(8), 1–11.

Prakash, S., Balaji, J. N., Joshi, A., & Surapaneni, K. M. (2022). Ethical conundrums in the application of artificial intelligence (AI) in healthcare—a scoping review of reviews. *Journal of Personalized Medicine*, *12*(11), 1914.

Rosemann, A., & Zhang, X. (2022). Exploring the social, ethical, legal, and responsibility dimensions of artificial intelligence for health-a new column in intelligent medicine. *Intelligent Medicine*, *2*(02), 103–109.

Sun, T. Q., & Medaglia, R. (2019). Mapping the challenges of artificial intelligence in the public sector: Evidence from public healthcare. *Government Information Quarterly*, *36*(2), 368–383.

Topol, E. J. (2019). High-performance medicine: The convergence of human and artificial intelligence. *Nature Medicine*, *25*(1), 44–56.

Vo, V., Chen, G., Aquino, Y. S. J., Carter, S., Do, Q., & Woode, M. E. (2023). Multi-stakeholder preferences for the use of artificial intelligence in healthcare: A systematic review and thematic analysis. *Social Science & Medicine*, *116*, 357.

Chapter 6

# Analysis and predicting sector data

## The role of health news, telemedicine, and remote patient monitoring

*Tarika Singh Sikarwar, Harshita Mathur, Abhay Singh Chauhan, Sher Singh Bhakar, Prashiksha Tiwari, and Vitan Sharma*

### 6.1 INTRODUCTION

In light of the COVID-19 epidemic, health news can significantly affect the bottom lines of automobile firms. Here are a few significant ways that health news affects how well auto firms perform [1].

Production disruptions: The automotive industry may experience production delays as a result of health-related news, such as pandemics or other disease outbreaks. For automotive companies, lower output and a loss of revenue can result from supply chain disruptions, factory closures, and labor shortages brought on by health issues.

Consumer trust: Public health news can affect consumer confidence and behavior. Consumers are prone to spend less overall, including on expensive products like vehicles, during a health crisis. Reduced demand for cars due to public health issues could hurt sales and profitability. Government rules, such as safety standards and emissions standards, can change as a result of health-related news. The manufacturing and development of vehicles are impacted by these legislative changes, which may have an impact on the costs and profitability of the automotive industry.

Demand changes: Consumer preferences may change due to health concerns. As a result of people trying to avoid using public transit during the COVID-19 pandemic, for instance, we observed a shift toward telecommuting and an increase in demand for private vehicles. This change in consumer preferences may favor particular car models, including smaller, more fuel-efficient ones.

Supply chain disruptions: Health emergencies may alter international distribution systems and influence the supply of major parts and materials required for the production of automobiles. This may result in higher expenses and delays, which could harm the financial health of the automotive industry.


DOI: 10.1201/9781003634089-6

Investor sentiment: The stock market and investor sentiment can both be impacted by health news. The stock price of an automobile manufacturer can increase in response to good news about the creation of a vaccine or an efficient therapy. On the other hand, unfavorable health news might cause market turbulence and stock price drops.

Marketing and messaging: In response to health news, automotive businesses may need to modify their marketing and messaging. For instance, businesses might highlight cleanliness and safety elements in their advertising during a pandemic to allay consumer fears.

Long-term trends: In the automotive business, long-term trends may be accelerated or reversed by health news. For instance, a focus on air quality and public health issues may stimulate interest in electric cars and other environmentally friendly transportation options, thereby affecting the tactics and product lines of automobile businesses.

It is crucial to remember that the effects of health-related news on automobile companies might change based on the particular circumstance, the type of health-related event, and how each company reacts. How health-related events affect a company's bottom line is significantly influenced by elements including its financial stability, agility, and capacity for risk management. Investors and industry experts should actively watch health-related trends and evaluate their possible impact on automobile manufacturers because this can be a dynamic and changing part of industry performance.

The study may seem unrelated to telemedicine and remote patient monitoring at first glance. However, the methodologies and insights presented in this chapter have far-reaching implications that transcend industry boundaries. As healthcare embraces digital technologies such as telemedicine and remote patient monitoring, the capacity to analyze and forecast patient outcomes, behavioral trends, and treatment efficacy becomes critical. By investigating the interaction of health news and automobile sector data, this research indirectly offers information on the possible applications of data analysis and predictive modeling in healthcare. Our goal is to bridge this gap by investigating how the study's findings might inform and improve telemedicine and remote patient monitoring services, hence improving patient care and outcomes. This introduction acknowledges the study's primary focus on the automotive industry while emphasizing its possible implications for healthcare and telemedicine. By recognizing the transferable approaches and ideas, a link may be made between the study and the field of telemedicine and remote patient monitoring, paving the way for additional investigation and research.

## 6.2 LITERATURE REVIEW: VARIOUS NEWS AND STOCK MARKET RETURNS

Numerous research initiatives have been undertaken to assess the influence of a particular event on the stock market. To illustrate, a particular study unveiled that the variability of returns is higher on days marked by news events compared to days without such events. Likewise, we can compute the effects of significant global events in a similar manner on the S&P 500 index. Even news related to corporate events, such as reward or stock split announcements, influence stock market fluctuations, and it has been established that these events serve as a complement to the other events that affect the stock market [2, 3]. The stock market is notably influenced by news associated with political events; for example, a study emphasized the stock market reactions during general elections, economic and other political events, and short-term inability to share prices [4]. In emerging nations, the impact of political risk is larger than in developed markets [5, 6].

Suleman [7] examined the effect of good and negative announcements on the stock market and discovered that positive news increased KSE100 index returns while reducing volatility. Unfavorable political news, on the other hand, has a negative influence on returns (lower returns) and increases volatility (favorable effect). Moreover, the data indicates that negative news affects volatility to a nearly twofold extent compared to positive news. The majority of sectors, including the KSE100 index, demonstrate sensitivity to both favorable and unfavorable news. Additionally, the study noticed that specific industries such as oil and gas, banking, and healthcare exhibited no statistically significant alterations in reaction to positive or negative political news. This suggests that such news had minimal impact on returns or volatility within these sectors.

Optimism in local news forecasts a short-run gain in local sectoral statistics of an automobile company, but pessimism in local news indicates a brief reduction in local returns. To separate the effects of local and global news, the authors recalculated the sentiment index for each nation after eliminating items that mentioned other countries. Over time, positive global news attracts permanent inflows and has a greater influence on returns. Surprisingly, the impact of global news emotion is four times larger in worldwide "bear" markets than in global "bull" markets, implying that investors are more sensitive to news tone during global market downturns [8].

Jain investigated the phenomena of short-term event demonetization news, utilizing closing price returns from private and public sector banks before and after demonetization [9]. Public sector banks (PSBs) reported increased returns immediately after demonetization. On the other hand, private banks did not register any immediate growth and subsequently declined during the period of demonetization. The extended reach of PSBs in rural regions gives these banks an edge over their private counterparts. When compared to private banks, PSBs have three times the number of branches in the country (Business Standard, 2016). PSBs have witnessed larger deposits due to lesser pressure on the cost of funds for future recapitalization and less reliance on the government, with 70% of Jan Dhan

Yojana accounts. This beneficial influence may be seen in the price fluctuations of all PSB equities. A rise in PSB returns is a one-time occurrence.

The effect of demonetization news on IT stocks was evaluated by using the stock prices of ten software companies listed on the BSE Sensex [10]. The impact of demonetization news was minor, and even the software sector reconfigured itself in a short amount of time. Among the chosen few, Oracle is the only software business that is unaffected by demonetization. According to these data, the market was highly turbulent during the early stages of the news of demonetization, which was an unexpected event, despite the large damage. The IT industry swiftly completed the necessary procedures and began to expand. The impacts of the demonetization announcement on the BSE and S&P BSE SENSEX indexes were assessed. Demonetization during the research had no discernible impact on stock values, according to data analysis. The initial effects of the demonetization declaration were transient, and over time, the market regained stability, returning to its usual state. The reliability of the study's findings is substantiated by its analysis of the enduring effects of demonetization through long-term data. As a result, the analysis revealed no evidence of a substantial impact of the demonetization announcement on stock market values [11].

COVID-19 outbreak news had effects on Indian financial markets. An analysis centered on the dynamic variations in sector-specific data for the automobile company sector, net foreign institutional investor (FII) inflows, and exchange rate volatility. The study compared the consequences of the coronavirus epidemic to recent important structural changes in the Indian economy, specifically demonetization and the installation of the Goods and Services Tax (GST). The researchers employed a nonlinear dynamic model known as the MSI (2) VAR (2) EVENT (3) MSVAR which stands for Markov-Switching Intercept (2) Vector Autoregression (2) Event-Driven (3) Markov-Switching Vector Autoregression model, utilizing various techniques such as maximum estimation, autoregressive coefficients, variance analysis, transition probabilities, and an expectation maximization technique, this model was used to forecast the projected lengths of various economic regimes. The following are the study's key findings: First, during the initial phase of the COVID-19 epidemic, the BSE Sensex share price fell by 22.6%, in contrast to the favorable increase seen during the demonetization and GST implementation periods. Second, throughout the COVID-19 period, all stock index returns were negative. Furthermore, in the period marked by the prevalence of COVID-19, the BSE Sensex benchmark exhibited a calculated stock price volatility of 2.77, in contrast to the figures of 0.51 and 0.59 witnessed during the times of demonetization and GST implementation, respectively. Fourth, the real estate business suffered the most dramatic impact during the epidemic, with share prices falling by 41.67% by December 2020. Bankex's sectoral data for automobile companies is the most volatile. Nonetheless, sectoral data of automobile companies are adversely affected due to setbacks in both the short and long terms [12].

Another study leveraged the global COVID-19 pandemic news as a means to examine the importance of health-related news. Salisu and Vo employed Google searches to predict stock returns [13]. The research focused on the nations that were most affected by the outbreak in terms of reported cases and fatalities [14–16–17]. Although the effect of health news in predicting withdrawal is unclear, it is the study's principal contribution. Given the short temporal dimension of data available since the advent of novel coronaviruses, panels utilize a data forecasting technique to assess the efficacy of health news for sectoral data of automobile companies. To ensure the resilience of the health news forecasting model, various variants are tested. Notably, the automobile company sector data series exhibits specific characteristics such as the time-of-day market sensitivity, as well as the "asymmetry" effect and the macro abnormal component in the predictive health news model for automobile sector data. Furthermore it was found that health benefits had a negative and statistically significant effect on the sectoral data of automobile companies, indicating that more information on health issues is sought after the epidemic has spread [18]. In another study it was demonstrated that standard model predictions of infectious disease change in total sectoral data of automobile companies in Hong Kong during the COVID-19 epidemic and SARS outbreaks in the United States [19].

Researchers used COVID-19, monetary and fiscal policies, the Super Tuesday Democratic primary election, and the March 9 oil price fall news and studied how the market reacted to this news. The analysis focused on 17 trading days from late February to March 2020, when the market experienced considerable volatility. Their approach, which is based on text-based models, was able to explain a considerable amount of the variances in firm-level returns on these specific days, accounting for up to half of the observed discrepancies [20]. Further, the pandemic-related news resulted in significant negative abnormal return responses among high-risk businesses in sectors such as news, travel, housing, traditional retail, energy, aircraft manufacturing, residential buildings, real estate investment trusts (REITs), and restaurants.

Conversely, businesses engaged in ventures like high-risk drug trials, e-commerce, essential food items, online services, video games, and financial administration, as well as the manufacturing of crucial metals and minerals for semiconductors, electrical devices, and cloud computing encountered favorable abnormal returns due to the crisis related announcements. These answers were linked to supply chain complexities. Other researchers presented a straightforward yet new statistical examination of the association between daily market returns, COVID-19 for FTSE 100 firms, and market liquidity. The rapid spread of this global epidemic has impacted the global community, due to both catastrophic economic and human tolls. The capital market, in particular, has received strong unfavorable criticism on a large chunk of the economy's magnitude. In brief, this study determined that the emergence of COVID-19 leads to an adverse effect on daily market returns and liquidity, underscoring the magnitude of the COVID-19 outbreak's influence on activities within the capital market. Furthermore, the statistics indicate that the majority of industries encountered significant uncertainty. Furthermore, the data show that market liquidity has decreased, which has harmed market returns [21]. Incorporating innovative empirical data, Cepoi's study delves into the connection between news associated with COVID-19 and stock market returns within the six countries significantly impacted by the outbreak [22]. A panel analysis using a quintile regression model demonstrates that stock markets have varying relationships with COVID-19-related data, including disinformation, media exposure, and contagion effects. The outcome shows that proper communication channels should be used more intensively to reduce COVID-19-related financial turbulence.

Another researcher presented an analysis of the distribution and timing properties of natural returns and the impact of news related to disasters in the Australian equity market. The findings imply that intraday return volatility in the Australian market is best captured by a GARCH-M analysis, the inclusion of variables for natural occurrences and catastrophes in the specification and mean equation, and the absence of any fluctuation found in daily market returns. One reason for these findings is the natural effect. At the market level, events and disasters are vastly different. Rather than being a systematically priced market component, these shocks and tragedies have an ineffectual or non-risky influence on certain enterprises or geographical sectors. Furthermore, the expected cost or benefits of these catastrophes and disasters may be unclear for an extended period, resulting in no immediate market impact [23].

Brien and Kryzanowski suggested that disasters associated with news significantly disturb sector-specific data. In contrast, certain research indicates that these events news do not impact returns [24, 25]. This research investigated if contradictory outcomes are caused by geographic or event period news. The findings of an investigation into the impact of US catastrophe news on the sector data of automobile companies located in affected areas are consistent with stories from both geographic and extended event periods. Firms located in the area of a disaster have, on average, received more unusual returns than headquarters in nearby states. In very short event periods (one to five days), disaster news does not produce abnormal returns after controlling for the expected percentage of incorrectly rejected hypotheses. However, when assessing abnormal returns over a medium-term event period of two to three months, between instances of severe weather events news, only a tiny proportion of 6% to 7% influences the data inside the automobile company sector [26].

Employing an innovative analytical approach, we showcase that conditional instability sees a significant surge following news of events like hurricanes, floods, elevated temperatures, and severe winters. Nonetheless, no corresponding alteration in the secondary moment of return is observed for other major storm events. Further other researchers examined an extensive collection of significant global political crisis news to evaluate the direct connection between shifts in catastrophe risk and alterations in stock market values. The primary influence on global stock market returns stems from fluctuations in the count of international crisis news within the disaster probability model across time. There is an economically large, negative impact on the sector data of automobile companies. Changes in the number of international crises that can be studied for volatility have quite a substantial impact on the worldwide market, the commencement of an international crisis raises the monthly variability of returns in the global market, and each crisis that ends reduces monthly volatility [27]

Furthermore, it is shown that when news related to more severe crises is there, markets tend to respond more strongly (in terms of average returns and volatility). By conducting cross-sectional analysis with US survey data, we reinforce a key presupposition of the time-bound disaster framework: namely, that disaster-related news regarding crisis probabilities has a negative influence on consumption growth.

Wang and Kutan conducted a study that delved into how natural disaster news affected both the insurance sector and the overall market presence in Japan and the United States [28]. Significantly, no discernible effects on property-related aspects have been observed in either the composite stock markets of the US or Japan. This is evident as the returns within these markets remain unaffected by any of the natural disasters news included in the dataset under investigation. However, both countries have significant wealth impacts on the insurance industry. The results for the Japanese insurance business support the "profit from loss theory" associated with earthquakes, tsunamis, and tropical storms. However, the evidence against this concept exists in the US insurance market. Except for the Japanese composites market, all returns are impacted by natural catastrophes as risk effects.

The link between macroeconomic factors and movements of the hospitality stock was assessed. This study focuses particularly on non-social economic variables, such as political developments, significant athletic events, financial meltdowns, natural disasters, military conflicts, and terrorist attacks showing that several of these variables could have a greater impact than macroeconomic influences. It is advised to use stock markets from other Asian nations across various continents, such as South Asia, Europe, and Africa, to verify the results [29].

## 6.3 RESEARCH GAP

While academic research and financial news analysis have looked into the relationship between health news and its impact on the stock market, there are substantial gaps in the existing literature. Understanding causality and directionality, distinguishing between long-term and short-term impacts, sector-specific analysis, sentiment and media analysis, global perspectives, behavioral and psychological factors, data and methodological improvements, the impact of regulatory changes, non-public information, and the role of various media channels and sources are all important areas of future research.

Furthermore, the emerging subject of telemedicine and its impact on stock market performance is an important yet understudied issue. Despite the substantial literature on the relationship between various types of news and the stock market, there are still many unanswered questions and possible research areas, specifically concerning health-related news. Understanding the complex interactions between health-related events, such as advances in telemedicine, and financial markets is critical for investors, governments, and the general public.

## 6.4 OBJECTIVE OF STUDY

The objective of this study was to find the difference in returns of the Auto Index, pre- and post-health news.

## 6.5 RESEARCH METHODOLOGY

The study was descriptive. Health-related news was used to evaluate the effect of health news on the return of the Auto Index. To investigate the differences among returns for the Auto Index in response to health news, seven days' worth of pre- and post-return news were taken.

The population of the study included all of the companies listed on the National Stock Exchange (NSE). The automobile sector index return was used for the study. The data collection of the daily closing value of the Automobiles Index (Nifty Auto) was from 1 April 2022 to 31 March 2023. The data intended for this research was collected from the NSE website (www.nseindia.com). The COVID case data considered as health news was taken from the official website of the Ministry of Health, Government of India. A paired t-test was applied to show the differences between the pre- and post-COVID-19 health news returns for Nifty Auto.

## 6.6 RESULTS AND ANALYSIS

We collected data through the NSE websites for Nifty Auto. During the time frame of 1 April 2022 to 31 March 2023, we looked for news related to health on the Ministry of Health Department website, and such news is considered as an event for study. Keeping the selected news date in mind, we took data seven days prior and seven days after closing of the stock prices for the automobile sector. We repeated the same process for multiple news events. After data collection, we applied the paired t-test for a better analysis of our research.

Table 6.1 is the summary of the paired test applied on pre- and post-seven days returns of Nifty Auto taking health news as an event. There is a mean difference between pre- and post-event returns for Nifty Auto, and the result is different for each news item considering the significance level of 5%. It can be seen that for the health news of April 2022, the 2-tailed result was 0.37, indicating no effect of the news on the auto sector return. In May 2022, the 2-tailed result was 0.119, indicating no effect of news on auto sector returns. We can see that for health-related news in May 2022, the 2-tailed result is 0.00, indicating a significant effect of health-related news on auto sector returns.

We can observe that the 2-tailed result for June 2022 was 0.18, showing that news had no effect on automobile sector returns. For July 2022, the

*Table 6.1* Summarized results for paired t-test

| *Date of news* | *Hypothesis* | *Mean* | *Standard deviation* | *t* | *df* | *Sig. (2-tailed)* | *Hypothesis rejected/not rejected* |
|---|---|---|---|---|---|---|---|
| 15-Apr-22 | 0.05 | –473.52 | 469.47 | –2.69 | 6 | 0.37 | Not rejected |
| 7-May-22 | 0.05 | –122.12 | 177.58 | –1.81 | 6 | .119 | Not rejected |
| 28-May-22 | 0.05 | –756.73 | 63.77 | –31.39 | 6 | .000 | Rejected |
| 17-Jun-22 | 0.05 | –197.55 | 162.69 | –3.21 | 6 | 0.18 | Not rejected |
| 8-Jul-22 | 0.05 | –125.47 | 241.69 | –1.37 | 6 | .219 | Not rejected |
| 29-Jul-22 | 0.05 | –129.28 | 121.92 | –2.08 | 6 | .031 | Not rejected |
| 19-Aug-22 | 0.05 | –253.16 | 111.20 | –6.03 | 6 | .001 | Rejected |
| 9-Sep-22 | 0.05 | –117.42 | 93.70 | –3.31 | 6 | .016 | Not rejected |
| 30-Sep-22 | 0.05 | –352.49 | 216.12 | –4.31 | 6 | .005 | Rejected |
| 22-Oct-22 | 0.05 | 72.10 | 88.15 | 2.16 | 6 | .074 | Not rejected |
| 12-Nov-22 | 0.05 | –516.45 | 89.14 | –15.32 | 6 | .000 | Rejected |
| 4-Dec-22 | 0.05 | –274.71 | 253.44 | –2.86 | 6 | .029 | Not rejected |
| 28-Dec-22 | 0.05 | –259.67 | 315.25 | –2.17 | 6 | .072 | Not rejected |
| 18-Jan-23 | 0.05 | –318.21 | 299.33 | –2.81 | 6 | .031 | Not rejected |
| 9-Feb-23 | 0.05 | –358.67 | 469.93 | –2.02 | 6 | .089 | Not rejected |
| 18-Feb-23 | 0.05 | 566.75 | 141.24 | 10.61 | 6 | .000 | Rejected |

2-tailed result was 0.219, demonstrating that the news had no influence on automotive sector returns. For news in July 2022, the 2-tailed result was 0.031, showing that news had a significant impact on automobile sector returns.

We can see that in August 2022, the 2-tailed result was 0.001 indicating no effect of news on the auto sector returns. We can see that in September 2022, the 2-tailed result was 0.016 and for other news it was 0.005, indicating a significant effect of news on auto sector returns.

We can see that in October 2022, the 2-tailed result was 0.074 indicating no significant effect of news on auto sector returns. We can see that in November 2022, the 2-tailed result was 0.00 indicating a significant effect of news on auto sector returns.

We can see that in December 2022, the 2-tailed result was 0.029 indicating a significant effect of news on auto sector returns. For news of December 2022, the 2-tailed result was 0.072 indicating no significant effect of news on auto sector returns.

We can see that in January 2023, the 2-tailed result is 0.031 indicating a significant effect of news on auto sector returns. For similar news in January 2023, the 2-tailed result is 0.089 indicating an insignificant effect of news on auto sector returns. We can see that in the event of February 2023, the 2-tailed result is 0.00 indicating a significant effect of the news on auto sector returns.

## 6.7 DISCUSSION

It can be understood that due to several interrelated elements and market dynamics, health news affects the returns in the automotive industry. The global supply chains can be disrupted by health-related problems like pandemics or outbreaks. Similarly, health news has a big impact on how people shop. For instance, consumers might be less willing to make discretionary expenditures like new cars amid a health crisis. Returns on the vehicle sector might be adversely impacted by a drop in customer demand. Health crises can result in economic unpredictability. Auto stocks may become less popular as investors become less risk-tolerant. The performance of the auto industry can be impacted by economic uncertainty, which can also have an impact on loan rates and how vehicles are financed. Further, government rules may change as a result of health-related news.

It can be inferred that the shifts in oil prices may be caused by health emergencies. The price of fuel has a substantial impact on the vehicle industry. Consumer preferences for fuel-efficient or electric vehicles may change when oil prices increase as a result of supply shortages related to illness or geopolitical causes. To a greater extent, the auto industry is impacted by investor sentiment, and bad health news might cause the market to be pessimistic. Panic or worry among investors might cause selling pressure on car stocks, which will impact their results.

As multinational corporations, many automakers depend on global trade for their day-to-day operations and financial success. The profitability of the vehicle industry can be impacted by health difficulties that impede international trade, particularly if there are tariffs, border closures, or import or export restrictions.

Governments may implement new car safety standards in response to health concerns. The profitability of the industry may be impacted by compliance expenses that arise as a result of these rules. During health emergencies, demand for autonomous automobiles and in-car health monitoring devices may increase.

In conclusion, because of its interdependence with other variables like supply chain disruptions, consumer behavior, governmental regulations, and economic uncertainty, health news can have an impact on auto sector returns. Changes in these areas can have an impact on the sector's overall performance and stock prices because it is susceptible to changes in them.

## 6.8 CONCLUSION

The present research is driven by the growing concerns regarding health after the current global pandemic (COVID-19) and seeks to investigate the role of health-related news in projecting the stock returns of the Auto Index. We collected information from the NSE website to examine the impact of health-related news on the Nifty Auto Index return statistics.

We employed the paired t-test to assess the COVID-19 impact and discovered a difference in returns for the automotive sector. The findings can be linked to a variety of factors, including industrial disruption, consumer behavior shifts, supply chain concerns, and economic challenges caused by the pandemic.

The empirical literature is replete with studies on news and information patterns and market reactions [14–16, 18, 29, 30]. We meticulously evaluated various previous articles and analyzed their results. There are studies that have looked at news about certain variables, such as oil prices and economic sector developments, as predictors of stock returns. The significance of health news is rarely understood, therefore this study is a crucial contribution to the field, where a void exists for studies focused on health news and market reaction.

In conclusion, news concerning health difficulties can have a range of effects on the Auto Index's return statistics and the economy as a whole. The nature and scope of health-related news, as well as how businesses and policymakers respond to these events, will determine their influence. Such news is closely studied by industry participants, policymakers, and investors to see how it may affect the auto sector and the entire economy. The Auto Index and the overall economy are susceptible to the domino impact of health-related news. It has the power to affect government policy, investor mood, production, customer behavior, and the auto industry's general course. These consequences can therefore affect the Auto Index's performance and have wider economic ramifications outside of the automobile industry. Investors, legislators, and other industry players must keep an eye on and react to health-related news in order to adjust to shifting consumer preferences and market conditions.

## 6.9 IMPLICATIONS

By recognizing these connections, researchers and healthcare professionals can:

- Apply data analysis techniques from other industries, such as the automotive sector, to healthcare to enhance patient outcomes and optimize services.
- Use predictive modeling to forecast disease progression, treatment effectiveness, and patient outcomes, thus improving telemedicine and remote patient monitoring.
- Consider the impact of health news on patient behavior and treatment adherence, thereby informing strategies for better healthcare outcomes.
- Draw insights from various sectors, including the automotive industry, to advance digital health services and enhance telemedicine and remote patient monitoring.

This summary highlights the potential for interdisciplinary approaches to drive innovation in healthcare and telemedicine.

## DATA AVAILABILITY STATEMENT

The dataset is available on request. It cannot be shared openly.

## REFERENCES

1. Gupta, S. "Pandemics, COVID-19 and India," *Indian Economic Review*, vol. 55, no. S1, pp. 1–12, 2020.
2. Kothari, S. P., & Shanken, J., "Book-to-market, dividend yield, and expected market returns: A time-series analysis," *Journal of Financial Economics*, vol. 44, no. 2, pp. 169–203, 1997.

3. Manning, N. "Common trends and convergence? South East Asian equity markets, 1988–1999," *Journal of international Money and Finance*, vol. 21, no. 2, pp. 183–202, 2002.
4. Prabu, A. E., Bhattacharyya, I., & Ray, P. "Impact of monetary policy on the Indian stock market: Does the devil lie in the detail?" *Indian Economic Review*, vol. 55, no. 1, pp. 27–50, 2020.
5. Beaulieu, M.-C., Cosset, J.-C., & Essaddam, N., "The impact of political risk on the volatility of stock returns: The case of Canada," *Journal of International business studies*, vol. 36, no. 6, pp. 701–718, 2005.
6. Lin, B. H., &. Wang, J. M. C. "Systematic skewness in asset pricing: An empirical examination of the Taiwan stock market," *Applied Economics*, vol. 35, no. 17, pp. 1877–1887, 2003.
7. Suleman, M. T. "Stock market reaction to good and bad political news," *Asian Journal of Finance & Accounting*, vol. 55, no. S1, pp. 299–312, 2012.
8. Fraiberger, R. R. "Media sentiment and international asset prices," *Journal of International Economics*, vol. 133, no. 103526, pp. 1–43, 2021.
9. Jain, R. "Is demonetisation a Windfall for the banking sector? Evidence from the Indian stock market," *Economics Bulletin*, vol. 37, no. 2, pp. 712–722, 2017.
10. Divya, S. S. "Impact of demonetization on stock market return," *Amity Journal of Finance, India. ISSN*, vols. 2456–1568, pp. 14–34, 2017.
11. Upadhyay, S. S. W. "Impact of demonetization on the Indian stock market: With special reference to Bombay stock exchange," *Paradigm*, vol. 22, no. 2, pp. 175–184, 2018.
12. Mishra, A. K., Rath, B. N., & Dash, A. K. "Does the Indian financial market nosedive because of the COVID-19 outbreak, in comparison to after demonetisation and the GST?" In *Research on Pandemics*. Routledge, pp. 30–48, 2021.
13. Salisu, A. A., & Vo, X. V. "Predicting stock returns in the presence of COVID-19 pandemic: The role of health news.," *International Review of Financial Analysis*, vol. 71, 101546, pp. 1–10, 2020.
14. Even-Tov, O. "When does the bond price reaction to earnings announcements predict future stock returns?," *Journal of Accounting and Economics*, vol. 64, no. 1, pp. 167–182, 2017.
15. Narayan, P. K. "Can stale oil price news predict stock returns?," *Energy Economics*, vol. 83, pp. 430–444, 2019.
16. Narayan, P. K., & Bannigidadmath, D. "Are Indian stock returns predictable?," *Journal of Banking & Finance*, vol. 58, pp. 506–531, 2015.
17. Salisu, A. A., Sikiru, A. A., & Vo, X. V. "Pandemics and the emerging stock markets," *Borsa Istanbul Review*, vol. 20, pp. S40–S48, 2020.
18. Calomiris, C. W., & Mamaysky, H. "How news and its context drive risk and returns around the world," *National Bureau of Economic Research Working Paper No. 24430*, 2018.
19. Alfaro, L., Chari, A., Greenland, A. N., & Schott, P. K. "Aggregate and firm-level stock returns during pandemics, in real time," *National Bureau of Economic Research*, 2020.

20. Davis, S. J., Hansen, S., & Seminario-Amez, C., "Firm-level risk exposures and stock returns in the wake of COVID-19," National Bureau of Economic Research, Working Paper No. 27867, 2020.
21. Tahat, Y., & Ahmed, A. H. "Stock market returns, liquidity and COVID-19 outbreak: Evidence from the UK," *Date of Access*, 12 August 2020.
22. Cepoi, C. O. "Asymmetric dependence between stock market returns and news during COVID-19 financial turmoil," *Finance Research Letters*, vol. 36, p. 101658, 2020.
23. Worthington, A. C. "The impact of natural events and disasters on the Australian stock market: A GARCH-M analysis of storms, floods, cyclones, earthquakes and bushfires," *Global Business and Economics Review*, vol. 10, no. 1, pp. 1–10, 2008.
24. Wang, L., & Kutan, A. M. "The impact of natural disasters on stock markets: Evidence from Japan and the US," *Comparative Economic Studies*, vol. 55, pp. 672–686, 2013.
25. Worthington, A. C. "The decline of calendar seasonality in the Australian stock exchange, 1958–2005," 2008. Available at SSRN 1290905. http://ssrn.com/abstract=1290905.
26. Bourdeau-Brien, M., & Kryzanowski, L. "The impact of natural disasters on the stock returns and volatilities of local firms," *The Quarterly Review of Economics and Finance*, vol. 63, pp. 259–270, 2017.
27. Berkman, H., Jacobsen, B., & Lee, J. B. "Time-varying rare disaster risk and stock returns," *Journal of Financial Economics*, 2010. http://dx.doi.org/10.2139/ssrn.1572042
28. Wang, L., & Kutan, A. M. "The impact of natural disasters on stock markets: Evidence from Japan and the US," *Comparative Economic Studies*, vol. 55, pp. 672–686, 2013.
29. Chen, M. H., Kim, W. G., & Chen, C. Y. "An investigation of the mean reversion of hospitality stock prices towards their fundamental values: The case of Taiwan," *International Journal of Hospitality Management*, vol. 26, no. 2, pp. 453–467, 2015.
30. Loughran, T., & McDonald, B. "Textual analysis in accounting and finance: A survey," *Journal of Accounting Research*, vol. 54, no. 4, pp. 1187–1230, 2016.

Chapter 7

# An industrial applications-based generalized model on the effect of trade credits on healthcare items under multivariate demand-based production with time-dependent deterioration and partial backlogging

*Sanjay Sharma, Anand Tyagi, Vidhi Agrawal, and Sachin Kumar*

## 7.1 INTRODUCTION

The healthcare system in India is a complex network comprising both the public and private sectors. The existing system offers a variety of medical services and healthcare facilities to the 1.4 billion people residing in India. Although the system was working well before the COVID-19 pandemic, the health crisis that came with the pandemic compelled the Indian government and private sector to rethink the investment patterns in healthcare systems. The challenges that were posed by the pandemic exposed the deficiencies in the existing healthcare infrastructure in India, making it apparent that robust investment in this sector is not just necessary but urgent.

To address the issue, the Indian government enacted several crucial initiatives for enhancing the healthcare capabilities across the nation. For example, the government has increased the budget allocation for expanding healthcare facilities. Additionally, the public health policies have also been revised with the primary focus on preparedness for emergency/crisis situations. With this proactive approach and active involvement of the policymakers in the healthcare sector, it is expected that in the future, medical services will be available in all rural and remote areas. The COVID-19 pandemic has been an eye-opener for all concerned stakeholders. The private sector is also playing a vital role in the healthcare ecosystem. Private hospitals, pharmaceutical companies, and the healthcare providers have enormously increased their investments in advanced medical technologies, telemedicine, and digital devices.

The COVID-19 pandemic shed light on the significance of keeping an effective supply chain for equipment and materials that can save lives. Issues like the shortages of ventilators, personal protective equipment

 DOI: 10.1201/9781003634089-7

(PPE), and necessary medications during the pandemic have highlighted the need for improved inventory management and logistics in the healthcare industry. The proper management of healthcare items is the demand of time. As was seen in the COVID-19 pandemic, the proper running of these lifesaving items is important. We have to work and develop updated models for such lifesaving items. The effect of demand actually plays a vital role in the proper running and manufacturing of pharmaceutical items as well as their supply. To confirm that there is smooth running and supply of the lifesaving items, we have to develop a critical model based on past experiences. The present model has been developed on pharmaceutical items.

In the current model, the role of the different patterns on the demand as per the different market situations on environmental conditions has been considered. Trade credit has always been considered as a helpful tool for growing businesses. Keeping this fact in mind, we have also considered trade credits effects in the developed model. When favorable terms are agreed with a business supplier, then this type of finance contributes to the reduction and the management of capital requirements of a business. A multivariate demand has been introduced in the model, as the pharmaceutical items deteriorate after a certain period of time. The market demand, its fluctuations, and its trends are totally changed. The strategies that were used before COVID-19 will not be applicable after COVID-19. So, as a result, the current model has been developed for multiple demand patterns. Spoilage of lifesaving items needs to be minimized as much as possible. Keeping this fact in mind, the current model also considered deterioration. In the past, deteriorated items were sold on discount. So to avoid this loss, we have planted the short life items in the warehouse that have to be used first to satisfy the demand of customers. Demand before COVID-19 will not be the same after COVID-19, and the storage facility and other costs will also be affected before and after COVID-19.

The number of new pharmaceuticals licensed for sale rose by 60% between 2010 and 2019 when compared to the preceding ten years, reaching a peak of 59 new drugs approved in 2018. The model was also developed considering partial backlog; the demand of customers has to be satisfied first when the stock of goods is received, as it improves the trust of the customers. Many research papers have attempted to get this updated form of the economic order quantity (EOQ) model. The model will play a vital role in managing the proper storage and manufacturing of lifesaving items.

The current study covered the issues of supply chain management of input materials, finished products, and precautions during storage in warehouses. This study is crucial and makes significant contributions to the healthcare sector, as the authors of this study have tried to address the critical issues that come in the supply chain management of lifesaving items by introducing an innovative model for pharmaceutical supply chain management.

The model proposed by the authors will facilitate enhancing the inventory and logistics management, and will ensure continuous and reliable access to essential medications. The model has been designed in context of the current realities and has been developed with the objective of efficient resource utilization and cost management. The proposed model has direct practical applications and can be utilized by policymakers and healthcare providers for making strategies that can improve the reliability and efficiency of healthcare services.

## 7.2 LITERATURE REVIEW

There is always uncertainty with lifesaving medical items, and their supply has become a very tough task to handle. Therefore, for hospitals to run smoothly, the demand and supply of such items become an important task. With this in mind, a model has been developed by Saha and Ray [1]. In this study, an optimization under uncertainty of the pharmaceutical supply chain in hospitals has been presented. Rastogi and Singh [2] presented an advanced model for the inventory system by considering varying deterioration on pharmaceutical items. The model considered a price-based demand, and the holding cost was considered as variable. Backlogging is also assumed and it has been taken as partial backlogged. Also, Woods and Hollnagel [3] developed a model on joint cognitive systems.

Weraikat et al. [] developed an inventory model to improve the sustainability for the pharmaceutical supply chain based on a two-level vendor-managed inventory system. COVID-19 has changed the medical policy of almost all countries of the world. We have to develop new models as per today's needs. The models must be capable of avoiding shortages of lifesaving items, and we have to be very responsive to the pandemic. Based on a multistage stochastic program, Tucker et al. [5] discussed a model in which drug shortages have been calculated, and an incentivizing resilient supply chain design method has been adopted for the presentation of the drug items.

Game theory can help the player to read the strategy of the opposing player. Using the concepts of game theory in pharmaceutical products, Priyan and Mala [6] presented an optimal inventory model for pharmaceutical products. The incorporating quality degradation of the items has been developed and the expiration date of the items is also assumed. Based on emerging markets, Cakmakli et al. [7] presented an inventory control epidemiological model with international production networks and capital flows. The model was suitable to understand the emerging demand of international customers. The main issue faced by most of the country was to find out the exact number of cases infected by the COVID-19 virus. Tracking systems were not up to the task during the initial stages. Leslie [8] developed a COVID-19 tracking system in which responsible AI innovation systems were used. Health issues became critical aspects during COVID-19. Schwab and Malleret [9] presented an implementation guide for health systems recovery in emergencies.

Bloom et al. [10] studied the impact of COVID-19 on productivity. The uncertainty of the pharmaceutical supply chain and its proper distribution in hospitals during and after COVID-19 was a challenge for the government, as medical facilities are not up to the task in most Asian countries. Franco and Alfonso-Lizarazo [11] developed a model based on uncertainty of the pharmaceutical supply chain in hospitals.

The major issue that has been faced by pharmaceutical distributors is to handle the supply chain of lifesaving items. Alkahtani et al. [12] presented a model on different approaches to handle the supply. The model was developed on variable production where the uncertain environmental conditions were also taken into consideration. Similarly, sustainable and resilient healthcare is also a point to be considered, and a non-cold pharmaceutical distribution supply chain model for the COVID-19 pandemic was developed. The stockout situation can also be seen after the pandemic. Illahi and Mir [13] presented maintaining efficient logistics and supply chain management operations during and after COVID-19.

Most of the aforementioned models target how to handle the critical situation and how to keep Supply Chain Management (SCM) in a proper way, but the wastage of medicines is also a very crucial part as the waste of medicines must also stop. Tat and Heydari [14] developed a model to avoid medicine waste by introducing a sustainable approach in the pharmaceutical supply chain. Abdolazimi et al. [15] developed a sustainable and resilient healthcare and non-cold pharmaceutical distribution supply chain model for the COVID-19 pandemic. As trade credits play a vital role in inventory models, their impact can also be extended to the medical sector. Poswal et al. [16] developed an integrated model on medicinal products and presented an economic ordering policy to control deterioration where medicinal products of uncertain demand with trade credit for healthcare industries have been assumed.

Uncertainty in production for manufacturing industries has become a very tough task to manage. In the same way, Sharma et al. [17] developed an EOQ model of uncertainty in demand and production for manufacturing industries during COVID-19. The main focus of most authors was during COVID-19, but things changed very drastically after COVID-19. Some researchers are continuing to study post-COVID effects and precautions. Blanco Izquierdo and Gázquez [18] presented a mathematical optimization model in which the main focus was to reallocate and share health equipment as per their requirement in pandemic situations.

Rafele [19] also developed a model of a calculation for materials management. Most of the available models aim to face any pandemic situations related to pharmaceutical products. But the effect of the COVID-19 pandemic can also be seen in almost every sector. Its effect on the engineering manufacturing sector was studied by Almaharmeh [20] who presented a model on the impact of the COVID-19 pandemic disruption on supply chain performance in the engineering manufacturing sector. A few more models on intelligent inventory management approaches for perishable pharmaceutical products, a sustainable-resilience healthcare network, and decision-making have been developed [21–23].

In this study, an EOQ model has been developed under uncertain demands and also provided the tools to control the deterioration of medicinal products. One team of researchers developed a new model that presents intelligent inventory management approaches [21]. Based on a network for handling COVID-19, a model for medical items has been developed [22]. In this model, sustainable-resilience techniques developed the network-based information on the COVID-19 pandemic. Most of the preceding studies have been developed to provide medicine on time, but some of the models have been developed to avoid medicine shortages. In one model, the unused medicine is collected to improve corporate social responsibility [23].

Dohale et al. [24] presented a model on COVID-19 and supply chain risk mitigation: A case study from India. Also, Çetindaş et al. [25] developed a model on effect of supply chain agility on firm performance during COVID-19 pandemic: the mediating and moderating role of demand stability.

Based on a fuzzy approach, Pant et al. [26] presented a channel financing policy for an EOQ model of fast-moving consumer goods. The effect of deterioration on the items is also assumed. The fuzzy approach makes the study relevant in the aspect of the fast-moving goods. Deterioration is a major issue in inventory, as it plays a vital role in the handling of the items in stock. There are so many models to minimize the deterioration in the past. In the same way, to avoid the spoilage of items in storage, many inventory control models have been developed. In addition, some models have been developed for deteriorated items where a small discount is offered on expiring items. Payment flexibility is also a new approach to benefit consumers. Palanivelu and Chandrasekaran [27] developed and presented a two-phase time-based demand model in which comparative analysis of an inventory management system was discussed. The model was developed under shortages with tolerable slack of payment for deteriorating goods.

To present the effects of the salvage value of the items, Sharma et al. [28] considered quadratic demand on Pareto-distributed decaying products and presented an economic order quantity model in which shortage and salvage value both were considered. At the end, applications and scope of Laplace in the inventory management have been considered by Haque et al. [29], who developed a model on neutrosophic Laplace transform and its application considering price and deterioration-dependent demand.

The use of artificial intelligence in the inventory has been introduced by Debnath et al. [30] and a supply chain management strategy during COVID-19 was presented. The pharmaceutical retail supply chain responses to the COVID-19 pandemic were presented by Schleifenheimer and Ivanov [31].

Many research papers have been developed in the area of the pharmaceutical industries, using various techniques, such as game theory, constant rate of the deterioration, and the time-dependent rate of the deterioration. Some studies are based on the evaluation of the drug supply chain management, which plays a major role in the medical sector. But as we have seen, the effects of the COVID-19 pandemic have led to changed strategies. In the present study we have developed an inventory control model for the pharmaceutical industry; the model has been developed under the time-dependent rate of deterioration.

The demand of the product has been assumed as stock-dependent as well as price-dependent, which makes this study more realistic as per the current stage of the pharmaceutical industries. The shortage of the items has been assumed and taken as partially backlogged and the rate of the backlogged taken as time dependent. The holding cost of holding the items in the stock is taken as a function of time. The sensitivity analysis in the model has been calculated for the validation.

### 7.2.1 Contribution to the current scenario

Models of the past were mainly developed under the same storage facility, either owned or rented. For the high demand of lifesaving items, especially during a drastic situation like COVID-19, we have to maintain the supply chain of items. We introduce a new concept of assuming rented warehouses, which makes this study more realistic in facing the unwanted ups and downs in the supply.

| *Reference* | *Stock-dependent demand* | *Selling price-dependent demand* | *Time-dependent demand* | *Time-dependent deterioration* | *Production-based on demand* | *Partial backlogging* | *Variable holding cost* | *Pharmaceutical items taken or not* |
|---|---|---|---|---|---|---|---|---|
| Saha and Ray (2019) | No | No | No | Yes | Yes | Yes | No | Yes |
| Rastogi and Singh (2019) | No | Yes | No | Yes | No | Yes | No | Yes |
| Weraikat et al. (2019) | Yes | No | Yes | No | No | Yes | No | Yes |
| Tucker et al. (2020) | Yes | No | No | Yes | No | Yes | Yes | Yes |
| Bloom et al. (2020) | Yes | No | No | Yes | No | Yes | No | No |
| Franco and Alfonso (2020) | Yes | No | No | Yes | No | Yes | No | Yes |
| Illahi and Mir (2021) | Yes | No | No | Yes | No | Yes | Yes | Yes |
| Tat and Heydari (2021) | Yes | No | Yes | Yes | No | No | No | Yes |
| Rafele et al. (2022) | No | Yes | No | Yes | No | No | Yes | No |
| Ahmadi et al. (2022) | No | Yes | No | Yes | No | Yes | Yes | Yes |
| Nematollahi et al. (2022) | No | Yes | No | No | No | Yes | No | Yes |
| Çetindaş et al. (2023) | Yes | No | No | Yes | No | Yes | No | Yes |
| Pant et al. (2023) | No | Yes | Yes | No | No | Yes | No | Yes |
| Sharma et al. (2024) | Yes | Yes | No | No | No | Yes | No | Yes |
| Haque et al. (2024) | Yes | Yes | No | Yes | Yes | Yes | No | Yes |
| Debnath et al. (2024) | No | Yes | Yes | No | No | Yes | No | Yes |
| Schleifenheimer and Ivanov (2024) | Yes | Yes | No | No | No | Yes | No | Yes |
| Current model | Yes | Yes | No | Yes | No | Yes | Yes | Yes |

Another contribution of the current study is to store the items in the warehouse from which the demand is going to satisfy. The assumption of storage makes this study more resolute. The model is also useful as far as the industry aspect is concerned. It will help the wholesaler and manufacturer to avoid the deterioration of the items.

## 7.3 COMPARISON TO THE PREVIOUS STUDIES

The present model has been developed as per the current market situation and current environmental conditions.

- The current model has been developed to help manufacturers avoid the loss of sales and unwanted deterioration. The model also helps to maintain the proper supply chain of lifesaving items. The model is compared to previous models.
- In most of the previous inventory control models, the main outcomes are to develop such models in which various parameters-based demand have been assumed. But the current model also presents the industrial aspect and application to the current market scenario developed.
- Due to high demand fluctuations, the author has assumed both warehouses as rented, which is a key approach in the direction toward the manufacturer's space-related restriction issues. Also, in most of the studies conducted on warehouse problems, the demand was mainly considered stock-dependent, so as a result there was no such need for extra rented warehouses.
- The present model has been developed on different demand rates in different warehouses. The demand has been assumed stock-dependent until a subsequent interval of time; after that it is assumed as constant.
- The present model was also developed to the maximum utilization of the inventory, to control and maintain market supply and demand of items, and shortage and overstock both have been managed. The model also developed under maximization techniques, which makes this study more realistic and feasible as far as market and COVID-19 effects on the stock are concerned.
- It is also assumed that the deterioration rate is considered different in both warehouses. Also, both warehouses have different storage facilities. Due to high ups and downs in demand, a shortage of items is also assumed where the shortage is treated as partially backlogged during the out-of-stock period. This study is mainly presented to find out the optimal total cost and shortage period in the case when both warehouses are rented and the product is deteriorating in nature.

## 7.4 ASSUMPTIONS AND NOTATIONS

### 7.4.1 Assumptions

In the current model, the following assumptions have been taken:

1. The models have been developed under two levels of demand pattern, the model has been developed under time-dependent demand during the initial stage of COVID-19, and demand has been assumed stock dependent during the peak stage of COVID-19.
   D(t) = $\left[ a + bI(t) 0 < t < t_1 \ \alpha p^{-\beta} \ t_1 < t < t_2 \right]$
2. The shortages of the items are considered and assumed as partially backlogged.
3. The lead time is zero.
4. The backlogging rate during the stockout period has been assumed, and it is considered as a function of waiting time up to the next arrival $\mu, \theta(\mu) = 1 - \frac{\mu}{T}, 0 \leq \mu \leq T$
5. The cost of holding the items has been considered as a variable function of time.
6. Backlog has not been assumed due to the pandemic situation.
7. There is no replacement of the deteriorated item considered.

### 7.4.2 Notations

The following notations have been applied:

| | |
|---|---|
| I(t): | Inventory level |
| D(t): | Demand rate |
| $a, b, \alpha, \beta, \gamma, \delta$: | Coefficient of demand |
| $\theta$: | Deterioration rate |
| Hc: | Holding cost |
| $Q_1$: | Back-ordered quantity |
| Q: | Ordering quantity |
| C(q): | Purchase cost per unit of time |
| $\theta(\mu)$: | Rate of backlog during stock out |
| T: | The duration of the production cycle |
| O: | Ordering quantity |
| $Q_2$: | Back-ordered quantity for stockout period |
| $\mu$: | Waiting time for the arrival of the next lot |
| $h_1, h_2$: | Holding cost parameters |
| S(c): | Shortage cost per unit |
| L(S): | Lost sale cost per unit |
| T.A.C.: | Total average cost |
| $t_1$*, Q*, and T.A.C.*: | Optimal values of $t_1$, Q, and T.A.C., respectively |

## 7.5 FORMULATION AND ANALYSIS OF THE MODEL

The model is presented graphically in Figure 7.1. It shows that the production starts with zero inventory. As the production starts, the increasing graph shows that the items in stock are increasing, and at the same time we have also satisfied the demand of the customers. It shows the linear trend in demand. However, when we stored most of the items in the inventory, an incident happened and the stock decreased during the uncertain demand and unavoidable situation in the market.

Initially, at time t = 0 as per graphical representation of the study, we have no items in the inventory. Production starts at time t = 0. As we get items in stock at a certain level, as a result, deterioration and demand take place. When we reach the maximum inventory level, the production stops.

As both demand and deterioration take place together, we drop to zero inventory in the stock. At this time, a shortage of items takes place and in time it reaches the maximum shortage level. Then fresh production starts to clear the backlog by the time. Graphical representation of the model is shown in Figure 7.1.

The differential equations governing the proposed model are:

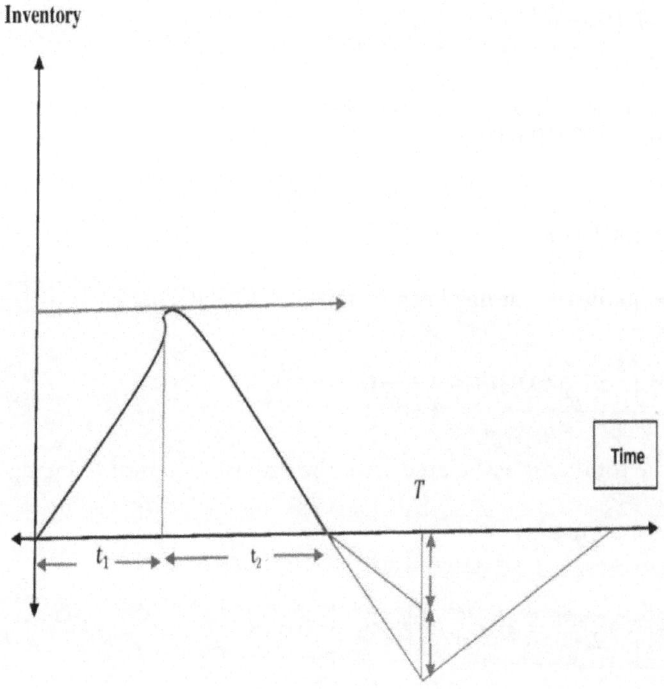


*Figure 7.1* Inventory cycle with respect to time.

$$\frac{dI_1(t)}{dt} + \theta t I_1(t) = -\left[a + bI_1(t)\right] \quad 0 \le t \le t_1 \tag{7.1}$$

$$\frac{dI_2(t)}{dt} + \theta t I(t) = -\alpha p^{-\beta} \quad t_1 \le t \le \tag{7.2}$$

Following are the boundary conditions: $I_1(t_1) = Q, \qquad I_2(t_2) = 0$ (7.3)

Solutions to the preceding equations under the boundary conditions are as follows:

$$I_1(t) = e^{bt_1} a\left[t_1 + \frac{b}{2}t_1^2 - \frac{\theta}{6}t_1^3 - \frac{b\theta}{4}t_1^4\right] \tag{7.4}$$

$$I_2(t) = \alpha p^{-\beta}\left[-t_1 - \frac{\theta}{6}t_1^3\right]e^{-\theta\frac{t_1^2}{2}} \tag{7.5}$$

The quantity that is initially ordered is

$$Q_1 = I_1(0) = e^{bt_1} a\left[t_1 + \frac{b}{2}t_1^2 - \frac{\theta}{6}t_1^3 - \frac{b\theta}{4}t_1^4\right] \tag{7.6}$$

The quantity that has been used to satisfy the demand of customers during peak time of COVID-19 is

$$Q_2 = \alpha p^{-\beta}\left[-t_1 - \frac{\theta}{6}t_1^3\right]e^{-\theta\frac{t_1^2}{2}} \tag{7.7}$$

Also, the quantity that has been ordered as a backorder is

$$Q_3 = \int_{t_2}^{T} -\frac{\gamma}{p^{\delta}}\theta(\eta)\,dt = \frac{\gamma}{2Tp^{\delta}}\left(T^2 - t^2\right) \tag{7.8}$$

Hence, the total cost associated with the ordering quantity, during [0, T] is

$$Q = Q_1 + Q_2 + Q_3$$

$$Q = \left\{e^{bt_1} a\left[t_1 + \frac{b}{2}t_1^2 - \frac{\theta}{6}t_1^3 - \frac{b\theta}{4}t_1^4\right] + \alpha p^{-\beta}\left[-t_1 - \frac{\theta}{6}t_1^3\right]e^{-\theta\frac{t_1^2}{2}} + \frac{\gamma}{2Tp^{\delta}}\left(T^2 - t^2\right)\right\} \tag{7.9}$$

Following are the different costs associated with the model.

1. **Ordering cost:** This is the cost that was initially made at the start of the inventory cycle:
   Ordering cost = O(c)
   As per the model, the shortage starts at point $t_2$and continues until the end of the cycle at T. So, the storage period $[t_2$, T] is consistent with two costs: First the shortage cost, which is associated with the backlogged items, and, second, the cost that has been paid due to lost sales.
2. **Shortage cost:** The shortage cost, S(c), during the period $[t_2$, T] is given by

$$\mathrm{S(c)} = \mathrm{S}\int_{t_1}^{T} -I_2(t)dt = \mathrm{S}\int_{t_1}^{T} -\frac{\gamma}{p^{\delta}}[t_1 - t]\mathrm{dt} = \mathrm{S}\frac{\gamma}{p^{\delta}}\left[(T-t)^2\right] \tag{7.10}$$

3. **Lost sale cost (LSC):** It is obvious from the graphical representation of the model that we have lost some items during the stockout period $[t_2$, T]. The lost sale cost is given by the following:

$$\mathrm{LSC} = \mathrm{L}\int_{t_1}^{T}\left[1-\frac{\mu}{T}\right]dt \quad 0 \le \mu \le T$$

$$= L\frac{\gamma}{2Tp^{\delta}}\left[T^2 - t_1^{\,2}\right] \tag{7.11}$$

4. **Holding cost:** The items in the stock are available in the period $[0, t_2]$. After a shortage occurs, the holding cost for holding the pharmaceutical items in the inventory is given by

$$\mathrm{H.C.} = \int_0^T [h_1 + h_2 t] I_1(t)dt$$

$$h_1 e^{bt_1} a\left[t_1 + \frac{b}{2}t_1^{\,2} - \frac{\theta}{6}t_1^{\,3} - \frac{b\theta}{4}t_1^{\,4}\right] + \alpha p^{-\beta} h_2 t\left[-t_1 - \frac{\theta}{6}t_1^{\,3}\right]e^{-\theta\frac{t_1^2}{2}} \tag{7.12}$$

5. **Deterioration cost:** For the calculation of the deteriorated inventory, we must take the difference of the maximum inventory and the number of units used to meet the demand. Also, the total demand during the period $[0, t_2]$ is given by
   Total demand =

$$\int_0^T\left\{e^{bt_1} a\left[t_1 + \frac{b}{2}t_1^{\,2} - \frac{\theta}{6}t_1^{\,3} - \frac{b\theta}{4}t_1^{\,4}\right] + \alpha p^{-\beta}\left[-t_1 - \frac{\theta}{6}t_1^{\,3}\right]e^{-\theta\frac{t_1^2}{2}}\right\}$$

The deterioration cost = $c\{I_1(0) - Total\,demand\}$

$$= \left\{I_1(0) - \int_0^{t_2}\left\{e^{bt_1}a\left[t_1 + \frac{b}{2}t_1^2 - \frac{\theta}{6}t_1^3 - \frac{b\theta}{4}t_1^4\right] + \alpha p^{-\beta}\left[-t_1 - \frac{\theta}{6}t_1^3\right]e^{-\theta\frac{t_1^2}{2}}\right\}\right\}$$

$$= c\left\{e^{bt_1}a\left[t_1 + \frac{b}{2}t_1^2 - \frac{\theta}{6}t_1^3 - \frac{b\theta}{4}t_1^4\right] + \alpha p^{-\beta}\left[-t_1 - \frac{\theta}{6}t_1^3\right]e^{-\theta\frac{t_1^2}{2}}\right\} \quad (7.13)$$

Now, the total average cost of the model can be obtained by

T.A.C. = $\frac{1}{T}$ [Ordering cost + Shortage cost þ + Lost sale cost + Holding cost þ + Deterioration cost] (7.14)

We can use various mathematical tools to get the optimal solution of Equation 7.14, the latest methods we can apply are Mathematica software and MATLAB.

## 7.6 NUMERICAL EXAMPLE

To check the validation of the developed model, a numerical calculation based on real values of different parameters has been carried out.

$\alpha = 500\,units$, $\beta = 1.5$, $\gamma = 1.4$, $\delta = 1.3$, $a = 1$, $b = 2$ $h_1 = 0.5\ Rs\,/\,unit$, $h_2 = 0.2\ Rs\,/\,unit$ ,$O = 500\,Rs\,/\,order$, $T = 60\,days, p = 30\,Rs\,/\,unit$, $S(c) = 7Rs\,/\,unit$, $L(s) = 6\,Rs\,/\,unit$, $C(q) = 10\,Rs\,/\,unit$

With the help of Mathematica software, the optimal values of $t_1$ and T.A.C. are found as follows:

$t_1^* = 29.789\ days, T.A.C^* = Rs.257.821$, and the optimal value of the ordering quantity is $Q^* = 295.493$ units.

## 7.7 SENSITIVITY ANALYSIS

Based on the different values of the parameters, the sensitivity of the optimal solution has been calculated. The sensitivity analysis of the model has been considered by noting the variation in the different variables.

The analysis has been done by taking ± 5%, ± 10%, and ± 15% of changes in the variables (see Figure 7.2, Figure 7.3, and Figure 7.4).

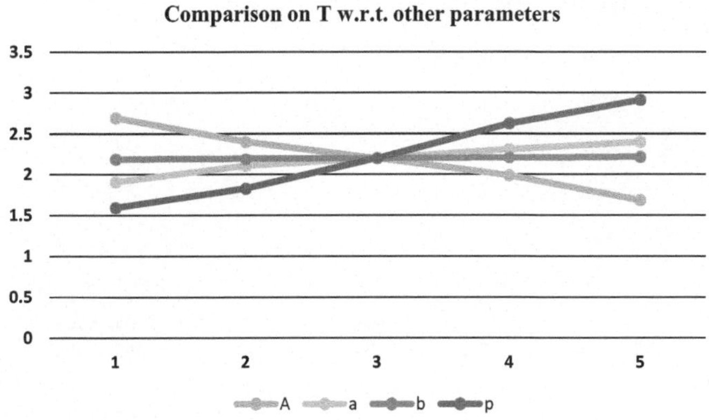


*Figure 7.2* Comparison of T with respect to other parameters.

## 7.8 RESULTS AND DISCUSSION

From the figures and tables, the following results were found:

1. From Tables 7.1 and 7.2, when the demand parameters $a$ and $b$ increase, the total average cost decreases where an increase has been noted in total average cost when the demand decreases.
2. From Tables 7.3 and 7.4, when the demand parameters and β increase, the total average cost decreases where an increase has been noted in total average cost when the demand decreases.

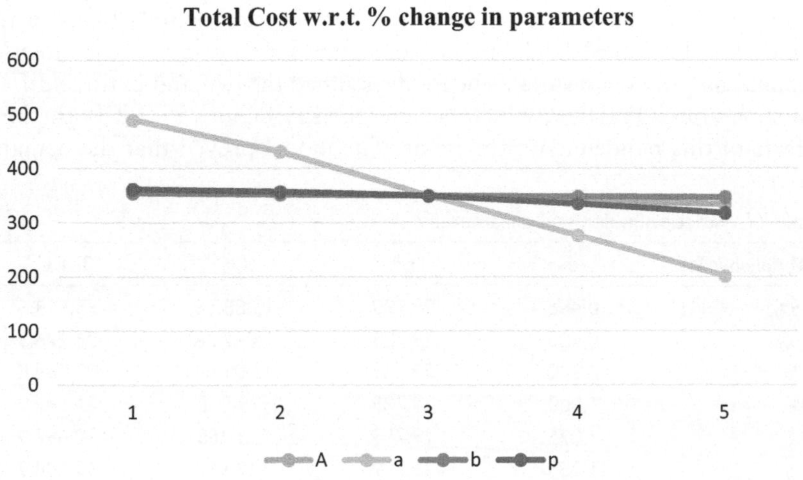


*Figure 7.3* Comparison of total cost with respect to parameters.

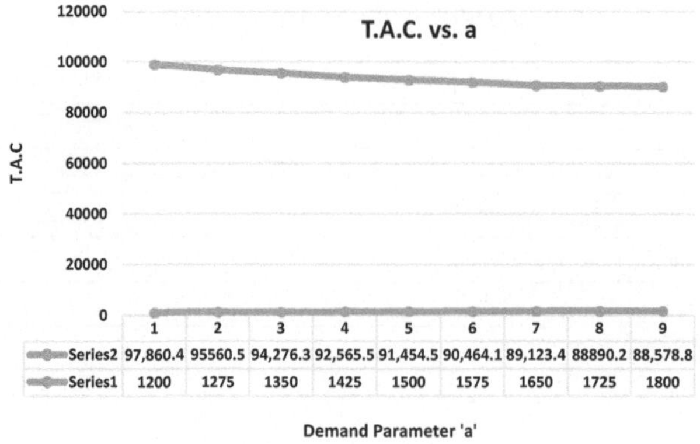


*Figure 7.4* Comparison of total cost with respect to parameter *a*.

3. From Table 7.5, when the deterioration parameter θ increases, the total average cost also decreases where a decrease has been noted in total average profit when the deterioration increases.
4. From Table 7.6, when the selling price parameter *P* increases, the total average cost decreases where an increase has been noted in total average profit when the selling price increases.
5. From Tables 7.7 and 7.8, when the holding cost parameters $h_1$ and $h_2$ increase, the total average cost decreases where an increase has been noted in total average cost when the demand decreases.

## 7.9 CONCLUSION

In the current study, we considered the different stages and effects of the demand on COVID-19. The model was extended to calculate the effect of demand on prices and stock. The model studied the demand in three different stages of COVID-19, which became the key factor to identify the long effects of this pandemic on the items. The model proved that the demand

*Table 7.1* Variation in demand parameter *a*

| *% Variation in W* | *a* | $t_1$* | Q* | T.A.C.* |
|---|---|---|---|---|
| –15% | 0.456 | 29.789 | 1,088.25 | 95,523.6 |
| –10% | 0.680 | 29.789 | 1,042.78 | 92,276.3 |
| –5% | 0.920 | 29.789 | 1,009.64 | 92,564.8 |
| –0% | 1.000 | 29.789 | 979.978 | 91,642.9 |
| 50% | 1.075 | 29.789 | 953.285 | 90,697.9 |
| 10% | 1.285 | 29.789 | 929.161 | 89,608.9 |
| 15% | 1.475 | 29.789 | 907.270 | 89,074.7 |

*Table 7.2* Variation in demand parameter *b*

| *% Variation in W* | ***b*** | $\mathbf{t}_l^*$ | **Q*** | **T.A.C.*** |
|---|---|---|---|---|
| −15% | 1,275 | 29.789 | 1,205.76 | 94,523.6 |
| −10% | 1,375 | 29.789 | 1,220.77 | 92,176.3 |
| −5% | 1,475 | 29.789 | 1,217.84 | 92,164.8 |
| −0% | 1,575 | 29.789 | 1,176.21 | 91,942.9 |
| 50% | 1,675 | 29.789 | 1,141.27 | 90,897.9 |
| 10% | 1,775 | 29.789 | 1,109.51 | 89,708.9 |
| 15% | 1,875 | 29.789 | 1,080.52 | 88,074.7 |

*Table 7.3* Variation in demand parameter $\alpha$

| *% Variation in W* | $\alpha$ | $\mathbf{t}_l^*$ | **Q*** | **T.A.C.*** |
|---|---|---|---|---|
| −15% | 1,175 | 29.789 | 1,212.06 | 96,860.4 |
| −10% | 1,275 | 29.789 | 1,088.25 | 93,176.3 |
| −5% | 1,375 | 29.789 | 1,042.78 | 92,164.8 |
| −0% | 1,475 | 29.789 | 1,176.21 | 91,942.9 |
| 50% | 1,575 | 29.789 | 1,141.27 | 90,897.9 |
| 10% | 1,675 | 29.789 | 1,109.51 | 89,708.9 |
| 15% | 1,775 | 29.789 | 1,080.52 | 88,074.7 |

and its price are found to be directly related to each other. The current model has been checked for all parameters with the help of the sensitivity analysis, where one parameter has been fixed and the corresponding changes in the other parameters have been noted. The assumption of taking multiple variable demands plays a vital role here.

From Tables 7.1 and 7.2, it is noted that as the demand parameter increases, the total average cost decreases, where an increase has been noted in total average cost when the demand is decreasing. It is also noted from

*Table 7.4* Variation in demand parameter $\beta$

| *% Variation in W* | $\beta$ | $\mathbf{t}_l^*$ | **Q*** | **T.A.C.*** |
|---|---|---|---|---|
| −15% | 1,275 | 29.789 | 1,205.76 | 97,860.4 |
| −10% | 1,375 | 29.789 | 1,190.25 | 95,476.4 |
| −5% | 1,475 | 29.789 | 1,102.74 | 93,864.8 |
| −0% | 1,575 | 29.789 | 1,095.20 | 92,942.4 |
| 50% | 1,675 | 29.789 | 1,000.27 | 90,997.9 |
| 10% | 1,775 | 29.789 | 9,909.51 | 89,908.9 |
| 15% | 1,875 | 29.789 | 9,580.52 | 88,974.7 |

*Table 7.5* Variation in demand parameter θ

| *% Variation in W* | θ | $t_l^*$ | $Q^*$ | T.A.C.* |
|---|---|---|---|---|
| −15% | 1,075 | 29.789 | 1,385.76 | 96,960.4 |
| −10% | 1,175 | 29.789 | 1,690.25 | 96,176.4 |
| –5% | 1,275 | 29.789 | 1,290.74 | 95,964.8 |
| –0% | 1,375 | 29.789 | 1,075.20 | 95,142.4 |
| 50% | 1,475 | 29.789 | 1,001.27 | 94,997.9 |
| 10% | 1,575 | 29.789 | 9,906.51 | 94,308.9 |
| 15% | 1,675 | 29.789 | 9,580.52 | 93,974.7 |

*Table 7.6* Variation on selling price *P* with respect to T.A.C.

| *% Variation in W* | P | $t_l^*$ | $Q^*$ | T.A.C.* |
|---|---|---|---|---|
| −15% | 1,175 | 29.789 | 1,205.76 | 95,523.6 |
| −10% | 1,275 | 29.789 | 1,220.77 | 92,276.3 |
| –5% | 1,375 | 29.789 | 1,217.84 | 92,564.8 |
| –0% | 1,475 | 29.789 | 1,176.21 | 91,642.9 |
| 50% | 1,575 | 29.789 | 1,141.27 | 90,697.9 |
| 10% | 1,675 | 29.789 | 1,109.51 | 89,608.9 |
| 15% | 1,775 | 29.789 | 1,080.52 | 89,074.7 |

the model that when the deterioration parameter θ increases, the total average cost also decreases, where a decrease has been noted in total average profit when the deterioration increases. The model has also been developed under partial backlog on shortages, which is also a very important assumption in the model. The proper supply of lifesaving items must be there, so the model also justifies the assumption on shortages that it should be a partial backlog.

At the end, the model has been developed to help the community and manufacturers to have the latest model for their businesses to run smoothly.

*Table 7.7* Variation on holding cost $h_l$ with respect to T.A.C.

| *% Variation in W* | $h_l$ | $t_l^*$ | $Q^*$ | T.A.C.* |
|---|---|---|---|---|
| −15% | 1,275 | 29.789 | 1,204.76 | 94,523.6 |
| −10% | 1,375 | 29.789 | 1,214.77 | 93,276.3 |
| –5 % | 1,475 | 29.789 | 1,214.84 | 92,564.8 |
| –0% | 1,575 | 29.789 | 1,170.21 | 91,642.9 |
| 50% | 1,675 | 29.789 | 1,140.27 | 89,697.9 |
| 10% | 1,775 | 29.789 | 1,108.51 | 88,608.9 |
| 15% | 1,875 | 29.789 | 1,090.52 | 87,074.7 |

*Table 7.8* Variation on holding cost $h_2$ with respect to T.A.C.

| *% Variation in W* | $h_2$ | $t_1^*$ | $Q^*$ | T.A.C.* |
|---|---|---|---|---|
| −15% | 1,275 | 30.987 | 1,304.45 | 95,623.6 |
| −10% | 1,375 | 30.987 | 1,230.76 | 95,176.3 |
| –5% | 1,475 | 30.987 | 1,194.84 | 94,864.8 |
| –0% | 1,575 | 30.987 | 1,070.21 | 94,12.9 |
| 50% | 1,675 | 30.987 | 9,940.27 | 93,697.9 |
| 10% | 1,775 | 30.987 | 9,608.51 | 93,120.9 |
| 15% | 1,875 | 30.987 | 9,390.52 | 92,074.7 |

The numerical examples from the model help to prove that the multiple variable demand pattern is the most powerful approach behind this study.

## 7.10 FUTURE SCOPE OF THE STUDY

Although the current study has been developed under the updated market requirement and application, there is always scope for improvement or upgradation. The present model can further be extended by applying many other environmental parameters on the demand as well as other factors. Some of the future explanations are as follows:

1. The current model deals with the unwanted spoilage of items due to improper warehouse storage. The model can be further extended by introducing the concept of trade credits on the deteriorated items.
2. Trade credits can also be used for the purchase of the items.
3. The model can also be extended by assuming other parameters on demand.

## REFERENCES


1. Saha, E., and Ray, P. K. 2019. Modelling and analysis of healthcare inventory management systems. *Opsearch*, *56*(4), 1179–1198.
2. Rastogi, M., and Singh, S. R. 2019. An inventory system for varying deteriorating pharmaceutical items with price-sensitive demand and variable holding cost under partial backlogging in healthcare industries. *Sādhanā*, *44*(4), 1–10.
3. Woods, D. D. and E. Hollnagel. 2012. *Joint cognitive systems*. Boca Raton: CRC Press/Taylor & Francis.
4. Weraikat, D., Zanjani, M. K., and Lehoux, N. 2019. Improving sustainability in a two-level pharmaceutical supply chain through Vendor-Managed Inventory system. *Operations Research for Health Care*, *21*, 44–55.

5. Tucker, E. L., et al. 2020. Incentivizing resilient supply chain design to prevent drug shortages: policy analysis using two-and multi-stage stochastic programs. *IISE Transactions*, *52*(4), 394–412.
6. Priyan, S., and Mala, P. 2020. Optimal inventory system for pharmaceutical products incorporating quality degradation with expiration date: A game theory approach. *Operations Research for Health Care*, *24*, 100245.
7. Cakmakli, C. et al. 2020. *COVID-19 and emerging markets: An epidemiological model with international production networks and capital flows.* https://doi.org/10.2139/ssrn.3670613
8. Leslie, D. 2020. Tackling COVID-19 through responsible AI innovation: Five steps in the right direction. *arXiv preprint arXiv:2008.06755.*
9. Schwab, K., and Malleret, T. 2020. *The great reset* (Vol. 22). Geneva, Switzerland: World Economic Forum.
10. Bloom, N., et al. 2020. *The impact of COVID-19 on productivity* (No. w28233), Working paper, National Bureau of Economic Research, Cambridge, MA, available at: https://www.nber.org/system/files/working_papers/w28233/revisions/w28233.rev0.pdf.
11. Franco, C., and Alfonso-Lizarazo, E. 2020. Optimization under uncertainty of the pharmaceutical supply chain in hospitals. *Computers & Chemical Engineering*, *135*, 106689.
12. Alkahtani, M., et al. 2021. A covid-19 supply chain management strategy based on variable production under uncertain environment conditions. *International Journal of Environmental Research and Public Health*, *18*(4), 1662.
13. Illahi, U., and Mir, M. S. 2021. Maintaining efficient logistics and supply chain management operations during and after coronavirus (COVID-19) pandemic: Learning from the past experiences. *Environment, Development and Sustainability*, *23*(8), 11157–11178.
14. Tat, R., and Heydari, J. 2021. Avoiding medicine wastes: Introducing a sustainable approach in the pharmaceutical supply chain. *Journal of Cleaner Production*, *320*, 128698.
15. Abdolazimi, O., et al. 2021. Development of sustainable and resilient healthcare and non-cold pharmaceutical distribution supply chain for COVID-19 pandemic: A case study. *The International Journal of Logistics Management*, *34*(2) 363–389.
16. Poswal, P., et al. 2022. An economic ordering policy to control deteriorating medicinal products of uncertain demand with trade credit for healthcare industries. *International Journal of Health Sciences*, 6(S2), 9392–9414.
17. Sharma, R., Singh, A. P., Arora, R., and Chauhan, A. 2022. Effect of uncertainty in demand and production for manufacturing industries during COVID-19. *International Journal of Services and Operations Management*, *43*(3), 378–400.
18. Blanco Izquierdo, V., and Gázquez, R. 2022. Mathematical optimization models for reallocating and sharing health equipment in pandemic situations. *Top (Berl)*, *31*(2):355–390.
19. Rafele, C. 2022. Development of a calculation model for materials management using DDMRP (Demand Driven MRP) (Doctoral dissertation, Politecnico di Torino).

20. Almaharmeh, M. Y. 2022. The impact of the covid-19 pandemic disruption on supply chain performance in the engineering manufacturing sector (Doctoral dissertation, The British University in Dubai (BUiD)).
21. Ahmadi, E., et al. 2022. Intelligent inventory management approaches for perishable pharmaceutical products in a healthcare supply chain. *Computers & Operations Research*, *147*, 105968.
22. Goodarzian, F., et al. 2022. A sustainable-resilience healthcare network for handling COVID-19 pandemic. *Annals of Operations Research*, *312*(2), 761–825.
23. Nematollahi, M., and Hosseini-Motlagh, S. M. 2022. A collaborative decision-making model for collecting unused medications in an environmentally responsible pharmaceutical supply chain. *International Journal of Environmental Science and Technology*, *19*(3), 1907–1924.
24. Dohale, V., Verma, P., Gunasekaran, A., and Ambilkar, P. 2023. COVID-19 and supply chain risk mitigation: A case study from India. *The International Journal of Logistics Management*, *34*(2), 417–442.
25. Çetindaş, A., Akben, İ., Özcan, C., Kanuşağı, İ., and Öztürk, O. 2023. The effect of supply chain agility on firm performance during COVID-19 pandemic: the mediating and moderating role of demand stability. *Supply Chain Forum: An International Journal*, 1–12. doi:10.1080/16258312.2023.2167465.
26. Pant, M., Rajput, N., Sharma, S., and Chauhan, A. 2023. A channel financing policy for an EOQ model of fast-moving consumer goods with fuzzy approach. In Panos M. Pardalos (ed.), *Operations research forum* (Vol. 5, No. 1, p. 1). Cham: Springer International Publishing.
27. Palanivelu, S., and Chandrasekaran, E. 2024. Comparative analysis of inventory management system with two-phase time-dependent demand and shortages under tolerable slack of payment for deteriorating goods. *Journal of Advanced Research in Applied Sciences and Engineering Technology*, *34*(1), 116–132.
28. Sharma, U. K., Mohan, V., Sindhuja, S., and Iqbal, P. 2024. Economic order quantity model for Pareto distributed decaying products with quadratic demand, shortage and salvage value. *International Journal of Mathematics in Operational Research*, *27*(4), 479–495.
29. Haque, R., Rahaman, M., Alam, S., Behera, P. K., and Mondal, S. P. 2024. Generalized neutrosophic Laplace transform and its application in an EOQ model with price and deterioration-dependent demand. *OPSEARCH*, *1*, 1–33.
30. Debnath, R., Majumder, P., Tarafdar, A., Bhattacharya, B., and Bera, U. K. 2024. Artificial intelligence-based supply chain management strategy during COVID-19 situation. *Supply Chain Forum: An International Journal*, *25*(4), 1–20.
31. Schleifenheimer, M., and Ivanov, D. 2024. Pharmaceutical retail supply chain responses to the COVID-19 pandemic. *Annals of Operations Research*, *1*, 1–26.

Chapter 8

# AI and ML based system for early detection of malignant cells of the brain through image processing pavingway for personalized treatment strategies

*Ruchira Goel, Rahul Sharma, Khushi Bansal, and Ashutosh Sirohi*

## 8.1 INTRODUCTION

One of the most difficult and dangerous adversaries that contemporary healthcare encounters is brain cancer. Cancer is essentially a disease characterized by the uncontrolled and unabated proliferation of abnormal cells. This fast growth is risky since it can interfere with regular biological processes and lead to serious health issues or even death. However, brain cancer presents a unique set of difficulties due to the sensitivity of brain tissue and the fact that it regulates so many vital bodily processes. Cancer is essentially caused by unchecked cell proliferation. This unregulated cell division leads to malignant cancers, the hallmark of this complex condition. These uncontrolled growths pose a major risk to one's life and health. They cannot only prevent tissues from working normally, but they can also infiltrate nearby tissues and spread to other organs. Tissues around the brain are the first to develop into brain cancer. This broad category encompasses a wide range of cancer types, including meningiomas, gliomas, and even metastatic cancers that start in other body areas before spreading to the brain.

The high death rate from brain cancer cruelly emphasizes how serious the disease is. Brain cancer continues to be the primary cause of cancer-related fatalities globally, even with advances in medical knowledge. In the United States during 2019, an estimated 70,000 people were battling brain tumours. While diagnoses reached a staggering 86,000, not all were cancerous. Out of these diagnoses, 60,800 were classified as benign, non-cancerous growths. The remaining 26,170 cases, however, were malignant, a more aggressive form of brain tumour. Unfortunately, the survival rate for malignant brain tumours in the US stands at only 35%. Global Cancer Observatory (GLOBOCAN) predictions for 2020 indicate that 19.3 million incident cases of cancer were reported globally [1]. India came in third place [2], behind the United States of America and China. In India, around


DOI: 10.1201/9781003634089-8

one in nine individuals will face cancer at some point in their lives [3]. India, which now ranks third in the world for cancer incidence after China and the US, has a serious and urgent public health concern, according to the Indian Council of Medical Research (ICMR). However, estimates from the GLOBOCAN indicate that between 2020 and 2040, there will be a significant 57.5% increase in cancer cases in India. The ICMR is preparing to introduce corrective measures because just a few districts in India are able to conduct cancer screening methods in accordance with Health Ministry regulations. Expressions of Interest [4] regarding the application of research to expedite cancer screening, early diagnosis, and treatment have been invited. The government estimates that the number of cancer cases in India will increase from 14.6 lakh in 2022 to 15.7 lakh in 2025.

These depressing figures emphasize the urgent need for innovative approaches to stop this incurable illness. The problem is made even more challenging by the obstacles to early detection and efficient treatment. The complexity of brain cancer frequently creates obstacles to an early diagnosis, even though this critical stage is essential for effective treatment and better patient outcomes. Early on, traditional diagnostic methods can be unreliable because they frequently rely on intrusive procedures, which are associated with risks. This emphasizes how urgently more effective and trustworthy detection techniques are needed.

The utilization of predictive analytics, especially machine learning techniques, in the diagnosis and research of cancer has increased significantly. These algorithms have the amazing capacity to uncover hidden patterns and produce remarkably accurate prediction courses of the disease. They are powered by enormous datasets that include genetic profiles, medical imaging data, and patient information. This has the potential to significantly transform the field of early diagnosis and prognostic assessment for brain cancer. By utilizing a wide range of input factors, research has demonstrated encouraging findings for machine learning models in predicting the prognosis of patients with brain cancer. These algorithms can categorize patients according to their unique risk profiles by examining genetic markers, radiological scans, and medical histories. With the use of this data, individualized treatment programs that are catered to the requirements of each patient may be created, greatly increasing the likelihood that their care will be successful. Furthermore, the iterative learning capabilities of machine learning provide a clear benefit. With every iteration, these algorithms learn and get better, making predictions that are increasingly accurate over time.

An important factor in raising the detection rate of brain cancer lesions is the application of image processing tools. The structural and functional characteristics of brain tumours can be better understood by using medical imaging modalities like magnetic resonance imaging (MRI), computed tomography (CT), and positron emission tomography (PET). However, because tumour forms can vary widely and because confusing imaging abnormalities might occur, evaluating these pictures can be difficult. These problems are tackled by image processing algorithms that extract important features from medical scans and identify anomalous locations. Medical practitioners can more precisely visualize and analyze tumour characteristics thanks to techniques like segmentation and feature extraction. These algorithms can greatly help medical professionals identify and characterize brain lesions by emphasizing areas that may host tumours and extracting pertinent information including size, shape, and texture.

In this chapter, we have leveraged the capabilities of TensorFlow, a convolutional neural network (CNN), Keras, and associated libraries to develop a robust cancer detection model. By combining the strengths of deep neural networks and traditional machine learning algorithms, the aim is to create a versatile and accurate system for identifying potential cancer cases.

## 8.2 LITERATURE REVIEW

An approach for identifying brain tumours in MRI brain images was proposed by Natarajan et al. [5]. The median filter is used as a preprocessing step for the MRI brain images. Threshold segmentation and morphological operations are then applied to the segmented image, and image subtraction is used to obtain the tumour region. This method provides the precise tumour shape in MRI brain imaging. The probabilistic neural network (PNN) is utilized for automated brain tumour classification in MRI scans, following the image segmentation technique [6] to identify brain tumours from MRI images. The PNN approach that has been suggested can classify brain tumours more precisely. Research by ZainEldin et al. suggested a CNN based on a brain tumour classification model (BCM-CNN) to increase the accuracy rate of detection and diagnosis [7]. The algorithm known as the adaptive dynamic sine-cosine fitness grey wolf optimizer (ADSCFGWO) was used to tune the CNN's hyperparameters. In the experiments, the BCM-CNN was employed as a classifier, and the findings show that it generated the best outcomes because the CNN's performance was improved during optimization with an accuracy rate of 99.99%. The primary drawback of the suggested approach is its high processing time, which is brought on by the additional optimization stages.

The machine learning models naive Bayes, random forest (RF), neural network, k-nearest neighbour (KNN), and decision tree (DT), along with a hybrid ensemble classifier (KNN-RF-DT), were proposed by Garg et al. [8] for the detection of brain cancers. Using 2556 pictures of brain tumours—85% for training and 15% for testing—they assessed the machine learning models. Thirteen features were found for the categorization as a result of SWT, PCA, and GLCM feature extraction. After evaluation, the suggested method for recognizing and classifying brain tumours was shown to have a 97.305% accuracy rate, a 97.73% precision rate, a 97.60% specificity rate, a 97.04% sensitivity rate, and a 97.41% dependability rate. For the early diagnosis of brain cancers, Stadlbauer et al. [9] combined nine distinct popular machine learning models with a physiological MRI technique. When assessing the model, a number of performance metrics were considered, such as classification error, AUROC, F-score, accuracy, and precision. They suggested in their study that machine learning-based radio physiomics could be useful in the clinical context for identifying brain cancers. An automated technique for MRI-based brain tumour detection was presented by Aamir et al. [10]. After testing the suggested machine learning model, they found that it outperformed previous methods in classification, with a 98.95% accuracy rate.

The purpose of the work by Sharma et al. [11] was to develop a very accurate model for identifying brain tumours from MRI pictures. The 253 brain MRI pictures in the dataset were adequate to assess the model's performance. The CNN machine learning technique serves as the foundation for the model. Resizing and decreasing the image without erasing any crucial information that will be utilized for prediction aids in prediction.

When applied to the training set, the developed model achieves an accuracy of 97.79%, and when applied to the validation set, it obtains an accuracy of 82.86%. When the number of epochs increases, the loss progressively begins to decrease. Siar and Teshnehlab's [12] research presents the usage of a CNN for brain tumour detection using MRI images that were initially applied to CNN. The Softmax Fully Connected layer achieved a classification accuracy of 98.67% for the images. Additionally, the radial basis function classifier yields a 97.34% accuracy rate, while the decision tree classifier yields a 94.24% accuracy rate for CNN. Sensitivity, specificity, and precision benchmarks and the accuracy criterion to assess network performance were employed. Based on the categorization results, CNN's Softmax classifier had the highest accuracy according to the network accuracy results for the picture testing. This is a novel approach to tumour diagnosis from brain imaging that combines feature extraction methods with CNN. On the test data, the proposed method's accuracy was 99.12%.

Yahyaoui et al. published a method for combining 2D and 3D MRI images [13]. They recommended using special 3D CNN architectures for multimodal picture segmentation and DenseNet for classification. The suggested approach demonstrated excellent performance on the test set, achieving 92% accuracy with DenseNet and 85% accuracy with customized 3D CNN models. Kang et al. [14] proposed the use of deep CNN feature ensemble and machine learning classifiers for brain cancer classification. The tests carried out by the authors made use of datasets of different sizes. Radial basis function kernel-based support vector machines (SVMs) outperformed other machine learning and deep learning classifiers. An automatic brain cancer classification method based on machine learning networks was created in a different study publication [15] to distinguish between photos of high- and low-grade glioma sickness. With accuracy rates of 90% and 95%, respectively, the researchers classified cancers of the central nervous system, which includes the brain, using an extreme gradient boosting model. "Adaptive Fuzzy Deformable Fusion," a completely novel ensemble model, was unveiled by Murthy et al. [16]. This model enhanced classification and segmentation by combining the deformable snake approach with the fuzzy C-means clustering strategy. The results of the experiment demonstrated that the ensemble approach performed better than individual models and achieved a 95% classification accuracy. To distinguish benign from malignant brain cancers, Mehrotra et al. [17] looked at several deep learning-based pretrained CNN algorithms. To accomplish the goals, a variety of optimizers were employed, such as Adam, RMSprop, and stochastic gradient descent (SGD). The study demonstrated that AlexNet performed exceptionally well at medical imaging tasks when calibrated correctly. Using VGGNet and a customized CNN architecture, Grampurohit et al. [18] were able to categorize 253 brain cancer pictures (155 cancers and 98 non-cancers). Preprocessing techniques and data augmentation were used to increase sample variety and reduce overfitting. The custom CNN model's validation accuracy was 86% overall, whereas VGGNet's on a single dataset was 97% accurate.

Rokhana et al.'s model [19] makes use of the CNN model without the normalization layer, which aids in removing non-trainable parameters from the dataset and improves the model's overall efficiency. The highest accuracy of 84.76% was attained using ten epochs and a dropout value of 20%, according to experiments they conducted with various epoch values and dropout values. Khalil et al. [20] described a study that classified the malignancy of breast cancer from digital mammograms using a variety of machine learning techniques, including support vector machine, logistic regression, decision tree, random forest, and deep neural network, which were implemented using the TensorFlow and Keras frameworks and Python programming. The study trained and tested machine learning using the Breast Cancer Wisconsin (Diagnostic) Data Set, which includes 30 mammogram features. This dataset's diagnosis results were used as a baseline. Sensitivity and specificity were used to gauge how well the machine learning models performed; the models achieved sensitivity rates of between 90.8% and 98.5% and specificity rates of between 90.5% and 94.6%.

The main goal of Srinivasa Rao et al. [21] was to preprocess the HAM10000 skin lesion dataset in order to find critical factors that will facilitate the accurate classification of skin cancer. In this study, CNN uses a sequential architecture to create the training model, and K-fold cross-validation is used for testing. To reduce the complexity, they proposed K-fold cross-validation as an alternative to several other methods. It has been observed that the dataset's K-fold method exhibits a maximum accuracy performance of approximately 97.88%.

The automated detection of breast mass abnormalities was made possible by adapting the region proposal network (RPN) and region of interest (ROI) sections of the faster R-CNN [22]. A CNN-based technique for breast mass detection was devised for the feature extraction step. This technique instantly distinguishes between benign and malignant abnormalities in mammography pictures based on detecting mass regions. The photos were subjected to various preprocessing phases, including bilateral, median, and Gaussian filters, to remove the breast region from the mammogram image's background. The test dataset yielded the following results for the model's performance: 91.86% detection accuracy, 94.67% sensitivity, and 92.2% AUC-ROC.

Using 3D MR images, Abiwinanda et al. [23] presented a modified two-step dragonfly algorithm for segmenting brain cancers. Variations in the size and shape of the cancer pose the most challenges to the identification and classification of brain cancers in their early stages. The researchers used a two-step dragonfly technique to precisely retrieve the original contour point in order to get around these difficulties. Utilizing the BRATS 2017 3D MR brain cancer dataset, they were able to derive the results. Their accuracy was around 5% greater than the previous researchers', who conducted a trial that was almost exactly the same. They also used a number of methods, such as random forest, SVM, and fuzzy C-means, to confirm their findings. They took into consideration the measures of accuracy, precision, and recall. They evaluated their suggested model and found that it performed better than the others, with accuracy of 98.20%, recall of 95.13%, and precision of 93.21%. This study's primary flaw was that the investigators only looked at the whole cancer section, failing to account for the large number of cancers in each slice. A CNN completed with the aid of Keras API and the Conv2D, MaxPool2D, ReLU, and ADAM optimizer make up the operational architecture for Rahi et al.'s model [24]. The CNN algorithm has also been used for VGG, ResNet, and DenseNet techniques. For models other than CNN, they have attained 79% accuracy with CNN with 50 epochs, 90% accuracy with both ResNet50 and DenseNet121, and ultimately 85% accuracy with VGG11 BN with 10 epochs.

## 8.3 RELATED WORK

With advancements in machine learning, genetics, and medical imaging, the diagnosis of malignant cells of the brain has evolved substantially over the years. The foundation of conventional methods was the pathologists' manual assessment of diagnostic pictures and materials. These models now assess enormous datasets using complex algorithms, which allows for the faster and more precise detection of patterns and signs suggestive of malignant cells.

### 8.3.1 Convolutional neural network

Deep learning and computer vision have significantly advanced with CNNs. These systems are specifically designed to extract meaningful information from complex visual data, such as images and videos. The basic structure of the CNN (shown in Figure 8.1) is composed of convolutional, pooling, and fully connected layers, which replicate how the human visual system interprets hierarchical structures and patterns. Convolutional layers use convolutional methods to discover local properties, and pooling layers abstract the information. Fully connected layers are useful for tasks involving categorization. With its remarkable success in a range of applications, including object detection and image classification, medical image analysis, and face recognition, CNN has fundamentally altered the area of image identification. The layers of the CNN are as follows:

i. **Input layer**: The architecture of the CNN is finely tuned to align with the dimensions of the preprocessed imagery. Take for example, image adjustments that render them to a 128×128 pixel framework, infused with the rich detail of RGB colour. In such a case, the CNN's input shape is precisely set to (240, 240, 3). This trio of numbers represents a picture with a 240-pixel span in both height and width, alongside three distinct channels that capture the vibrancy of the red, green, and blue hues.
ii. **Convolutional blocks**: CNN's convolutional blocks are its fundamental building components. Usually, these blocks include:
   a. **Convolutional layer**: This layer extracts spatial elements such as edges, forms, and textures from the input data by applying filters to it. To capture different levels of information, we can utilize

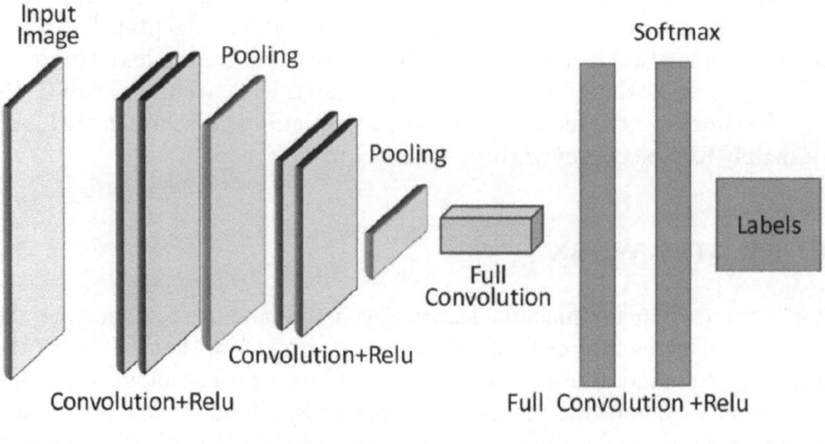


*Figure 8.1* Architecture of a convolutional neural network.

multiple convolutional layers with variable filter sizes and number of filters.

b. **Batch normalization:** By normalizing the activations of the preceding layer, this approach aids in increasing training stability and speed.
c. **Activation function:** To add non-linearity to the network, an activation function is added after each convolutional layer and batch normalization layer. Rectified Linear Unit, or ReLU, is a popular activation function that aids in solving the vanishing gradient issue and enables the network to pick up intricate patterns.
d. **Pooling layer:** By reducing the dimensionality of the data, this layer improves the computational efficiency of the network. Methods such as max pooling summarize the activation maps by determining the maximum value within a certain window.

iii. **Dense layer:** We flatten the retrieved features into a one-dimensional vector after the convolutional blocks. After that, this vector is fed into dense, fully connected layers. By multiplying matrices, these layers are able to learn higher-level abstractions from the combined characteristics.
iv. **Output layer:** One neuron with a sigmoid activation function is present in the last layer. This neuron's probability score ranges from 0 to 1, signifying the presence or absence of a malignant lesion in the image (positive class) or negative class.

### 8.3.2 Keras

Keras, a cutting-edge open-source software library for neural networks crafted using Python, stands as a beacon of innovation in the medical imaging field, especially in the nuanced area of brain cancer detection and scrutiny. Its user-friendly high-level API democratizes the creation of sophisticated deep learning architectures, inviting both scholars and medical practitioners to the table. A standout feature of Keras is its harmonious integration with robust frameworks like TensorFlow, which offers the computational horsepower needed to navigate the intricate landscape of medical imagery. When it comes to pinpointing brain cancers, Keras proves indispensable in forging CNNs that pinpoint and categorize malignancies in MRI imagery with remarkable precision. Its modular design and intuitive operation make for swift prototyping and continual refinement of models—a critical process for crafting cutting-edge diagnostic instruments. Furthermore, Keras provides an arsenal of layers, optimizers, and activation functions, empowering developers to sculpt neural networks that rise to the specialized challenges of medical image evaluation. This adaptability is a key asset in addressing the complex and varied signatures of brain cancer. Beyond its technical prowess, Keras boasts a vibrant community and extensive documentation, propelling a swift ascent up the learning curve and nurturing a spirit of collective progress in medical exploration. In summary, Keras is a potent tool that propels the medical field forward by applying the most avant-garde deep learning methods, thereby sharpening the precision, and streamlining the process of diagnosing and plotting the course for brain cancer treatment.

## 8.4 METHODOLOGY

Brain cancers are accurately detected and classified using machine learning algorithms in combination with advanced imaging techniques like CT and MRI scans. These methods (shown in Figure 8.2) offer thorough insights into the characteristics and progression of malignancies, enabling earlier diagnosis and more effective treatment planning.

### 8.4.1 Proposed architecture

Medical research is always working to combat cancerous cells of the brain. Improving patient outcomes depends critically on their early and accurate detection. Within this framework, scientists are investigating the possibility of using deep learning methods, specifically CNNs, to automatically identify them from medical imaging such as MRI scans. This examination explores the design parts, training details, and general process of a CNN

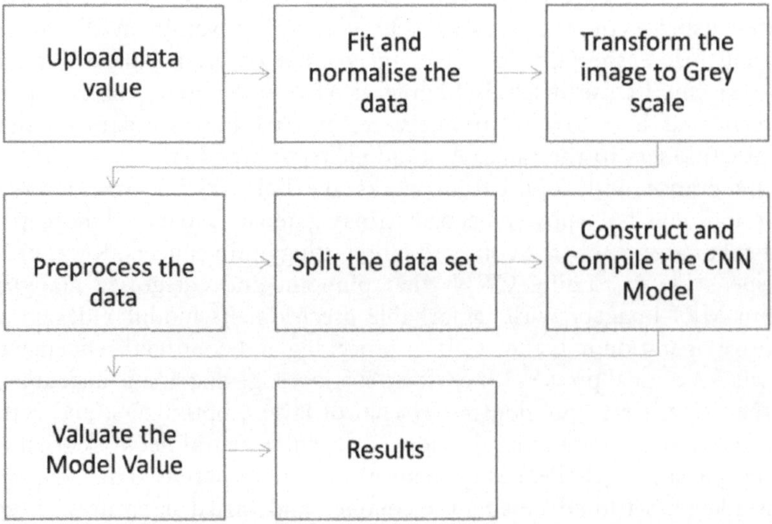


*Figure 8.2* Flowchart for detection of malignant brain cells.

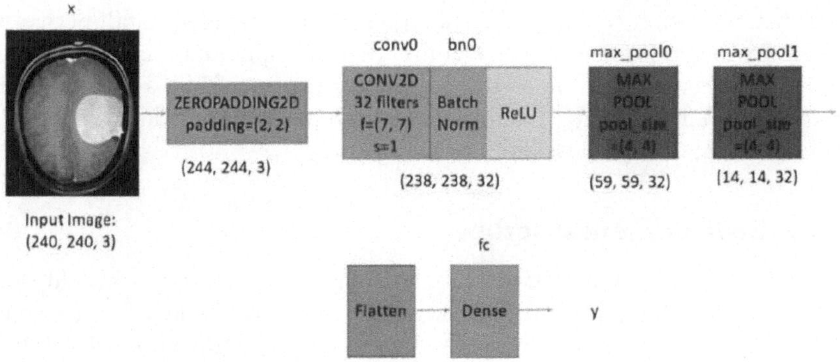


*Figure 8.3* Neural network architecture.

architecture (shown in Figure 8.3) created specifically for this purpose. MRI scan-specific CNN architecture for brain cancer detection is detailed in this given description. The input layer starts the process by receiving an MRI scan image that has been preprocessed. This image has been resized to the industry standard of 32×32 pixels to make it work with the network layout.

The convolutional layers are the key component of this architecture. Extracting significant features from the input image falls to these layers. Every convolutional layer uses a collection of filters, referred to as kernels. These filters are essentially tiny 3×3 matrices that examine the image pixel by pixel to find patterns and traits. This architecture's initial convolutional layer makes use of sixteen 3×3 filters which are good at picking up on subtle details that are present in an entire picture. The number of filters rises as we move through the convolutional layers in order to gradually extract more complex and advanced characteristics from the MRI data. This enables the network to discover intricate connections between pixels, which are essential for identifying healthy tissues.

Max pooling layers have been placed in between the convolutional layers. These layers are essential for lowering the dimensionality of the data and giving little spatial variations in the image, creating some degree of invariance. The functionality of these layers is as follows: the input data, which are feature maps, are divided into predetermined grids by the max pooling layer. The pixel with the maximum value (highest) within each grid is chosen.

As a result of the down sampling technique, the network is less vulnerable to minute changes in the locations of features within the images. This also lowers the computational cost of training the network. Moreover, prognosis and treatment planning are included in the integration of image processing and machine learning, escaping simple detection. The output layer, the last layer of the network, is made up of a single neuron with a Softmax activation function. The neuron's output will always fall between 0 and 1, which represents the probability that the input image belongs to the malignant class, according to the Softmax function. While a result closer to 0 would reflect healthy brain tissue, a high probability value of nearly 1 would indicate a high possibility of malignancy.

### 8.4.2 Environmental setup

We used the fully cloud-based Google Colab Pro+ software to build our environment. This platform is powered by NVIDIA Tesla K80, T4, and P100 GPUs, which provide powerful processing capabilities. Additionally, we employed a 52 GB high-RAM runtime memory. This configuration ensures a faster and more efficient machine learning model training procedure due to its great degree of customization. Google Colab Pro+ offers an advanced and flexible platform suited for complex computing operations. Using the power of NVIDIA's top-tier GPUs, the platform significantly accelerates machine learning algorithm testing and training. Performance is further enhanced by the addition of a 52 GB high-RAM runtime, which enables the handling of big datasets and intricate models without experiencing bottlenecks. This customized environment may be used to construct and enhance complex machine-learning models. Because of its cloud-based design, Google Colab Pro+ is an excellent choice for large-scale machine learning projects since it is both accessible and scalable. Strong GPUs and gobs of RAM combine to speed up and improve training efficiency, leading to more accurate and consistent model output. Consequently, this highly personalized platform encourages state-of-the-art machine learning research and applications, advancing productivity and creativity in the sector.

### 8.4.3 Dataset used

One of the cornerstones of medical imaging is magnetic resonance imaging, especially in the field of neuroimaging, which is used to identify and describe brain cancers. Doctors can see abnormalities in the brain with unprecedented clarity via MRI's great spatial resolution and precise anatomical information. The MRI scans used in this study were obtained from individuals who had diagnostic imaging performed as a part of their medical examination. The dataset includes MRI scans from healthy people (shown in Figure 8.4). The fact that no neurological abnormalities were present at the time of the pictures' acquisition guaranteed that the characteristics taken from the malignant tissue could be separated from the normal structure of the brain. Gliomas, meningiomas, metastatic tumours, and other forms of brain cancer were among the verified diagnoses for patients in the dataset (shown in Figure 8.5). The inclusion criteria made strong analysis

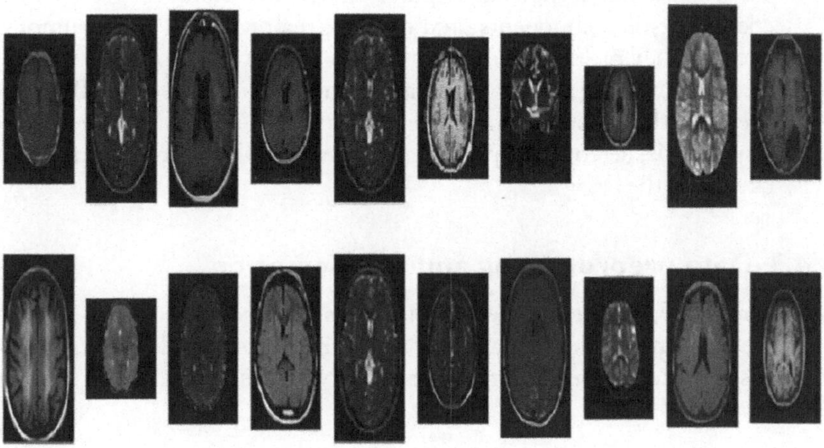

*Figure 8.4* MRI scans with no tumours.

and classification possible, which guaranteed a thorough representation of the various tumour kinds and pathological features.

The collection is made up of MRI pictures obtained with various sequences, each of which provides a different perspective on the composition and properties of brain tissue. Among these sequences are:

i. **T1-weighted imaging:** T1-weighted pictures offer superior contrast between the cerebral fluid, white matter, and grey matter, making it easier to see anatomical features and improve the identification of lesions that enhance contrast.

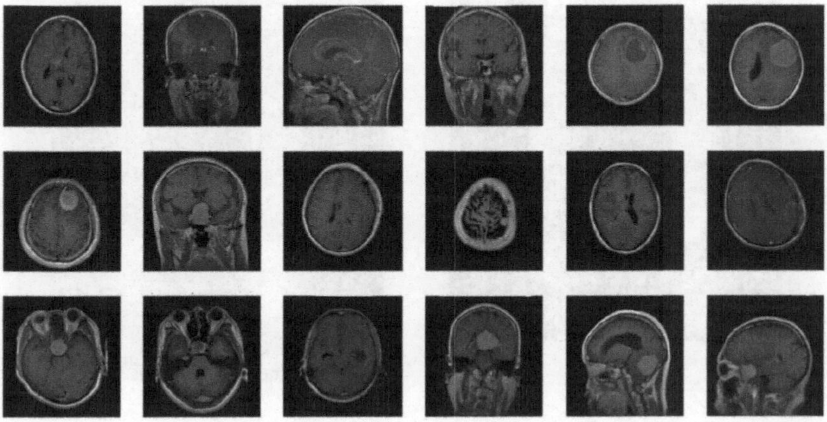

*Figure 8.5* MRI scans with tumours.

ii. **T2-weighted imaging:** T2-weighted images are useful for recognizing edema, cystic components, and necrotic regions inside brain tumours because they are sensitive to changes in tissue water content.
iii. **FLAIR imaging (fluid-attenuated inversion recovery):** By suppressing the signal from the cerebrospinal fluid, FLAIR sequences improve tissue contrast preservation and the ability to identify clinical anomalies.

### 8.4.3 Data preprocessing and augmentation

An essential step in getting the MRI pictures prepared to be input into the machine learning models is data preprocessing. This includes a number of methods designed to improve the data quality and make feature extraction easier.

i. **Image cropping:** A cropping technique is used in each MRI image to isolate the brain region. By doing this, unnecessary background data is eliminated (shown in Figure 8.6), allowing the model to concentrate on the pertinent characteristics linked to brain tumours. The model can perform much better by cropping the photos to only include the region of interest.
ii. **Resizing and normalization:** Once the MRI pictures have been cropped to the proper dimensions, they are then uniformly scaled to a consistent size, which brings consistency to the entire collection of data.

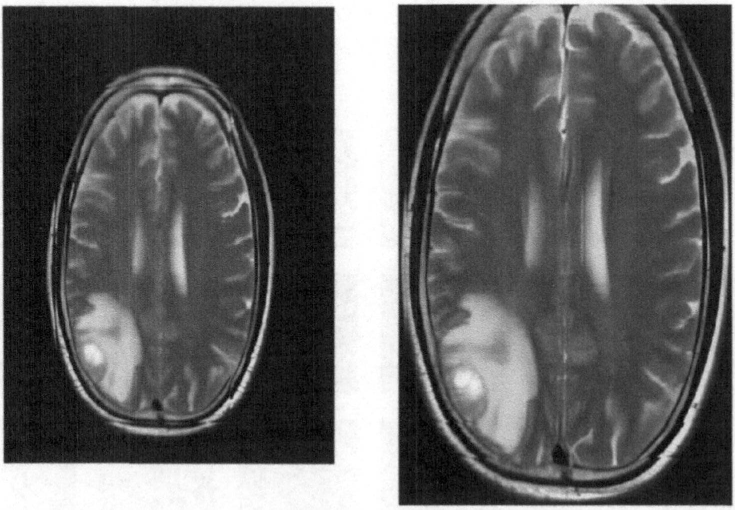

*Figure 8.6* Original image versus cropped image.

This step of resizing not only simplifies the calculations needed but also streamlines the learning phase for the algorithms. Furthermore, we apply specialized methods to even out the intensity levels across all images, which effectively counteracts any discrepancies caused by varying machine configurations and scanning procedures. This process of normalization significantly improves the reliability of the data when analyzing and comparing features from diverse MRI examinations.

iii. **Data augmentation:** By using data augmentation approaches, the dataset is made larger and more diverse, which enhances the machine learning models' capacity to generalize. MRI pictures are rotated at random angles to replicate differences in head posture during image acquisition. The model becomes more resilient to spatial transformations by rotating the images, which enables it to identify tumours from various orientations. Also, MRI images are randomly zoomed in to mimic changes in imaging resolution and magnification (shown in Figure 8.7). By enlarging the image, the model becomes more sensitive to minute irregularities and can identify cancers of all sizes and scales.

The MRI dataset is prepared for training and assessment following preprocessing and augmentation. Annotated with a label designating whether or not a brain tumour is present, the augmented dataset consists of a variety of MRI pictures (yes or no). The cornerstone for creating precise and efficient machine learning models for brain cancer diagnosis is this carefully selected dataset.

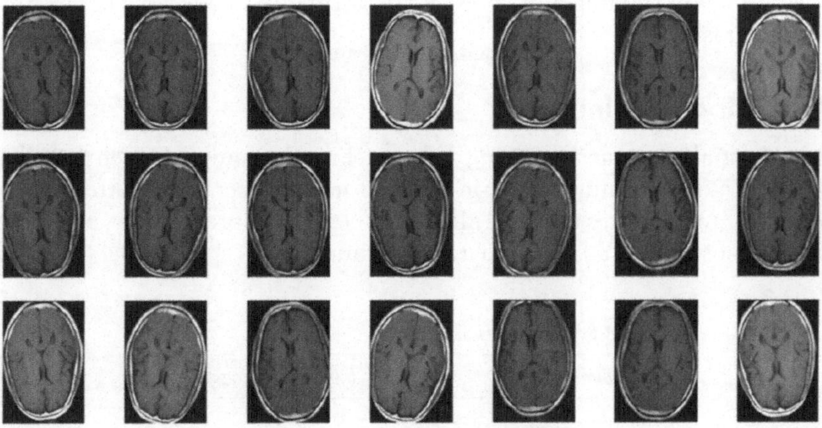

*Figure 8.7* Augmented images.

### 8.4.4 Data splitting

To make it easier to train, tune, and evaluate the model, divide the dataset into training, validation, and testing sets. Provide roughly 70% of the total for training, 15% for validation, and 15% for testing to guarantee that the sets contain an equal number of tumour-positive and tumour-negative samples.

### 8.4.5 Model compilation

Setting up the neural network architecture for training is an essential stage in the compilation of models. CNNs are assembled with a number of critical parameters adjusted to maximize their performance. By modifying learning rates for every parameter separately, the Adam optimizer, renowned for its flexible learning rate qualities, makes gradient descent more effective during training. For binary classification problems, the binary cross-entropy loss function selection is especially appropriate since it guarantees that the model's predictions closely match the true binary labels. Furthermore, accuracy is a basic assessment statistic that sheds light on the model's overall performance during validation and training.

Additional callbacks are set up to improve and monitor the training process. TensorBoard, a visualization tool, provides a graphical representation of numerous metrics over epochs, making it easier to analyze the model's behaviour. In order to prevent overfitting and facilitate the recovery of the best model for deployment or additional research, the Model Checkpoint callback helps to guarantee that the top-performing model is regularly saved during training, based on predetermined parameters like validation loss or accuracy. Overall, thorough model compilation with proper optimizers, loss functions, evaluation measures, and callbacks is required for effective CNN training and improved performance in a variety of machine learning tasks.

### 8.4.6 Model training

An essential step in developing any machine learning or deep learning model is model training. To train the algorithm to recognize patterns, correlations, and features that will allow it to classify or predict new, unknown data, it must be fed a labelled dataset (training set).

*Table 8.1* Division of images

| *Folder directory* | *Number of images* |
|---|---|
| Training | 1445 |
| Testing | 310 |
| Validation | 310 |

The batch size is a crucial factor to take into account when training a model. The training process's memory efficiency and convergence speed can be affected by selecting the right batch size. While more frequent model updates are possible with smaller batch sizes, there may be an increase in variance in parameter adjustments. On the other hand, although they might need more memory, higher batch sizes can offer more consistent updates. The number of epochs also controls the number of times the model iterates across the whole training dataset. By increasing the number of epochs, the model is able to examine the training data more often, which may help it learn more intricate patterns. But if the model is trained for an excessive number of epochs, it may become overfit, which prevents the model from learning patterns that are applicable to a larger set of data. It is crucial to keep an eye on the model's performance on a different validation set as it is being trained. This validation set aids in evaluating the model's generalizability to previously unobserved data. Through monitoring measures like loss, accuracy, or other pertinent assessment metrics, developers can identify instances of overfitting or underfitting and modify the hyperparameters of the model correspondingly.

Moreover, overfitting can be avoided and the effectiveness of the training process increased by putting early stopping mechanisms in place, depending on the validation performance. To avoid wasting computational resources, early stopping entails terminating the training process if the model's performance on the validation set does not improve after a predetermined number of epochs.

### 8.4.7 Model evaluation

A crucial step in determining the reliability and efficiency of machine learning models is model evaluation. It uses a variety of methods to gauge a model's effectiveness, especially concerning untested data. Evaluating accuracy and loss on the test set is a key component that sheds light on how well the model generalizes to new, unobserved cases (shown in Figure 8.8 and Figure 8.9). The percentage of correctly categorized cases is represented by accuracy, while the gap between the anticipated and actual values is measured by loss. However, depending only on loss and accuracy could not give a whole picture of a model's performance, particularly when dealing with unbalanced datasets. To assess the model's capacity to achieve a balance between precision and recall, other metrics are computed, such as the F1 score.

Because the F1 score considers both false positives and false negatives, it is especially helpful when deciding between recall (the percentage of true positives among all actual positives) and accuracy (the percentage of true positives among all projected positives). Model evaluation, which takes all these measures into account, offers a comprehensive analysis of the model's capability, and helps with decision-making regarding its implementation and future improvement.

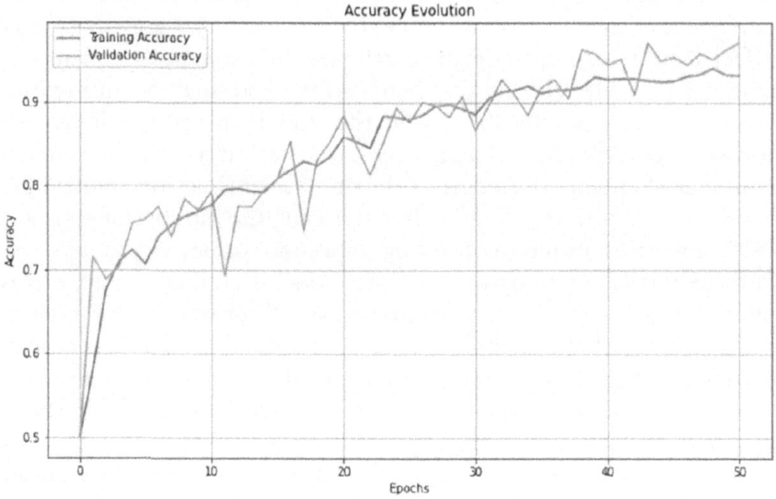


*Figure 8.8* Accuracy evolution graph.

## 8.5 RESULTS

A remarkable 98.37% accuracy rate in the field of cancer detection is encouraging and indicates that the model can correctly classify cases into cancerous and non-cancerous groups. This high accuracy suggests that the model is accurately classifying a large majority of cases, which is important for cancer-related scenarios including early identification and intervention.

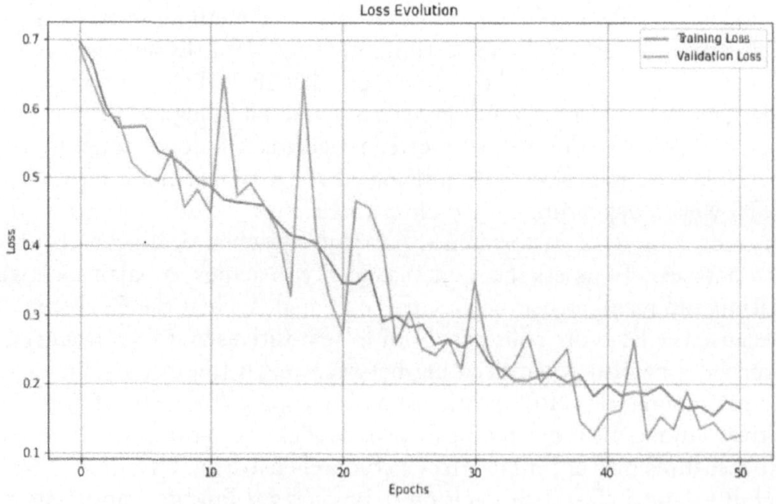


*Figure 8.9* Loss evaluation curve.

*Table 8.2* Comparative analysis of machine learning models

| *Model* | *Accuracy* |
|---|---|
| CNN using Keras (proposed) | 98.57% |
| Xception | 98.15% |
| VGG16 | 97.24% |
| MobileNet | 95.13% |
| Inception V3 | 95.3% |
| ResNet-50 | 82.0% |

## 8.6 CONCLUSION AND FUTURE WORK

The potential of deep learning models—specifically, CNNs—for early brain cancer (malignant cells) identification using MRI scans is investigated in this work since variable size, shape, and structure makes proper diagnosis difficult. Still when it comes to clinical diagnosis and therapy choices, magnetic resonance imaging is essential. A CNN model with promising results that was trained on a large dataset of MRI images is presented. Also, a variety of indicators to assess the model's efficacy with other existing models is shown here. This study can enable clinical professionals to customize treatment regimens for each patient individually, which can maximize different treatment benefits by forecasting malignant cells' (cancerous) aggressiveness. The possible response to different treatments can pave the way to individualized and successful treatment plans, thereby reducing side effects.

The training period was one of the research's limitations. Longer training times were caused by the CNN's several layers and our computer's constrained GPU capabilities. When dealing with much bigger datasets (thousands of photos), this duration would expand even further. We improved our GPU system to solve this, which greatly shortened the training period. In order to improve the accuracy of brain cancer identification, future research might concentrate on utilizing other data sources, such as specific patient information. This individualized technique might transform early detection and enhance patient treatment.

## REFERENCES

1. Sung, H., Ferlay, J., Siegel, R. L., Laversanne, M., Soerjomataram, I., Jemal, A., & Bray, F. (2021). Global cancer statistics 2020: GLOBOCAN estimates of incidence and mortality worldwide for 36 cancers in 185 countries. *CA: A Cancer Journal for Clinicians*, *71*(3), 209–249. https://doi.org/10.3322/caac.21660

2. Ferlay, J., Colombet, M., Soerjomataram, I., Parkin, D. M., Piñeros, M., Znaor, A., & Bray, F. (2021). Cancer statistics for the year 2020: An overview. *International Journal of Cancer*. https://doi.org/10.1002/ijc.33588
3. Sathishkumar, K., Chaturvedi, M., Das, P., Stephen, S., & Mathur, P. (2022). Cancer incidence estimates for 2022 & projection for 2025: Result from national cancer registry programme, India. *The Indian Journal of Medical Research*, *156*(4&5), 598–607. https://doi.org/10.4103/ijmr.ijmr_1821_22
4. https://main.icmr.nic.in/sites/default/files/seminars/EOI_on_Cancer_Screening.pdf
5. N Natarajan, P., Krishnan, N., Kenkre, N. S., Nancy, S., & Singh, B. P. (2012, December). Tumor detection using threshold operation in MRI brain images. In *2012 IEEE International Conference on Computational Intelligence and Computing Research* (pp. 1–4). IEEE.
6. Varuna Shree, N., & Kumar, T. N. R. (2018). Identification and classification of brain tumor MRI images with feature extraction using DWT and probabilistic neural network. *Brain Informatics*, *5*(1), 23–30.
7. ZainEldin, H., Gamel, S. A., El-Kenawy, E. M., Alharbi, A. H., Khafaga, D. S., Ibrahim, A., & Talaat, F. M. (2022). Brain tumor detection and classification using deep learning and sine-cosine fitness grey wolf optimization. *Bioengineering (Basel, Switzerland)*, *10*(1), 18. https://doi.org/10.3390/bioengineering10010018
8. Amin, J., Sharif, M., Haldorai, A. *et al.* (2022). Brain tumor detection and classification using machine learning: A comprehensive survey. *Complex & Intelligent Systems, 8*, 3161–3183. https://doi.org/10.1007/s40747-021-00563-y
9. Stadlbauer, A., Marhold, F., Oberndorfer, S., Heinz, G., Buchfelder, M., & Kinfe, T. M. (2021). Radiophysiomics: Brain tumors classification by machine learning and physiological MRI data. *Cancers*, *14*(10), 2363. https://doi.org/10.3390/cancers14102363
10. Aamir, M., Rahman, Z., Dayo, Z., Abro, W., Uddin, M. I., Khan, I., Imran, A., Ali, Z., Ishfaq, M., Guan, Y., & Hu, Z. (2022). A deep learning approach for brain tumor classification using MRI images. *Computers and Electrical Engineering*, *101*, 108105. https://doi.org/10.1016/j.compeleceng.2022.108105.
11. Sharma, M., Sharma, P., Mittal, R., & Gupta, K. (2021). Brain tumour detection using machine learning. *Journal of Electronics*, *3*(4), 298–308.
12. Siar, M., & Teshnehlab, M. (2019, October). Brain tumor detection using deep neural network and machine learning algorithm. In *2019 9th international conference on computer and knowledge engineering (ICCKE)* (pp. 363–368). IEEE.
13. Yahyaoui, H., Ghazouani, F., & Farah, I. R. (2021, July). Deep learning guided by an ontology for medical images classification using a multimodal fusion. In *2021 International congress of advanced technology and engineering (ICOTEN)* (pp. 1–6). IEEE.
14. Kang, J., Ullah, Z., & Gwak, J. (2021). MRI-based brain tumor classification using ensemble of deep features and machine learning classifiers. *Sensors*, *21*(6), 2222.

15. Bhatele, K. R., & Bhadauria, S. S. (2022). Machine learning application in glioma classification: review and comparison analysis. *Archives of Computational Methods in Engineering*, *29*(1), 247–274.
16. Murthy, M. Y. B., Koteswararao, A., & Babu, M. S. (2022). Adaptive fuzzy deformable fusion and optimized CNN with ensemble classification for automated brain tumor diagnosis. *Biomedical Engineering Letters*, *12*(1), 37–58.
17. Mehrotra, R., Ansari, M. A., Agrawal, R., & Anand, R. S. (2020). A transfer learning approach for AI-based classification of brain tumors. *Machine Learning with Applications*, *2*, 100003.
18. Grampurohit, S., Shalavadi, V., Dhotargavi, V. R., Kudari, M., & Jolad, S. (2020, October). Brain tumor detection using deep learning models. In *2020 IEEE India council international subsections conference (INDISCON)* (pp. 129–134). IEEE.
19. Rokhana, R., Herulambang, W., & Indraswari, R. (2020, September). Deep convolutional neural network for melanoma image classification. In *2020 International electronics symposium (IES)* (pp. 481–486). IEEE.
20. Khalil, H. A., Darwish, S., Ibrahim, Y. M., & Hassan, O. F. (2020). 3D-MRI brain tumor detection model using modified version of level set segmentation based on dragonfly algorithm. *Symmetry*, *12*(8), 1256.
21. Srinivasa Rao, B., Sri, V. N. B., Pamarthi, U. K., & Khan, P. F. (2023, June). Enhancing Local Feature Detection Performance with Sequential CNN Architecture in Keras. In *International conference on data analytics & management* (pp. 371–387). Springer Nature Singapore.
22. Hadush, S., Girmay, Y., Sinamo, A., & Hagos, G. (2020). Breast cancer detection using convolutional neural networks. *arXiv preprint arXiv:2003.07911.*
23. Abiwinanda, N., Hanif, M., Hesaputra, S. T., Handayani, A., & Mengko, T. R. (2019). Brain tumor classification using convolutional neural network. In *World Congress on Medical Physics and Biomedical Engineering 2018: June 3–8, 2018, Prague, Czech Republic* (Vol. 1, pp. 183–189). Springer Singapore.
24. Rahi, M. M. I., Khan, F. T., Mahtab, M. T., Ullah, A. A., Alam, M. G. R., & Alam, M. A. (2019, December). Detection of skin cancer using deep neural networks. In *2019 IEEE Asia-Pacific Conference on Computer Science and Data Engineering (CSDE)* (pp. 1–7). IEEE.

Chapter 9

# Advancing healthcare AI with federated learning

*Lokpriya Gaikwad, Vinod Surange, Sandip Kanase, and Agung Sutrisno*

## 9.1 INTRODUCTION

Healthcare artificial intelligence (AI) has demonstrated enormous potential for improving patient outcomes, increasing diagnostic accuracy, and optimising treatment approaches. The delicate nature of medical data, along with rigorous privacy regulations, offers substantial obstacles to standard centralised AI training methodologies. Federated learning (FL), a decentralised machine learning technique, provides a possible answer by allowing for collaborative model training across several universities without sharing raw data.

As a result of the proliferation of information technology (IT), particularly remote health monitoring, there has been a major improvement in the quality of healthcare services (Li et al., 2019). The use of physical sensor networks has two primary objectives, the first of which is the avoidance of illness, and the second is the early diagnosis of high-risk disease impairments (Mohammadzadeh et al., 2020). Due to its ability to quickly monitor and control patient difficulties through continuous vital sign evaluation and immediate access, smart wireless and wearable sensors, along with other advanced technology, have witnessed a significant spike in popularity in recent years (Gries et al., 2018).

Data storage and transfer capabilities of such smart devices are crucial in numerous healthcare contexts and treatments, including telemedicine (Da Costa et al., 2018). Wearable sensors are crucial for tracking patient health concerns (Li et al., 2019; Mohammadzadeh et al., 2020). Health also involves many other duties. Vital signs show the patient's health, organ function, and illness progression. The examination of these symptoms affects nursing care, diagnosis, treatment, and illness prevention (Fan et al., 2019). If properly and quickly evaluated, medical records can provide a wealth of information that can enhance care. Smart devices like the Internet of Things (IoT) and artificial intelligence can improve real-time patient health monitoring.

Over the past decade, smart gadgets, especially wearable sensors, have received attention, mostly from healthcare businesses. These devices monitor

 DOI: 10.1201/9781003634089-9

vital signs like pulse, respiration rate, temperature, and blood pressure to improve user health in therapeutic situations (Majumder et al., 2017). With the right wearable sensors and networks, crucial health data may be collected and shared. Wearable sensor networks (WSNs) for health monitoring involve many sensors (Mohammadzadeh et al., 2020). Patients may have these sensors implanted or worn. The networks use sensors put in various body parts. These sensors must meet particular requirements to recognise and record symptoms, which make up health data (Mohammadzadeh et al., 2020; Fan et al., 2019; Majumder et al., 2017). However, regular patient monitoring is needed for early medical intervention and delivery. This is because several diseases and disabilities exist (Mohammadzadeh et al., 2020; Gries et al., 2018). Patient monitoring via wireless sensor networks (WSNs) is a game-changer in smart wearable devices for healthcare. AI-healthcare collaboration has enhanced patient care in several ways. These include efficient (Lee et al., 2013), secure (Alotaibi and Federico, 2017), and high-quality medical treatment (Jamal et al., 2009).

AI is crucial to healthcare administration for interpreting and providing patient data (Sittig and Singh, 2011). Artificial intelligence studies have often shown positive effects on healthcare (Garcia et al., 2019). Recent studies have shown that medical professionals and patients utilise and oversee medical apps and games (Garcia, 2019; Mosa et al., 2012). The main uses of these apps and games are evidence-based therapy and remote patient monitoring. Both medical professionals and patients have this tendency. AI may help patients and healthcare providers communicate more fairly, supporting patient empowerment. AI and cloud computing can improve healthcare resource management and data availability (Chung and Park, 2019). Medical records are needed to create personalised treatment plans.

It is also possible to employ big data analytics (BDA) to identify illnesses and to provide information on healthcare policies (Islam et al., 2018). To enhance and facilitate the delivery of high-quality healthcare, it is feasible to integrate IoT as a tool with platforms or technologies based on AI (Aceto et al., 2020).

The success of IoT in various application areas is a sign of how widely used it is, especially when combined with wearable sensors and artificial intelligence, to provide high-quality healthcare. Controlling wearable sensors has become possible through the use of Bluetooth, Wi-Fi, and, more recently, the Internet. You might think of these sensors as IoT components or goods.

The introduction of IoT into the healthcare sector has made it possible for some devices, specifically sensors, to connect with one another and do data analysis (Jones, 2014). The burden of continually profiling health examination data has been relieved from physicians as a result of this development, which has made it feasible for basic health-related data to be collected in part or totally autonomously. A distributed platform is utilised by IoT in order to process and store data (Li et al., 2015). In order to better manage healthcare resources and anticipate patients' health problems, this platform aims to simplify the development and use of machine learning (ML) approaches (Ayodele, 2010; Janiesch et al., 2021). In order to accomplish this, we anticipate the needs and demands of our patients.

Federated learning is a game-changing strategy to improve healthcare AI by allowing collaborative model training while protecting data privacy. Despite its hurdles, federated learning has the potential to significantly improve medical imaging, electronic health record (EHR) analytics, and genomics. Continued research and development, combined with interdisciplinary collaboration, will be critical to realising the full potential of federated learning in healthcare.

Figure 9.1 presents a concise overview of a healthcare delivery system that utilises both IoT and machine learning technologies.

## 9.2 LITERATURE SURVEY

It was investigated by Kamruzzaman et al. (2022) how healthcare delivery in ubiquitous contexts can be aided by AI, edge computing, and the Internet of Medical Things (IoMT). Yang and colleagues (2022) examined the smart healthcare management system (HMS) and various types of sensor components used in each IoT framework.

### 9.2.1 Key technologies in healthcare

#### 9.2.1.1 Sensors

From simple devices like thermometers to intricate precision-based equipment, sensing technology is used in almost every aspect of hospital-based treatment. Diagnostic medicine has undergone a major shift thanks in large

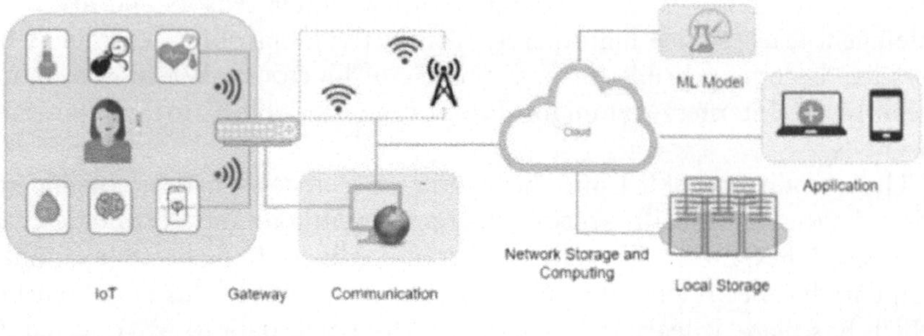


*Figure 9.1* A high-level illustration of the IoT–ML-powered healthcare delivery system (Sworna et al., 2021).

part to these sensors. Doctors can use this information, in instance, to undertake microsurgical treatments, identify damaged or aberrant areas, and assess the results of a procedure (Maurya et al., 2021). In hospital labs, pathologists also employ contemporary sensing technology for haematology, immunology, biochemistry, histopathology, and microbiology tasks. Additionally, sensors can be crucial to medical treatment. For instance, they are able to recognise occurrences like absent heartbeats. By determining the ideal time to give medication, they can also be used to enhance the pharmaceutical delivery process (Majumder et al., 2017).

The following are some notable examples of sensor application fields in HMS as shown in Table 9.1 (Dhanvijay and Patil, 2019): physiological, movement and trajectories, screening and diagnostics, and medical imaging.

Wearable and ambient (environmental) sensors are the two broad categories into which sensors can be divided.

#### *9.2.1.2 Wearable sensors*

From location to health status, wearable sensors are starting to emerge, providing patients with continuous, low-cost assessment of their medical problems. By 2018 (Majumder et al., 2017), 5 million of these sensors should be on the market. As they become more practical and inconspicuous, wearable sensors play a vital role in evaluating a patient's health or well-being without interfering with their daily activities. The sensors can track a number of vital signs as well as a patient's behaviour and mobility by being inserted into different body parts. In the end, low-power, compact, and affordable gadgets, along with the state of IT infrastructure, are opening the door for low-cost, covert, and long-lasting wearable sensors as shown in Table 9.2.

#### *9.2.1.3 Ambient sensors*

To identify and quantify changes in the physical environment, ambient or environmental sensors are used. Lung cancer and asthma are two physical

*Table 9.1* Sensor application fields in HSM

| *Type of sensor* | *Type of biosignal* | *Measured data* |
|---|---|---|
| Pulse oximeter | Oxygen saturation | Quantity of oxygen carried by human blood |
| Temperature | Body temperature | Ability of body to generate and get rid of heat |
| Accelerometer | Body movements | Measurement of acceleration forces in 3D spaces |
| Chest electrodes | Electrocardiogram | Measurement of waveform showing contraction and relaxation of cardiac cycle |
| Phonocardiograph | Heart sound | Measurement of heart sound by use of stethoscope |

*Table 9.2* Categorisation of wearable sensors

| *Type of Sensor* | *Subcategory* | *Examples* |
|---|---|---|
| Wearable sensors | Inertial sensors | Accelerometer |
| | | Gyroscopes |
| | | Pressure sensors |
| | | Magnetic field sensors |
| | Location sensors | Global Positioning System (GPS) |
| | | Blood pressure cuff |
| | | Electrocardiogram (ECG) |
| | Physiological sensors | Spirometer |
| | | Esophagogastroduodenoscopy (EDG) |
| | | Galvanic skin response (GSR) |
| | Image sensors | SenseCam |

health disorders that are made worse by air pollution (Sood and Mahajan, 2018). These environmental sensors can measure air pollution, temperature, and humidity. Additional subcategories and tags for ambient sensors are provided in Table 9.3, along with examples.

### 9.2.2 Frequently used sensors in the medical field

As far as the HMS is concerned, the health monitors are paramount. A variety of health concerns can be identified with their help in tracking relevant medical records. Another name for health sensors is biosensors, which describes devices that detect changes in biological parameters through implantation or skin-based sensing (health data).

*Table 9.3* Categorisation of ambient sensors

| *Type of sensor* | *Subcategory* | *Examples* |
|---|---|---|
| Ambient sensors | Environmental sensors | Thermometer |
| | | Hygrometer |
| | Binary sensors | Window contact |
| | | Door contact |
| | | Light switch |
| | | Remote control switch |
| | Location sensors | Infrared |
| | Physiological sensors | Zigbee |
| | | Active radio-frequency identification (RFID) |
| | | RFID tags |
| | Tags | Near field communication (NFC) tags |

Numerous health sensors are being created to identify various vital indicators in patients' bodies under the framework of an IoT-enabled, ubiquitous healthcare environment. Depending on how they are used, various devices may function differently. Accordingly, the following sections address a range of biosensors that are fundamental to widespread healthcare systems.

#### 9.2.2.1 Blood pressure sensor

Blood pressure (BP) is the measurement of the force exerted on the artery wall by the blood flowing through the blood channels. A sphygmomanometer is typically used to measure blood pressure. The blood pressure is normal if the artery's blood flow is normal. Blood pressure increases if there is a blockage in blood flow. Serious health problems could result from high blood pressure (Beevers et al., 2001). Two pressure points are found in the blood channels during the BP measuring procedure: the diastolic pressure point is found between two heartbeats, and the systolic pressure point is found during a heartbeat. Many common BP testing methods are available nowadays. A mercury sphygmomanometer is considered the gold standard.

Based on the oscillometric concept, the digital manometer measures blood pressure using an electronic pressure sensor. The results are subsequently displayed digitally on a screen (Mukkamala and Hahn, 2017). When connected to a smart hub like a smartphone, this simple method of taking blood pressure can improve an all-encompassing healthcare system.

#### 9.2.2.2 Body temperature sensor

Human body temperature (BT) is a valuable biomarker since it often falls within the normal range of 37 degrees Celsius. Blood pressure readings over the normal range are a hallmark of vascular shock and other conditions caused by inadequate blood flow (Wang et al., 2017). Time of day and thermometer placement could affect results even for healthy individuals. This is why it is so important to calibrate the thermometer before taking any readings.

#### 9.2.2.3 Electrocardiogram

Sensor electrocardiography (Yang et al., 2022) was one of the first and simplest techniques used in the diagnosis of heart problems. An ECG, or electrocardiogram, is a graph showing the cardiac muscles' generated electrical impulses in response to an electrical discharge.

#### 9.2.2.4 Electroencephalogram

The electroencephalogram (EEG) is a technique that uses tiny electrodes positioned at several places on the scalp to measure the electrical impulses in a person's brain (Mukhopadhyay, 2014). It's a safe, non-invasive treatment that can be frequently performed on patients, healthy adults, and kids. Electric impulses in the microvolt (mV) range, with frequency varying between 8 Hz and 50 Hz, are produced by nerves that can stimulate the brain. In many different medical and non-medical contexts, EEG is used.

#### *9.2.2.5 Oxygen pulse*

The amount of oxygen in the blood is an important factor for human health. The heart and brain can get tired from extremely low oxygen levels, and the human body has trouble functioning properly when there isn't enough oxygen. Blood oxygen saturation can be calculated by dividing the percentage of oxygen-saturated haemoglobin molecules by their maximum absorption value. Saturation levels of oxygen are typically higher than 89%. A pulse oximeter can be used to find the level of blood-oxygen saturation (Luks and Swenson, 2020). The pulse oximeter captures red and infrared light and uses that data to calculate the amount of oxygen bound to haemoglobin.

#### *9.2.2.6 Heart rate monitor*

The human heart is tasked with both collecting carbon dioxide-filled deoxygenated blood and pumping oxygenated blood along with nutrients to various organs and tissues in the body.

The steps taken by the heart to pump oxygenated blood via the aorta after it has been converted from deoxygenated blood in the lungs are known as the cardiac cycle (Porter et al., 2021). Beats per minute (BPM) are used to measure heart rate (HR), which is the frequency of the cardiac cycle. An important metric for assessing a patient's physical and mental health is their HR. An average healthy adult's heart rate ranges from 60 to 100 beats per minute. Improved heart fitness, cardiovascular health, and efficient heart function are generally indicated by a low HR value.

#### *9.2.2.7 Activity and motion sensor*

Exercise is essential to keeping your body and physique in good condition. Moreover, during a patient's hospital stay for rehabilitation, their mobility is an essential factor that needs to be constantly monitored. The three most popular sensors for evaluating a patient's motions and physical activity are an accelerometer, pedometer, and actometer.

## 9.3 INTERNET OF THINGS FRAMEWORK

The utilisation of IoT and related mechanisms in healthcare is driven by two main factors: patients' reluctance to physically visit doctors and the demand for immediate medical attention and support. As a result, people's reactions to physical illnesses are prompted by omnipresent healthcare technology. There isn't a single, widely accepted IoT architecture that scientists can agree upon. IoT frameworks were provided by different researchers in different methods. Three layers make up the most basic IoT architecture: network, application, and sensor. The IoT concept is presented in an extremely simplified manner, which does not provide enough detail for research needs. Consequently, our four-layer design includes a communication layer and a network storage layer beneath the network layer.

### 9.3.1 IoT layers

The four main parts of IoT are the application layer, the connection layer, the sensing layer, and the network storage layer. The sensor is installed right next to the patient in the layer that houses it. Getting data is what this layer is in charge of. In order to monitor a patient's vitals, it employs a network of several wearable or portable sensors (Wan et al., 2018).

The human body can be monitored by a network of sensors, as shown in Figure 9.2. These sensors assess glucose, ECG, EEG, GPS, BT, and BP. Various techniques and technologies are used to transmit the data collected by the sensors to the storage level of the network within the communication layer. At this level, many protocols are utilised according to the data type and type of sensor. Many more are among them, such as Zigbee, Wi-Fi, Bluetooth, near field communication (NFC), and radio-frequency identification (RFID). The network storage layer, the third tier of IoT architecture, is utilised by humans. Increased data transmissions are a direct result of the proliferation of users made possible by developments in IoT technology.

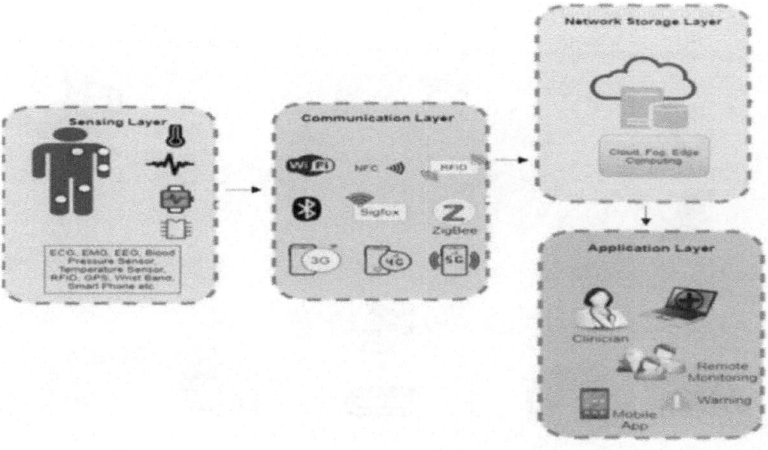


*Figure* 9.2 The HMS's four-layer IOT structure (Sworna et al., 2021).

The idea of cloud-based architecture for IoT was spurred by this issue. Large volumes of data are typically handled and stored by this layer. Additionally, it helps to lessen the load on a sensor apparatus (Yang et al., 2016). Data visualisation is the main focus of the application layer.

The IoT framework can serve as an application unit for a variety of use cases, such as health prediction, activity detection, smart cities, smart transportation, and smart home monitoring (Sworna et al., 2021). IoT architecture relies on sensors, actuators, and development boards.

### 9.3.2 Internet of Things in healthcare

The healthcare industry has made large IT investments, yet despite this, businesses in the field still use traditional (paper) medical procedures to facilitate communication between physicians and patients. Consequently, there is limited and challenging data sharing between departments and physicians, with physicians acquiring information only through physical examinations conducted during hospital visits. However, by integrating IoT with HMS, this issue can be resolved. Doctors and other healthcare professionals can freely, conveniently, and readily access patient information and status by utilising IoT in healthcare. Additionally, it may be more convenient and economical to monitor, treat, and diagnose public health issues. Stated differently, IoT can establish an efficient HMS by connecting people, machines, and smart devices (Al-Dhief et al., 2020) as shown in Figure 9.3.

## 9.4 ARTIFICIAL INTELLIGENCE

AI is further broken down into ML and BDA in the context of HMS. A better conceptual grasp of AI's role in HMS is the intended outcome of this

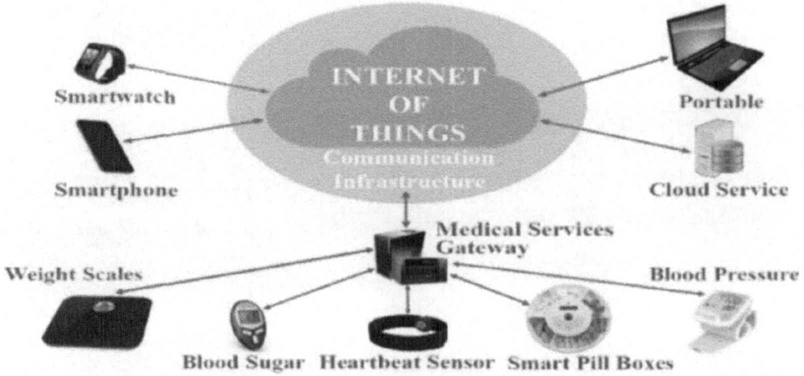


*Figure 9.3* Internet of Things devices in medicine (Al-Dhief et al., 2020).

categorisation. The ensuing sections include specifics on ML, BDA, and how each is used in HMS.

## 9.4.1 Machine learning

Artificial intelligence has a significant technical impact in the healthcare sector. With wearable sensors and other devices being used to periodically collect massive amounts of health-related data, ML is becoming increasingly valuable for data analysis in the healthcare industry (Adewole et al., 2021). The knowledge gained from these data could be essential to providing high-quality medical care and supporting the development of a good rapport between the patient and the physician. ML has many uses in the healthcare industry, including helping physicians find more specialised medications and focused medical procedures.

## 9.4.2 Analytics for big data

Text files, imaging, and narrative data are only a few of the many data sources that make up health data that describe patient features and treatments; these sources are all underutilised and have much more potential to be exploited than is currently the case (Mao et al., 2015). The potential for improving healthcare through the use of diverse data analytic technologies to medical data is widely recognised (Yang et al., 2015). Data mining and information retrieval are the predominant techniques employed for leveraging medical records. It is important to note that these tools serve two purposes: firstly, they can be utilised to gather comprehensive demographic data about the study populations, and secondly, they can be employed to gather intricate information about specific individuals. Both data-driven technologies exhibit significant differences, yet their ultimate objectives are opposite.

### *9.4.2.1 Blockchain*

Blockchain is a data-holding decentralised network of nodes. It is an excellent way to protect private information within the system. This technology protects sensitive information while facilitating the flow of necessary information. It is the best option for safely keeping all related documents in one location (De Aguiar et al., 2020). Blockchain expedites the process of searching for individuals that fulfil certain trial conditions by utilising a unified patient database. A peer-to-peer (P2P) network of individual computers called "nodes" that maintains, stores, and records transaction history is called the blockchain (Varshney et al., 2021).

This technology can provide insights on the value of individual therapy and connect disparate networks. A blockchain might thus be known for its

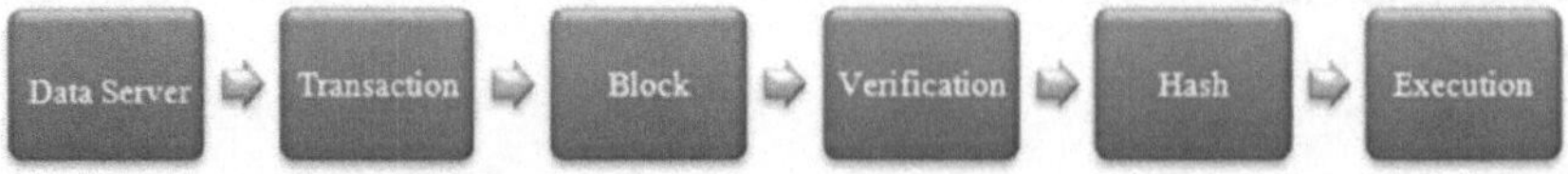


*Figure 9.4* Basic stages of blockchain technology functioning.

security and immutability. The three main ideas of blockchain are miners, nodes, and blocks. A blockchain keeps all of its data in separate locations. A computer network replicates and spreads the blockchain. Whenever a new block is added to the blockchain, every computer connected to the internet updates its version of the blockchain. Figure 9.4 shows the basic levels at which blockchain technology operates.

## 9.5 ISSUES WITH EMERGING TECHNOLOGIES IN THE PROVISION OF HEALTHCARE

Researchers have already done a great deal of important work on AI-powered IoT applications in the healthcare industry; yet, there are still certain limitations, as the unresolved issues show. As the concepts of IoT and advanced machine learning techniques such as deep learning and reinforcement learning continue to grow, there will be many new opportunities for research and exploration. Consequently, this investigation has led to the discovery of research difficulties and open topics, which are covered in the following sections.

### 9.5.1 Data acquisition

A well-curated dataset is essential to an AI-based HMS's performance. Several attempts have been made to use real-time data to train supervised ML methods (Aceto et al., 2020). However, the majority of the studies made use of datasets that were obtained from open sources that were provided by unaffiliated people or groups. These datasets frequently contain missing values, lack of variety, and unintentional bias. Compiling datasets is an important task, especially in the medical field. Moreover, modifications to the environmental control elements could vary the dataset's efficacy and character.

### 9.5.2 Managing streams of data

A method for obtaining useful information from fast-moving, continuous data streams is called data stream mining. Since the advent of remote HMS, the contemporary healthcare industry has made use of real-time components to obtain critical physiological data in real time. This idea deals with managing massive and continuous data streams (Mrozek et al., 2020). The volume, velocity, diversity, and veracity of the sensor data that passes through the IoT architecture are all quite high (Syed et al., 2019). This constant influx of data presents a number of obstacles, including but not limited to adaptive model selection, concept drift, imbalanced class labelling, high dimensionality, and model retraining. We need to go more into this new area in regard to healthcare management systems based on IoT because of these reasons.

### 9.5.3 Safety

To ensure patients receive the necessary care, it is essential to gather, share, and safeguard health-related information from them, which can be obtained either voluntarily or involuntarily. Safeguarding the confidentiality of patients' medical records is therefore of paramount significance.

At each point in the data lifecycle—during transmission, processing, collection, and storage—security measures are in place to prevent unauthorised access or modification (Selvaraj and Doraikannan, 2019). Better security measures should also be put in place at the level immediately adjacent to the sensor to protect user data. If data security is your top priority, an HMS powered by AI could be the way to go.

### 9.5.4 Ethics and privacy

The confidentiality of a patient's information is guaranteed by the governing body (Selvaraj and Doraikannan, 2019). It should additionally delineate the precise location and explicitly identify the individuals who are permitted to access the patient's medical records. Typically, exclusive access to this information is granted solely to healthcare professionals such as doctors and nurses. To receive the right care or attention, though, in some situations it is also necessary to disclose this private information to other people (Sworna et al., 2021). In addition, patients could be reluctant to disclose too much personal information to anybody outside of their family, such as an early pregnancy. Thus, such information shouldn't be disclosed to the public. Moreover, the sensing layer needs extra defence against outside threats because it is the layer nearest to the user (Kaur et al., 2021).

When a patient is being monitored remotely, their personal information is safely kept in the storage unit. Therefore, it is critical to prevent unauthorised access to such sensitive information (Vijayakumar et al., 2019). It should be mentioned that providing individualised service and protecting privacy must be balanced. The increasing volume of health-related data raises ethical questions about AI–HMS's capacity for making decisions. AI models' predictability is frequently overstated, and their lack of empathy is a serious issue for the healthcare industry.

## 9.6 EXPERIMENTAL FINDINGS

Following are a few experimental findings on recent technologies in the healthcare sector:

1. **Telemedicine and remote patient monitoring:** Clinical trials utilising these two healthcare technologies have shown notable gains in patient outcomes and accessibility to care. In comparison with conventional care, nowadays hospital readmission and mortality rates among patients with heart failure are decreased due to telemedicine interventions.
2. **Robotics in surgery:** Experimental studies show that compared to conventional surgical methods, robotic-assisted surgery has shown to have better accuracy, agility, and minimally invasive capabilities. Research has demonstrated a decrease in the frequency of complications and a speedier recuperation period for patients receiving robotic procedures in urology, gynecology, and orthopedics.
   Trials are currently looking into how virtual reality (VR) and augmented reality (AR) technologies can be used with robotic surgery systems to help surgeons see better, understand their surroundings better, and plan their procedures better.
3. **Genomic medicine:** Research results in this field demonstrate the potential of next-generation sequencing technology in elucidating the genetic underpinnings of pharmacogenomics, cancer subtypes, and uncommon disorders. It helps to develop individualised treatment plans based on the genetic profiles of specific individuals.
4. **Blockchain for healthcare data management:** Research is ongoing to look into how blockchain technology might be used to manage patient records, securely trade healthcare data, and provide transparency about clinical trials. Blockchain-based systems guarantee data honesty and interoperability while providing decentralised, impenetrable storage for critical health data.
5. **Wearable health technologies:** Research has shown how wearable devices like fitness trackers and smart watches can monitor health and spot illness symptoms early to encourage a healthy lifestyle.
6. **3D printing in personalised medicine:** With the help of 3D printing, medical gadgets and even human tissues that are specifically customised to the patient's needs are possible. Improved surgical outcomes and shorter operating times could result from the use of 3D-printed patient-specific anatomical models for surgical planning and medical education.

## 9.7 CONCLUSION

Digital technologies have already created a plethora of opportunities for influencing primary healthcare and guaranteeing successful public health initiatives. They have also sparked new forms of empowerment, engagement, and communication, as well as a number of changes in policy, practice, and education.

Blockchain, IoT, AI, and sensors have all been widely used in numerous fields in recent years. The purpose of implementing these cutting-edge technologies in healthcare is to improve HMS. As a result, scientists are closely monitoring how these technologies are being used in healthcare.

In healthcare systems, blockchain and artificial intelligence make it possible to make intelligent decisions, while sensors and IoT frameworks are responsible for data transmission and collection. It was observed that several HMSs had sensors and IoT technologies that worked effectively together. Specifically, IoT and related gadgets have enabled smarter and faster disease diagnosis, tracking, and treatment. Because of this, HMS is now significantly more efficient.

Although we have integrated sensors and IoT into HMS, we have yet to tackle many major challenges. Simple usage, interoperability with sensing and IoT devices, scalability, data synchronisation, data privacy and security compliance, and procedure streamlining are all part of this.

AI and blockchain are also growing in healthcare. Blockchain and AI platforms store, analyse, and visualise data, which is ideal for human resource management. Artificial intelligence has enabled modern health data analysis. Healthcare management systems could use these solutions now and in the future. Blockchain technology lets healthcare professionals create decentralised patient record storage systems. Only legitimate users of sensitive data are allowed access to these platforms. Blockchain may also solve data theft and security breaches. One of the biggest obstacles to HMS AI deployment is cost, end-user consent, and regulatory laws. The privacy, ethics, and quality of data must also be addressed.

## REFERENCES


Aceto, G., Persico, V., Pescapè, A., "Industry 4.0 and health: Internet of things, big data, and cloud computing for healthcare 4.0", *J. Ind. Inf. Integr.* 2020, 18, 100129. http://wpage.unina.it/giuseppe.aceto/pub/aceto2020industry40eHealth__JII.pdf

Adewole, K.S., Akintola, A.G., Jimoh, R.G., Mabayoje, M.A., Jimoh, M.K., Usman-Hamza, F.E., Balogun, A.O., Sangaiah, A.K., Ameen, A.O., "Cloud-based IoMT framework for cardiovascular disease prediction and diagnosis in personalized E-health care", In *Intelligent IoT Systems in Personalized Health Care*. Elsevier: Amsterdam, The Netherlands, 2021, pp. 105–145.

Al-Dhief, F.T., Latiff, N.M.A.A., Malik, N.N.N.A., Salim, N.S., Baki, M.M., Albadr, M.A.A., Mohammed, M.A., "A survey of voice pathology surveillance systems based on internet of things and machine learning algorithms", *IEEE Access* 2020, 8, 64514–64533. https://api.semanticscholar.org/CorpusID:215817930

Alotaibi, Y.K., Federico, F., "The impact of health information technology on patient safety", *Saudi Med. J.* 2017, 38, 1173. https://doi.org/10.15537/smj.2017.12.20631

Ayodele, T.O., "Machine learning overview", *New Adv. Mach. Learn.* 2010, 2, 9–18. https://doi.org/10.5772/9374

Beevers, G., Lip, G.Y., O'Brien, E., "The pathophysiology of hypertension", *BMJ* 2001, 322, 912–916. https://doi.org/10.1136/bmj.322.7291.912

Chung, K., Park, R.C., "Chatbot-based healthcare service with a knowledge base for cloud computing", *Cluster Computing* 2019, 22, 1925–1937. https://doi.org/ https://api.semanticscholar.org/CorpusID:10701424

Da Costa, C.A., Pasluosta, C.F., Eskofier, B., Da Silva, D.B., da Rosa Righi, R., "Internet of Health Things: Toward intelligent vital signs monitoring in hospital wards", *Artif. Intell. Med.* 2018, 89, 61–69. https://doi.org/10.1016/j.artmed.2018.05.005

De Aguiar, E.J., Faiçal, B.S., Krishnamachari, B., Ueyama, J. "A survey of blockchain-based strategies for healthcare", *ACM Comput. Surv. (CSUR)* 2020, 53, 1–27. https://doi.org/10.1145/3376915

Dhanvijay, M.M., Patil, S.C., "Internet of Things: A survey of enabling technologies in healthcare and its applications", *Comput. Netw.* 2019, 153, 113–131, https://doi.org/10.1016/j.comnet.2019.03.006

Fan, Y., Xu, P., Jin, H., Ma, J., Qin, L., "Vital sign measurement in telemedicine rehabilitation based on intelligent wearable medical devices", *IEEE Access* 2019, 7, 54819–54823, https://doi.org/10.1109/ACCESS.2019.2912410

Garcia, M.B., "A speech therapy game application for aphasia patient neurorehabilitation—A pilot study of an mHealth app.", *Int. J. Simul. Syst. Sci. Technol.* 2019, 20, 1–8, https://doi.org/https://doi.org/10.5013/IJSSST.a.20.S2.05

Garcia, M.B., Pilueta, N.U., Jardiniano, M.F., "VITAL APP: Development and user acceptability of an IoT-based patient monitoring device for synchronous measurements of vital signs", Proceedings of the 2019 IEEE 11th International Conference on Humanoid, Nanotechnology, Information Technology, Communication and Control, Environment, and Management (HNICEM), Laoag, Philippines, 29 November–1 December 2019, pp. 1–6, https://doi.org/10.1109/HNICEM48295.2019.9072906.

Gries, A., Seekamp, A., Wrede, C., Dodt, C., "Zusatz-Weiterbildung Klinische Akut- und Notfallmedizin in Deutschland", *DerAnaesthesist* 2018, 67, 895–900. https://doi.org/10.1007/s00101-018-0515-5

Islam, M.S., Hasan, M.M., Wang, X., Germack, H.D., "A systematic review on healthcare analytics: Application and theoretical perspective of data mining", *Healthcare* 2018, 6, 54. https://doi.org/10.3390/healthcare6020054

Jamal, A., McKenzie, K., Clark, M., "The impact of health information technology on the quality of medical and health care: A systematic review", *Health Inf. Manag. J.* 2009, 38, 26–37, https://doi.org/10.1177/183335830903800105

Janiesch, C., Zschech, P., Heinrich, K., "Machine learning and deep learning", *Electronic Markets* 2021, 31, 685–695. https://link.springer.com/article/10.1007/s12525-021-00475-2

Jones, N., "Computer science: The learning machines", *Nat. News* 2014, 505, 146. https://doi.org/10.1038/505146a

Kamruzzaman, M., Alrashdi, I., Alqazzaz, A., "New opportunities, challenges, and applications of edge-ai for connected healthcare in internet of medical things for smart cities", *J. Healthc. Eng.* 2022, 2950699, https://doi.org/10.1155/2022/2950699

Kaur, J., Verma, R., Alharbe, N.R., Agrawal, A., Khan, R.A., "Importance of fog computing in healthcare 4.0", In *Fog Computing for Healthcare 4.0 Environments*. Springer: Berlin/Heidelberg, Germany, 2021, pp. 79–101. https://doi.org/10.1007/978-3-030-70130-6_5

Lee, J., McCullough, J.S., Town, R.J., "The impact of health information technology on hospital productivity", *RAND J. Econ.* 2013, 44, 545–568. https://doi.org/10.1111/1756-2171.12030

Li, J., Ma, Q., Chan, A.H., Man, S., "Health monitoring through wearable technologies for older adults: Smart wearables acceptance model", *Appl. Ergon.* 2019, 75, 162–169. https://doi.org/10.1016/j.apergo.2018.10.006.

Li, S., Da Xu, L., Zhao, S., "The internet of things: A survey", *Inf. Syst. Front.* 2015, 17, 243– 259. https://doi.org/10.1007/s10796-014-9492-7

Luks, A.M., Swenson, E.R., "Pulse oximetry for monitoring patients with COVID-19 at home: Potential pitfalls and practical guidance". *Ann. Am. Thorac. Soc.* 2020, 17, 1040–1046. https://doi.org/10.1513/AnnalsATS.202005-418FR

Majumder, S., Mondal, T., Deen, M.J., "Wearable sensors for remote health monitoring", *Sensors* 2017, 17, 130. https://doi.org/10.3390/s17010130 (MDPI)

Mao, R., Xu, H., Wu, W., Li, J., Li, Y., Lu, M., "Overcoming the challenge of variety: Big data abstraction, the next evolution of data management for AAL communication systems", *IEEE Commun. Mag.* 2015, 53, 42–47, https://api.semanticscholar.org/CorpusID:206455176

Maurya, M.R., Riyaz, N.U., Reddy, M., Yalcin, H.C., Ouakad, H.M., Bahadur, I., Al-Maadeed, S., Sadasivuni, K.K., "A review of smart sensors coupled with Internet of Things and Artificial Intelligence approach for heart failure monitoring", *Med. Biol. Eng. Comput.* 2021, 59, 2185–2203. https://doi.org/10.3390/life14010145

Mohammadzadeh, N., Gholamzadeh, M., Saeedi, S., Rezayi, S., "The application of wearable smart sensors for monitoring the vital signs of patients in epidemics: A systematic literature review", *J. Ambient Intell. Humaniz. Comput.* 2020, 1–15, https://doi.org/10.1007/s12652-020-02656- x.

Mosa, A.S.M., Yoo, I., Sheets, L., "A systematic review of healthcare applications for smartphones", *BMC Med. Inform. Decis. Mak.* 2012, 12, 67. https://doi.org/10.1186/1472- 6947-12-67

Mrozek, D., Koczur, A., Małysiak-Mrozek, B., "Fall detection in older adults with mobile IoT devices and machine learning in the cloud and on the edge", *Inf. Sci.* 2020, 537, 132–147. https://doi.org/10.1016/j.ins.2020.05.133.

Mukhopadhyay, S.C., "Wearable sensors for human activity monitoring: A review", *IEEE Sens. J.* 2014, 15, 1321–1330. https://doi.org/10.1109/JSEN.2014.2370945

Mukkamala, R., Hahn, J.-O., "Toward ubiquitous blood pressure monitoring via pulse transit time: Predictions on maximum calibration period and acceptable error limits", *IEEE Trans. Biomed. Eng.* 2017, 65, 1410–1420. https://doi.org/10.1109/TBME.2017.2756018

Porter, P., Muirhead, F., Brisbane, J., Schneider, B., Choveaux, J., Bear, N., Carson, J., Jones, K., Silva, D., Neppe, C. "Accuracy, clinical utility, and usability of a wireless self-guided fetal heart rate monitor", *Obstet. Gynecol.* 2021 April 1, 137(4), 673–681. https://doi.org/10.1097/AOG.0000000000004322

Selvaraj, P., Doraikannan, S., "Privacy and security issues on wireless body area and IoT for remote healthcare monitoring", *Intell. Pervasive Comput. Syst. Smarter Healthc.* 2019, 227–253, https://doi.org/10.1007/978-3-030-34025-3_11.

Sittig, D.F., Singh, H., "Defining health information technology–related errors: New developments since to err is human", *Arch. Intern. Med.* 2011, 171, 1281–1284, https://doi.org/10.1097/PTS.0b013e31823d8df0

Sood, S.K., Mahajan, I., "IoT-fog-based healthcare framework to identify and control hypertension attack", *IEEE Internet Things J.* 2018, 6, 1920–1927, https://api.semanticscholar.org/CorpusID:69689572.

Sworna, N.S., Islam, A.M., Shatabda, S., Islam, S., "Towards development of IoT-ML driven healthcare systems: A survey", *J. Netw. Comput. Appl.* 2021, 196, 103244. https://doi.org/10.1016/j.jnca.2021.103244

Syed, L., Jabeen, S., Manimala, S., Alsaeedi, A., "Smart healthcare framework for ambient assisted living using IoMT and big data analytics techniques", *Future Gener. Comput. Syst.* 2019, 101, 136–151. https://doi.org/10.1016/j.future.2019.06.033.

Varshney, A., Garg, N., Nagla, K., Nair, T., Jaiswal, S., Yadav, S., Aswal, D., "Challenges in sensors technology for industry 4.0 for futuristic metrological applications", *MAPAN* 2021, 36, 215–226. https://doi.org/10.1007/s12647-021-00453-1

Vijayakumar, V., Malathi, D., Subramaniyaswamy, V., Saravanan, P., Logesh, R., "Fog computing-based intelligent healthcare system for the detection and prevention of mosquito-borne diseases", *Comput. Hum. Behav.* 2019, 100, 275–285, https://doi.org/10.1016/j.chb.2018.12.009

Wan, J., Al-awlaqi, M.A.A.H., Li, M., O'Grady, M., Gu, X., Wang, J., Cao, N., "Wearable IoT enabled real-time health monitoring system", *EURASIP J. Wirel. Commun. Netw.* 2018, 298. https://doi.org/10.1186/s13638-018-1308-x

Wang, Z., Yang, Z., Dong, T., "A review of wearable technologies for elderly care that can accurately track indoor position, recognize physical activities and monitor vital signs in real time", *Sensors* 2017, 17, 341. https://doi.org/10.3390/s17020341

Yang, J.-J., Li, J., Mulder, J., Wang, Y., Chen, S., Wu, H., Wang, Q., Pan, H., "Emerging information technologies for enhanced healthcare", *Comput. Ind.* 2015, 69, 3–11. https://doi.org/10.1016/j.compind.2015.01.012

Yang, Y., Wang, H., Jiang, R., Guo, X., Cheng, J., Chen, Y., "A review of IoT-enabled mobile healthcare: technologies, challenges, and future trends", *IEEE Internet Things J.* 2022, 9, 9478–9502. https://doi.org/10.1109/JIOT.2022.3144400

Yang, Z., Zhou, Q., Lei, L., Zheng, K., Xiang, W., "An IoT-cloud based wearable ECG monitoring system for smart healthcare", *J. Med. Syst.* 2016, 40, 286. https://doi.org/10.1007/s10916-016-0644-9

Chapter 10

# A systematic review of applications, challenges, data collection and academic research in healthcare using IoT

*Divya Srivastava, Vansh Budhiraja, Ashutosh Srivastava, and Madhushi Verma*

## 10.1 INTRODUCTION

Today, the world faces numerous troubles associated with serious health issues in view of challenging diseases like COVID. Recently, there has been a noticeable shift in how we use subtle movements, such as those tracked by smartwatches, to manage emotional responses to pain and enhance overall well-being. The field of IoT (Internet of Things) [1] has broadened our normal outcomes and expanded our lifestyles. With streaming displays and evaluations, IoT has risen as a tool for limitless receptivity, reliable communication, distant sensors, nearby devices, and electrical devices connected to the Internet. IoT works by linking various certified devices and sharing data and insights.

Forward-thinking and leaders have come about due to best-in-class advancements in the constantly changing healthcare environment. IoT separates itself as an ever-evolving technology that affects the way in which clinical benefits are received and experienced. IoT involves data from the healthcare network, from wearable sensors to remote sensing devices, offering better accessibility, accuracy, and capability in examination, treatment, and patient commitment.

Clinical monitoring is one of the areas where IoT in healthcare is making the most difference. By utilizing sensors that are worn from a distance or on the body, clinical specialists could accumulate countless physiological data continuously. Fundamental indicators like temperature, heartbeat, electrocardiogram (ECG), and electroencephalogram (EEG) are recorded by these sensors, providing a lot of information about the patient's well-being. Additionally, standard measurements like temperature, humidity, date, and time may be tracked by IoT-enabled devices, giving a complete picture of the patient's state and environmental components.

Ensuring reliable data and accessibility are fundamental for the smooth networking of IoT devices into healthcare systems. Importing data becomes fundamental while overseeing different data streams coming from many sources, like sensors, mobile phones, messages, programming, and applications. Access to this data is central for health specialists, carers, and

DOI: 10.1201/9781003634089-10

organizations to aid in informed clinical choices and give individualized treatment. In this way, IoT establishment is urgent for guaranteeing secure and suitable data sharing.

A user interface that is capable as a healthcare worker dashboard is a focus of various IoT systems. Healthcare specialists could see data, track patients' vitals, and do continuous assessment. These dashboards allow carers to upgrade patient outcomes, further foster self-governing direction, and smooth out processes through customizable components and straightforward controls. IoT-driven data visualization instruments clarify healthcare data, empowering experts to see connections, peculiarities, and examples that they would have missed. Beyond the constraints of clinical perception, IoT might conceivably change healthcare. The realities affirm that integrating IoT might change healthcare communication, support patient diagnoses, and increase decisions for care overall. Because of IoT affiliation, telehealth organizations engage patients to screen continuous ailments, partake in programs for virtual reconstruction and remotely meet from the comfort of their own homes. By enabling patients to successfully participate in their care, IoT-engaged devices advance a sense of obligation, reinforcing, and freedom. There are various issues with IoT-driven healthcare systems, ignoring the wonderful progress made. The biggest challenge is ensuring that IoT networks are secure and of the highest grade. To guard patient confirmation, information validity, and association network quality components, for example, information sharing assertion, security principles, cost effectiveness, constancy, and connection should be considered. Moreover, as a smooth mix is fundamental to thoroughly include IoT in the healthcare network, interoperability of IoT designs and devices continues to be a major test.

Big data assessment and IoT getting together is a game-changing improvement for healthcare advancement. Healthcare specialists could get useful insight into patient behavior, effective treatment, and disease development by utilizing big data. Early identification of possible ailments is made possible by careful evaluation of the data, which allows proactive mediation and individualized treatment programs. Likewise, IoT-enabled big data assessments make it possible to monitor patients in an effective way, share information, and lessen the workload on healthcare organizations.

The Internet of Medical Things (IoMT) [2] has obtained pervasiveness as a potential perspective for remote healthcare. IoMT development offers a total method for managing individualized clinical benefits by uniting specific devices and coordinated clinical sensors. Also known as the Healthcare Internet of Things, this nascent field consolidates a wide variety of purposes, for instance, drug adherence, teleconsultations, remote monitoring, and patients with chronic conditions. HIoT systems aim to change healthcare organizations by using the knowledge and relationship of the IoT to make clinical benefits more effective, engaged, capable, and accessible. The requirement for careful survey and examination is more obvious as IoT use in healthcare increases. Systematic literature reviews (SLRs) are important for recognizing research openings, sharing information, and proposing future assessments. SLRs contribute essentially to how we could analyze the capacity of IoT in healthcare by analyzing the examples, progression, and difficulties of HIoT research. This helps with coordinating evidence-based routes. Also, SLRs advance coordinated efforts and improve medical benefits development by sharing data among research organizations (Table 10.1).

With an ultimate objective to assist IoT's use in healthcare decision structures, a couple of nations have encouraged new projects and undertakings. Hence, healthcare data research was changed into a worthy area to investigate. This study means to give a layout of the state-of-the-art appraisals of IoT-based clinical networks and to give an examination of the affiliations, improvements, and applications that are appropriate to this field.

Different devices, sensors, and actuators that communicate online are associated with IoT. RFID innovations, wireless sensor networks (WSN), sensors for information assortment, complex calculations for information handling, and communication connection points are undeniably included. Additionally, cloud interfaces are included for accessing services [3].

Issues and arrangements: The Internet of Things faces various issues, like device heterogeneity, normalization, protection, security, and versatility. Clients now have the ability to pursue successful choices and conduct ongoing research closer to the framework thanks to haze processing, making it a potential solution for idleness, reliability, and asset limitations issues.

Participation: For consistent availability and communication between different gadgets and user frameworks, smart device collaboration is fundamental. Simple interoperability ensures economy and adaptability, easing future interactions with other users. 10.1

## 10.2 LITERATURE REVIEW

### 10.2.1 IoT in medical fields

The possibility of IoT was first introduced in 1999 by Kevin Ashton, who intended to relate things to the internet using RFID tags to work with more clear organization by laptops [4, 5]. IoT has been described in various ways as a hard copy. A couple of definitions highlight the accessibility strategies (e.g., RFID, remote sensor networks) that interface different things, while others revolve around the possibility of the genuine things (e.g., organizations and applications) and their application spaces, which consolidate magnificent city networks, traffic, trash, leaders, basic prosperity, safety, emergency services, factors that are composed, retail, current control, and medical care

*Table 10.1* Advantages and disadvantages of the categorization methods

| | *Sensor driven* | *Resource oriented* | *Communication oriented* | *Utilization driven* | *Security oriented* |
|---|---|---|---|---|---|
| Advantages | Better execution | Improved optimization | Improved performance | Better precision | Superior protection |
| | Increased output | Enhanced performance | Improved reliability | Enhanced inertness | More accuracy |
| | Improved cost | Improved vitality | Enhanced latency | Improved versatility | Reduced delay |
| Disadvantages | Bad protection | Inadequate flexibility | Dissatisfied cost | Dissatisfied interoperability | Inadequate flexibility |
| | Inadequate adaptability | Unsatisfactory protection | Dissatisfied with security | Dissatisfied with cost | Unsatisfactory protection |

While IoT is entrenched in various fields, it is at this point emerging in the healthcare industry, conceivable given the stringent rules managing healthcare affiliations. The advancement of wearable and phone technology has essentially impacted healthcare, changing customary systems into more tolerant and motivated models. This shift uses IoT improvements to make some separation from crisis facilities zeroed in, offering a more modified method for managing patient thought. IoT has modified the healthcare industry by setting out new entryways for reformed eHealth and mHealth organizations [2].

In healthcare, IoT implies an association of smart devices and real things connected to accumulate, screen, and control healthcare data. Sensors embedded in wearable articles (e.g., gloves, watches, glasses) networked through wired or wireless connections to tablets or phones, allowing fast access to patient data by the two experts and individuals [6].

A couple of researchers have featured the basic impact of IoT in healthcare. Authors have inspected how IoT has redesigned the board from a broad market survey, including supplier examination, advancement drivers, industry supply chains, and comparative assessments. Farahani et al. [7] saw that IoT has worked with computerization in clinical starters, giving significant experiences into healthcare. Holler et al. [8] fought that IoT has diminished healthcare expenses and incited new healthcare systems (Table 10.2).

Moreover, IoT has dealt with the utilitarian capability of healthcare affiliations. By using IoT advancements, clinical facilities have further developed information streams, overhauled communication with patients and their families, and facilitated patient data from various sources inside the organization.

*Table 10.2* The inspiration and studies questionnaire

| | *Question* | *Justification* |
|---|---|---|
| Q1 | What are the reasons why healthcare systems must incorporate IoT? | The article is to acquire understanding into what are the fundamental clarifications behind applying IoT in healthcare structures. |
| Q2 | What opportunities for IoT-based healthcare system research are currently available? In addition, what significant advancements in this field have been made? | The article is to have an impression of what research degrees are open in HIoT and the advantages and disadvantages of each. |
| Q3 | Which methods are currently being utilized to integrate the Internet of Things into the medical field? | The expectation is to recognize and examine existing components, methodologies, and contraptions that help HIoT. |
| Q4 | Which methods are currently being used to connect IOT to the medical field? | The plan is to uncover the investigation of open entryways and future opportunities in this field. |

### 10.2.2 Science-based investigation of exploration and patent fronts

The meaning of IoT in healthcare is projected to increase, with Gartner evaluating that the IoT device market will increase twofold [6]. HIoT can be developed for a fairly broad range of applications.

Ardito et al. [2] examined advancements in IoT and suggested that organizations, particularly in the telecom and information and communications technology sectors, tend to be more innovative than academic institutions, although the collaborative efforts between them are significant. Ceipek et al. [9] found that neglecting to measure up to expectations, firms will undoubtedly participate more in the emerging internet of things space.

Interest from specialists in IoT is also developing. Regardless, a transparent and reciprocal development of research and data among academics is creating progress in this domain.

At this point, there is no extensive review organizing what investigation has achieved so far from both spearheading and regulatory perspectives. This chapter hopes to address this opening using scientometric methodologies to analyze educational disseminations and patent data. Scientometrics incorporates the quantitative examination of intelligent data, including research, patents, clinical fundamentals, and grants. Salatino et al. [10] suggested a strategy that combines speech patterns and artificial intelligence to look at, monitor, and predict data flow among academia and industry. This chapter ponders designs in disseminations and patents to eliminate the investigation front.

The Bibliometrix R pack was used as the scientometric programming instrument [11]. Another audit of bibliometric programming instruments assumed that Bibliometrix stands separate for its scope of examinations and the convenience of its Biblioshiny web application. It continuously reviews the impact estimations of journals, makers, and records, and creates bibliometric associations to envision hypothetical, academic, and organizational structures. Bibliometrix carries out a long-term assessment (sudden recognition and effective progression), academic examination (spectroscopy/RPYS and historiography), and geospatial examination.

## 10.3 HEALTHCARE SYSTEMS

Healthcare systems are required in many areas, including remote medical monitoring, onsite monitoring, and verbal consultations. The following sections explore a few major areas where the healthcare system is much in demand.

### 10.3.1 Remote medical monitoring

The need for remote clinical testing has become increasingly obvious because of several factors, including the coronavirus pandemic, financial constraints, geographical limitations, and quarantine guidelines. For vulnerable groups, such as the elderly, and those with disabilities and chronic illnesses, it is difficult or impossible to visit medical facilities for routine examinations and treatment.

The necessity for easy-to-use and thorough PC-assisted development plans that can consistently monitor over the long term is rising as a result of these challenges. Medical services experts can utilize these advancements to screen their patients' important bodily functions, prescription intake, and well-being status from a distance, decreasing the requirement for in-person visits to clinics. Patients will be able to receive ongoing care and support from the comfort of their own homes with these remote monitoring systems, which will increase patients' overall satisfaction with their healthcare experience. In addition, remote clinical observation reduces medical care costs, increases asset productivity, and improves the arrangement of medical care's cost-effectiveness by reducing the need for subsequent clinic stays and ER visits.

### 10.3.2 IoT's function in healthcare

The way healthcare data is stored, analyzed, and used has undergone significant transformations due to the integration of IoT. Two of the essential utilizations of IoT in the medical care area are to work with the advancement of smart, prescient frameworks and to improve on the handling of immense amounts of information.

IoT makes it more straightforward to coordinate hardware, sensors, and gadgets in medical services settings. A connected network of devices that can gather, send, and process physiological data in real time is created as a result. Other vital signs and health indicators included in this data are breathing rate, heart rate, body temperature, blood sugar levels, and blood pressure. IoT-enabled devices can provide medical professionals with important insights into the state of health and trends of patients by continuously monitoring important physiological data. Clinical professionals can swiftly move, make early judgments, and begin treatment programs when atypical examples or deviations from benchmark values are identified right away.

In addition, ongoing observation enables patient-tailored therapies and lifestyle modifications to enhance outcomes and quality of life, making proactive treatment for chronic conditions possible. Notwithstanding its utilization, continuously checking IoT in medical services makes it conceivable to screen patients from a distance from patients' homes or networks as opposed to simply in conventional clinical settings. By cutting down the necessity for reiterated crisis facility stays and visits, this provides with steady comfort and convenience.

#### *10.3.2.1 IoT applications in healthcare*

The healthcare industry has seen a flood in creative applications that impact IoT development to move clinical investigation, improve your capacity to understand concepts and practical viability. Hospital management systems, home healthcare, and mobile healthcare (e-healthcare) are among the most widely used IoT applications in the healthcare industry [6]. Healthcare facilities can streamline administrative procedures, optimize resource allocation, and enhance patient flow by utilizing IoT-powered hospital management systems (Figure 10.1).

Functional productivity is improved by IoT-powered innovations that provide continuous information on clinic bed accessibility, staff and patient areas, and the utilization of clinical equipment like smart beds, resource global positioning systems, and constant area frameworks [7]. IoT is imperative for home healthcare since it makes telehealth, continuous monitoring, and remote monitoring possible. From the comfort of their homes, patients can screen their vitals, follow treatment regimens, and talk with healthcare providers because of related clinical devices, wearable sensors, and versatile applications. By reducing the need for clinic visits and readmissions, this

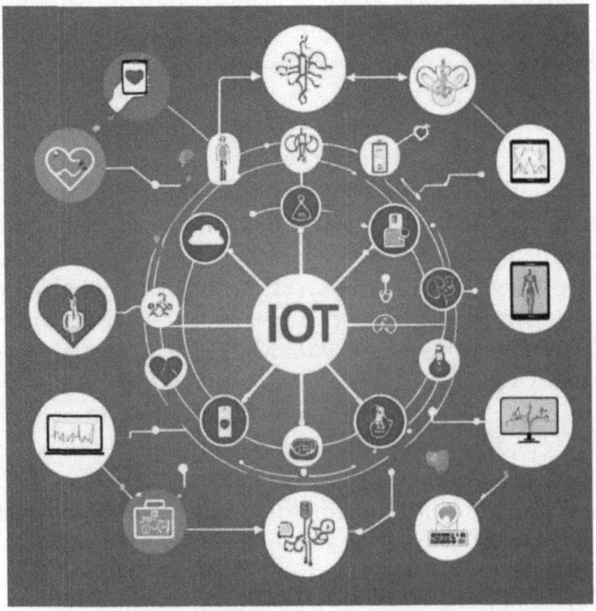


*Figure 10.1* IoT in healthcare use cases.

reduces the cost of medical care. IoT technology is used to provide medical services and information on mobile devices like smartphones and tablets in mobile healthcare. Clients can participate in telemedicine meetings with healthcare providers using portable health apps, access clinical records, make plans, and receive treatment updates wherever they are.

#### *10.3.2.2 Challenges in IoT healthcare*

Protection and security concerns are pivotal because medical services information is delicate and vulnerable to hacks, unapproved access, and cyberattacks. Several HIoT use cases are shown in Figure 10.2. Confounding issues further are standardization concerns, which thwart interoperability between IoT devices and structures due to the shortfall of uniform standards. Despite providing valuable health data, wearable technology and embedded sensors lack precision, consistency, and convenience. Due to compatibility issues and legacy systems, integrating IoT devices with existing hardware systems in healthcare facilities is difficult and costly. In addition, IoT structures need to adapt consistently to new determined prerequisites, clinical developments, and regulatory impediments. To overcome these obstacles, technology suppliers, regulatory agencies, and healthcare stakeholders must collaborate.

#### *10.3.2.3 Security procedures*

In the medical care area, with private patient information, areas of strength for critical conventions are fundamental for safeguarding delicate clinical information inside IoT frameworks. Among the many security methods used are k-anonymity, public-key crypto systems, encryption techniques, authentication protocols, and additional security features like access controls and intrusion detection systems.

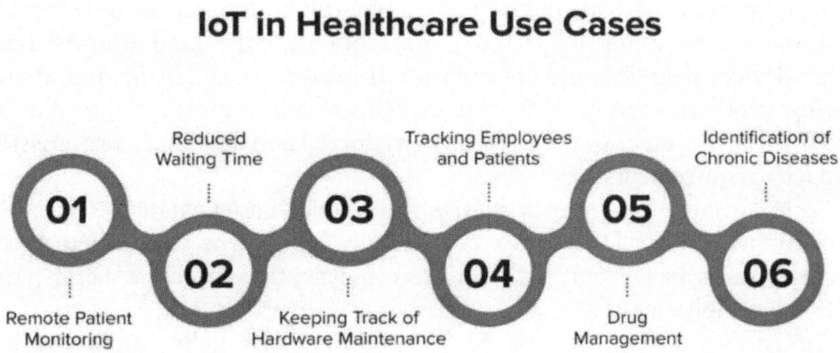


*Figure 10.2* IoT in healthcare use cases.

While k-anonymity anonymizes sensitive data to protect patient confidentiality, public-key cryptography ensures a secure connection and data transmission involving IoT devices and healthcare systems. Healthcare data is encrypted using techniques like AES to stop data leaks and illegal access. Additionally, authentication procedures verify the identities of users who access healthcare systems and IoT devices.

### 10.3.3 IoT devices and methods in healthcare

IoT devices and methods for HIoT projects are made up of various components, technologies, and procedures tailored to specific applications. With IoT in medical services, coming up next are a few fundamental components.

*Sensors and gadgets.* Countless sensors and gadgets for gathering information continuously are essential parts of HIoT. Wearable devices such as fitness trackers and smartwatches, medical devices such as glucose monitors and blood pressure cuffs, environmental sensors such as temperature, humidity, and air quality sensors, and even ingested sensors that can be used to monitor medication compliance or internal conditions are examples. Reliable connectivity is required for IoT devices to send data to centralized systems for analysis and processing. Wi-Fi, Bluetooth, Zigbee, and cellular networks are frequently utilized for this purpose. Using edge computing or gateway devices, data can also be preprocessed locally before being sent, reducing latency and bandwidth consumption.

*Conventions for information transmission.* To make it possible for IoT to be utilized in medical care, proficient conventions for information transmission are fundamental. To make communication between IoT gadgets and backend frameworks less complex, conventions like MQTT (Message Queuing Telemetry Transport), CoAP (Constrained Application Protocol), and HTTP (Hypertext Transfer Protocol) are oftentimes used. Cloud computing is used by a lot of IoT medical care applications for data storage, management, and analysis. Medical care associations can oversee gigantic measures of information and gain significant bits of knowledge on account of cloud frameworks' availability and adaptability. In circumstances where ongoing handling and low latency are required, edge computing is used. Edge devices near IoT sensors preprocess local data by sifting and aggregating it before sending it to frameworks. While improving information security and protection, this method reduces inertness and transmission capacity requirements.

*Security and protection of information.* Since patient data is so important to medical services, secure access points should be established. HIoT security relies heavily on authentication, encryption, access controls, and HIPAA compliance.

*Integration with electronic health records (EHRs).* By combining IoT data with existing electronic health record systems, healthcare providers can access comprehensive patient information through a unified interface. This integration facilitates care continuity across multiple healthcare facilities, simplifies clinical decision-making, and enhances care coordination.

### 10.3.4 Data collection using IoT devices

IoT changed data grouping in the healthcare industry, considering steady, reliable checking of assets, patients, and normal factors. Related with networks and furnished with sensors, IoT devices accumulate a large amount of data that is influencing the way in which health benefits are communicated, dealing with test results, and growing final sufficiency. Remote monitoring is a key use case for the HIoT. Health-related data is continuously collected by IoT devices like wearables, implanted sensors, and home monitoring systems. Medical services experts can utilize this continuous information to remotely screen patients' well-being, recognize abnormalities early, and attempt to lower emergency clinic readmission rates and work on understanding patient satisfaction.

Additionally, IoT-engaged clinical staff members work on caregiving and enhance assignments in crisis centers. Smart medication pumps, for example, can screen drug dose and organization and alert doctors to any errors or abnormalities. For instance, ventilators and cardiovascular screens that are connected to IoT can send data directly to EHRs, providing current and accurate data for clinical navigation. Patient care in healthcare facilities is made simpler by IoT. RFID tags and IoT sensors track the whereabouts and conditions of medications, clinical supplies, preventing thefts and errors, and guaranteeing brief maintenance and restocking.

Environmental monitoring is yet another crucial component of IoT in healthcare. Temperature, humidity, and air quality can be monitored by sensors in healthcare facilities to maintain optimal conditions for patient comfort, infection control, and the storage of sensitive goods like pharmaceuticals and vaccines. However, as IoT devices develop, so does the difficulty of managing and protecting the enormous amounts of data they generate in healthcare. In order to ensure that information is safeguarded, secure, and compliant with regulations like HIPAA, healthcare organizations ought to have administration rules for their areas of strength. In addition, healthcare organizations must invest in data analytics capabilities in order to gain useful insights from the vast amount of data generated by IoT. This will allow for decision-making and customized care to individual patients.

### 10.3.5 Data analysis using IoT devices

Information examination in IoT medical services involves handling and deciphering the huge amounts of information created by IoT gadgets to deliver significant bits of knowledge for improving decisions, well-being, and medical services results. A description of IoT healthcare data assessment is given next.

*Information assortment.* In the medical services area, IoT gadgets continually gather various information, including patient vitals, drug adherence, encompassing factors, and action levels. With the end goal of investigation and capacity, this information is transmitted through networks.

*Information preprocessing.* Preprocessing is frequently performed to clean, channel, and standardize the crude information from IoT gadgets before they are analyzed. Preprocessing procedures include fixing missing values, getting rid of outliers, and formatting the data so that it is ready for analysis.

The process of analyzing and displaying data in order to identify past patterns and trends is known as descriptive analytics. Strategies like information perception, dashboards, and run-down measurements are used in medical care settings to provide an unmistakable picture of past events and current circumstances.

*Prescient investigation.* Prescient investigation projects future occasions by using AI calculations and verifiable information. In IoT medical care, prescient examination can be utilized to anticipate disease spread, recognize patients in danger, estimate asset interest, and foresee hardware failures.

*Prescriptive examination.* This sort of investigation goes beyond determining and prescribing activities or medicines to take advantage of results. Prescriptive analytics provides relevant insights to healthcare professionals that help them make better decisions and provide better patient care by combining domain expertise, business principles, and historical data.

*Alarms and continuous monitoring.* IoT data analysis constantly takes natural and patient well-being status monitoring into account. Calculations can continuously break down web-based information from IoT devices to identify irregularities, send alarms for critical events (such as falls or abnormal vital signs), and initiate appropriate medications. Personalized medicine is made possible by data analysis in HIoT, which helps to identify distinct patient characteristics, preferences, and treatment responses. To alter treatment regimens, drug dosages, and interventions for additional created results and patient satisfaction, computer-based intelligence models break down persistent data. IoT data analysis powers clinical decision support systems (CDSS), which provide physicians with guidelines and recommendations based on evidence during care. CDSS helps medical professionals analyze ailments, select the most effective treatment plans, and avoid clinical errors. In HIoT, data analysis, which identifies population-level trends and patterns, and aids population health management initiatives. Healthcare organizations use analytics to target interventions, identify populations at high risk, and segment the population to improve patient outcomes and cut costs.

*Nonstop improvement.* Medical services offices can assess the viability of their processes, strategies, and therapies by persistently gathering and dissecting IoT information. By assessing execution measurements and results, associations can recognize areas for development, smooth out techniques, and steadily increase the expectation of care given.

#### *10.3.5.1 Scientific output*

The huge ascent in IoT use in the medical care area throughout recent years is an indication of the developing interest in using IoT innovations to address medical care issues. It is easier to advance knowledge and innovations in this sector thanks to the efforts of researchers and practitioners from a variety of fields, such as public health, computer science, engineering, and medicine.

*Research papers.* There has been a steady increase in the number of IoT-related research papers, publications, and conference proceedings. These are important components of the scientific output in IoT healthcare. IoT-powered clinical gear, remote monitoring, prescient examination, security and protection, and medical services framework improvement are only a couple of the numerous points canvassed in these papers.

*Interdisciplinary cooperation.* The interdisciplinary joint effort of designers, information researchers, strategy specialists, and medical services professionals is a typical part of IoT medical care research. Researchers can approach difficult healthcare issues from various perspectives and offer comprehensive solutions when they collaborate across disciplines.

*Novel advances.* The production of novel advancements and cures is aided by logical examination of IoT medical services. This covers advancements in edge computing, wearable development expected for healthcare applications, remote meetings, sensor advances, and artificial intelligence. To determine whether IoT-based healthcare therapies are user-friendly, safe, and effective, researchers conduct clinical trials and evaluations. The effect of IoT innovation on understanding results, medical care communication, and affordability is upheld by these investigations.

*Policy and regulation in healthcare.* Policy and regulatory aspects like data security, privacy, interoperability, and reimbursement are also covered in scientific research on IoT healthcare. To guarantee that IoT technologies are used in a responsible and ethical manner in healthcare, researchers are involved in the development of rules, standards, and laws.

*Contextual analyses and best practices.* These assets feature IoT applications that have been carried out effectively in medical services settings. These examples demonstrate how IoT technology could improve patient care, streamline medical service delivery, and improve clinical work processes.

*Preparation and instruction.* To instruct scientists, specialists, and medical care professionals about IoT advancements and applications, the logical development of IoT medical services incorporates instructional materials such as course readings, courses, and studios.

*Coordinated effort and global systems administration.* The logical outcome of IoT medical services is driven by global systems administration and establishment-to-school collaboration. Collaboration, skill sharing, and dissemination of research findings are made simpler by international groups, consortiums, and research networks.

*Emerging trends and future directions.* Through scientific production, IoT healthcare research and innovation can identify emerging trends and future directions. Edge simulated intelligence, blockchain, telemedicine, and accurate medication are standing out enough to be noticed by scholars as they research new IoT medical care applications and potential outcomes.

#### 10.3.5.2 Trending subject

The integration of IoT, artificial intelligence (AI), and machine learning (ML) technologies is one of the most popular IoT topics in the healthcare industry. This union is driving development and modifying the communication of medical services in various ways. By looking at the data that has been collected from IoT devices, prescient examination and ML calculations can identify examples and patterns that highlight early signs of illnesses or declining health. Because of this, medical professionals can go to great lengths to avoid or minimize negative health effects. Many patient-specific data, such as vital signs, medication adherence, and lifestyle choices, are generated by IoT devices, which can be used for personalized medicine and treatment optimization. By looking at this data, PC-based knowledge and ML estimations can smooth out suitability and diminish coincidental impacts by modifying treatment regimens, drug estimations, and interventions to resolve the issues of each and every patient.

AI-powered IoT devices make it easier for healthcare providers to remotely monitor their patients' health status in real time, making telemedicine and remote patient monitoring easier. With the help of artificial intelligence algorithms, streaming data from IoT devices can be analyzed to find anomalies, set off alarms, and aid in the decision-making process for remote consultations and interventions. IoT devices and sensors with AI capabilities improve the sustainability and effectiveness of healthcare facilities. Smart healthcare facilities and operational efficiency AI can be used by predictive maintenance algorithms to analyze data from IoT devices to anticipate issues, plan maintenance ahead of time, and optimize energy use, all of which cut down on downtime and operating costs.

Two examples of IoT devices that are transforming patient care and rehabilitation are smart prosthetics and robotic assistants. Medical care robots with artificial intelligence fueled assistive advances. Using IoT information and artificial intelligence calculations, these gadgets improve the freedom and personal satisfaction of patients by helping them with day-to-day errands, versatility, and recovery workouts. Data security and assurance are fundamental since progressively more IoT devices are gathering private health information. Anomaly detection and behavioral analytics are two AI-driven technologies that help to identify and mitigate cybersecurity risks in IoT healthcare ecosystems, safeguard patient data, and comply with legal requirements.

*Morals and guidelines.* Various moral and administrative issues emerge when artificial intelligence and IoT are joined in the medical care area. Informed consent, responsibility, straight-forwardness, and decreasing inclination are some of these issues. Research and discussions are being conducted to establish administration structures, moral standards, and authoritative standards to address these issues and ensure capable human knowledge in medical services.

#### 10.3.5.3 Conceptual framework

A calculated system for IoT gives a coordinated strategy to grasp, sort out, and put IoT innovations and applications into utilization in the medical services area. It provides a guide for thinking about, creating, and evaluating IoT-enabled healthcare systems while considering a wide range of things, including technology, stakeholders, procedures, and outcomes. An overview of the essential components of an IoT healthcare conceptual framework can be found next:

> *Objectives.* The structure ought to begin by defining the precise objectives of incorporating IoT into the medical care industry. This could incorporate cutting down healthcare, raising utilitarian practicality, growing patient outcomes, and dealing with consistent experience. Examine techniques for consolidating, joining, and incorporating information from different sources, for example, clinical imaging frameworks and electronic EHRs [12], and IoT gadgets. Consider data formats, data governance guidelines, and interoperability standards to ensure seamless integration and high-quality data.

*Stakeholders and roles.* Find out who's important to IoT healthcare projects. These organizations consolidate directors, IT prepared experts, patients, carers, and managerial associations. In the IoT system, depict their connections, obligations, and capabilities. Examine the different medical services IoT applications and use cases, for example, telemedicine, drug adherence monitoring, smart medical care offices, prescient investigation, and remote monitoring. Give scenarios and examples of how IoT technologies could be used to deal with specific healthcare issues and enhance patient care delivery. Discuss the role that information analysis and information from IoT-generated data play in the decision-making process for medical services. To comprehend health trends, predict outcomes, direct therapeutic treatments, and emphasize the importance of descriptive, predictive, and prescriptive analytics.

*Security and insurance.* Examine the security and security issues connecting with IoT healthcare systems. Talk about the requirements for information security, such as HIPAA and GDPR, consistency, access control, validation, encryption of data in transmission and storage, and device security for IoT. Examine the legal requirements and moral quandaries associated with IoT in healthcare and other aspects of ethics and regulation. Discuss issues such as patient consent, information possession, accountability, simplicity, and reducing predisposition in AI-based decisions. Assess the effectiveness, sufficiency, and proficiency of medical care frameworks enabled by IoT by characterizing appraisal models and execution indicators. Consider regulatory compliance indicators, clinical process efficacy, cost savings, user satisfaction, and patient outcomes. Communicating with IoT medical services, discuss the latest advancements in edge computer-based intelligence, blockchain, interoperability, adaptability, supportability, and different areas of interest. Deciding the areas where IoT for medical services requires imagination, coordinated effort, and extra exploration.

## 10.4 PROPOSED WORK

The proposed work hopes to address the essential openings and troubles recognized in current HIoT structures through a systematic literature review. The fundamental spotlight is on redesigning the process, security, adaptability, and energy efficiency of HIoT systems by using state-of-the-art advancements and creative ways of thinking. This assessment means to make a strong, secure, and useful HIoT climate that can deal with the needs of present-day healthcare organizations.

### 10.4.1 Further developing security and protection

Security and assurance are priorities in HIoT structures in light of sensitive healthcare data. This work will focus on making broad security plans to further develop trust, assurance, access control, protection, and data authenticity. A trust that the chief build is capable of changing trust levels considering the approach to acting and the participation history of devices to ensure a safeguarded environment. Significant level encryption procedures and fine-grained permission control parts will be executed to safeguard sensitive healthcare data from unauthorized access. Also, security saving computations will be expected to restrict data transparency, ensuring that relevant components can access or deal with health information. This will assist with manufacturing a strong HIoT structure that clients and healthcare providers can trust.

### 10.4.2 Further developing execution and flexibility

Execution upgrade and flexibility are vital for the overall gathering of HIoT structures. This assessment will focus on brainstorming capable resource task strategies and workload estimations to improve system execution. By changing the functions among IoT devices, bottlenecks can be thwarted, and response times quickened. Load changing estimations will be made to disperse tasks consistently across the association, ensuring ideal execution fundamentally under changing problems. Likewise, methodologies to lessen latency in data transmission will be completed to ensure consistent responsiveness in essential healthcare applications. These upgrades will make HIoT structures more trustworthy and fit for managing extended loads, thus chipping away at their flexibility and accommodation in healthcare settings.

## 10.5 EXPERIMENTAL FINDINGS

IoT devices make it possible to continuously monitor patients' vital bodily functions and health status from a distance. Remote monitoring has been shown to work with the management of chronic conditions, lessen clinic readmission, help in the early diagnosis of medical problems, and increase patient cooperation in taking care of oneself.

*Prescient investigation for diseases.* By combining advanced research with data from the IoT, it is possible to predict whether patients are infected. By identifying patients at high risk, predicting the progression of a disease, and optimizing treatment plans, studies indicate that predictive analytics can enhance clinical outcomes and resource allocation. IoT advancements are making medical service offices into smart environments by giving robotized frameworks to resource following, health checking, and office management. Research shows that smart healthcare facilities simplify workflow procedures, use less energy, work more efficiently, and make patients safer.

*Wearable health devices.* Smart watches, fitness trackers, and medical wearables are examples of wearable IoT devices that continuously monitor users' activity levels and health indicators. Wearable well-being gadgets, as indicated by research, work with early disease intervention, alert precaution medical services, support active work, and work with behavior change.

*Telemedicine and remote meetings.* Stages for telemedicine enabled by the IoT enable patients and healthcare specialists to communicate from a distance. According to the findings, telemedicine increases patient satisfaction, lowers healthcare costs, broadens access to healthcare services, and enables prompt interventions, particularly in disadvantaged areas.

*Issues with information protection and security.* In spite of IoT's advantages for medical services, worries about information protection and security persist. Research highlights that to protect private health information and diminish organization well-being risks, it is fundamental to put strong internet-based insurance confirmations, encryption procedures, access controls, and authoritative consistency into place. The integration of IoT data with EHRs improves patient information interoperability and accessibility across healthcare frameworks. When EHR integration provides comprehensive and current patient data, clinical decision-making, patient outcomes, and care coordination benefit. Concerns about patient consent, data ownership, accountability, and transparency are raised by IoT in healthcare. Research emphasizes the significance of patient empowerment, ethical data use, and informed consent in IoT-driven healthcare projects.

### 10.5.1 Publications and patents in IoT in healthcare

Indicators of innovation, research effort, and technological advancement in IoT in healthcare are patents and publications. An understanding of the scope, complexity, and patterns in this quickly developing field can be gained by looking at both articles and patents (Figure 10.3 and Table 10.3).

#### *10.5.1.1 IoT patents in the medical field*

*Mechanical developments.* Patents cover new devices, systems, estimates, and methods as well as extraordinary manifestations and advancements in HIoT. Data assessment stages, wearable innovations, clinical sensors, and remote checking systems are only a couple of instances of these progressions.

*Trends in the market and commercialization.* Patent applications demonstrate that businesses are investing in IoT healthcare and are interested in it. To protect their innovations and gain an advantage, new companies, educational establishments, and organizations submit patent applications. Through examination of patent information, designs in the IoT medical care market, key parts, and advancements in assembling are found. IoT clinical patent applications are recorded in many countries. The distribution of patent activity in IoT healthcare can reveal innovation clusters, collaboration networks, and regional strengths.

*Partnerships and collaboration.* Jointly filed patents and co-authored patents are two clear examples of collaboration between organizations. Progress is accelerated, and academic institutions, government organizations, advancement organizations, and healthcare providers are advancing the new development and use of HIoT. HIoT research is based on emerging

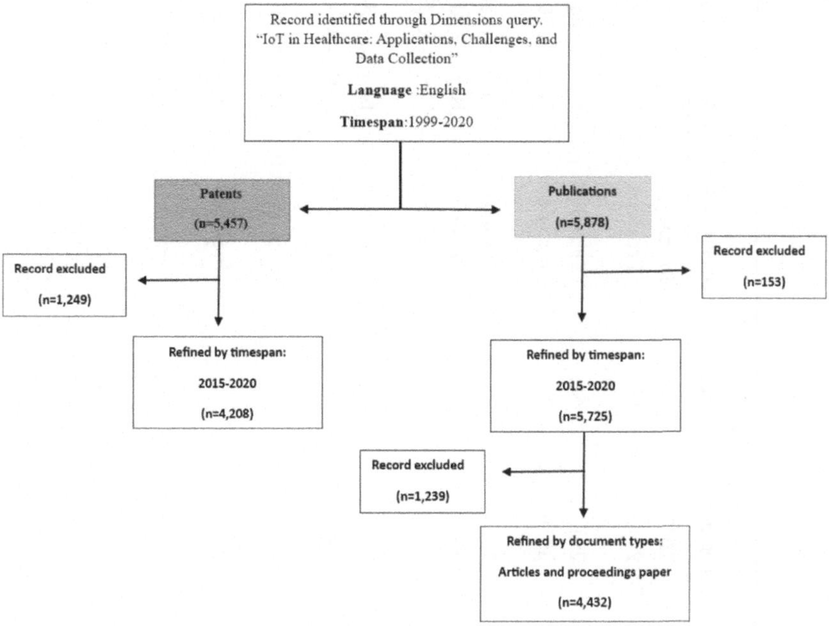


*Figure 10.3* Record of publications and patents.

advances and areas highlighted by patent data. Several examples of these upgrades integrate wearable sensor development, machine learning-driven assessment, edge computing, blockchain for health data, and IoT-engaged clinical devices for diagnosis and treatment.

#### *10.5.1.2 IoT publications in the healthcare field*

Academic papers provide significant perspectives on the state of examination, the availability of new devices, and mechanical advancements in IoT medical care. Researchers share their findings and spread data to increase the knowledge of IoT in healthcare by dispersing their research in educational correspondence, collecting techniques, and peer-reviewed journals (Figure 10.4).

*Collaboration across disciplines.* Research of IoT in healthcare incorporates knowledge from public health, engineering, computer science, medicine, and data analytics. Scientists from different fields team up to improve the research environment, encourage development, and accelerate the interpretation of study discoveries into common-sense applications. Inspecting the distributed information uncovers an assortment of IoT medical care to concentrate on subjects and areas of need. A few examples of models include personalized medicine, telemedicine, the smart medical care

*Table 10.3* Summary of HIoT-related surveys

| *Sort of review* | *Reference* | *Primary subject* | *Year of publication* | *Classification process* | *Open problem* | *Year covered* |
|---|---|---|---|---|---|---|
| Surveys | Farahani et al. (2018) | e-Health powered by fog in IoT | 2017 | No | Not provided | Not stated |
| | Darwish et al. (2017) | Cloud computing and internet of things | 2017 | No | Provided | Not stated |
| | Qi et al. (2017) | IoT for custom medical care | 2017 | No | Provided | Not stated |
| | Qi et al. (2018) | IoT healthcare: Identifying and tracking physical activity | 2018 | No | Provided | 2008–2018 |
| | Dhanvijay and Patil (2019) | IoT-based medical technology | 2019 | Yes | Provided | Not stated |
| | Habibzadeh et al. (2020) | IoT for healthcare | 2019 | No | Provided | Not stated |
| | Alam et al. (2018) | Connectivity tools in IoT for Healthcare | 2019 | No | Provided | Not stated |
| | Ray et al. (2019b) | HIoT edge computing | 2019 | Yes | Provided | Not stated |
| | Qadri et al. (2020) | New developments in the field of IoT | 2020 | Yes | Provided | Not stated |
| | Somasundaram and Thirugnanam (2020) | HIoT security problems | 2020 | No | Not provided | Not stated |
| | Kadhim et al. (2020) | IoT based patient health monitoring system | 2020 | No | Provided | Not stated |
| SLRs | Ahmed et al. (2018) | IoT security cloud-based electronic healthcare | 2018 | Yes | Provided | 2009–2017 |
| | Ahmadi et al. (2018) | IoT applications in healthcare | 2018 | Yes | Provided | 2000–2016 |
| | Saheb and Izadi (2019) | Fog computing and big data analytics in IoT | 2019 | Yes | Provided | 2014–2018 |

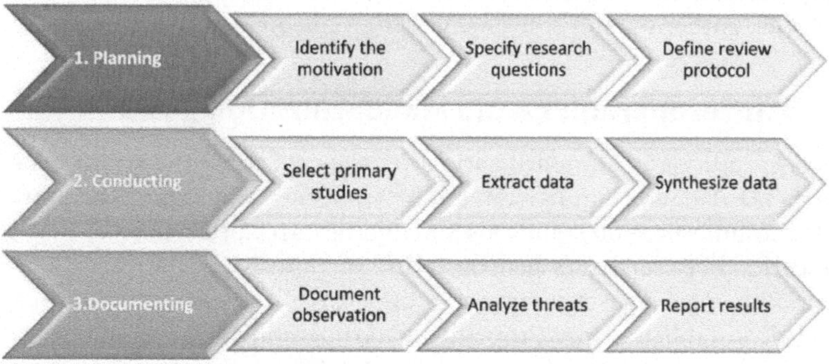


*Figure 10.4* An overview of proposed methodology.

framework, tests for sick patients, remote patient observation, and moral issues with IoT reception.

*Knowledge sharing and open access.* By enabling researchers to collaborate more effectively and openly share their findings, the open-access movement has made it easier for people to learn about science. Open-access journals, preprint articles, and websites all work with logical dispersal, speed up logical revelation, and advance exploration openness.

## 10.6 INFERENCES

### 10.6.1 Security and insurance concerns

The investigation shows that security and assurance are major concerns in HIoT systems. The sensitive thought of healthcare data requires the execution of strong security frameworks to shield against unapproved access and data breaches. Trustworthy networks, secure level encryption, and fine-grained access control are fundamental to ensuring data grouping and integrity. The progress of assurance shielding computations is key to restrict data receptiveness, highlighting the meaning of staying aware of patient trust in HIoT systems.

### 10.6.2 Execution and flexibility challenges

Execution improvement and versatility are fundamental for the successful working of HIoT structures. Resource allocation and workload distribution are essential to prevent bottlenecks and improve response times. The investigation features the prerequisite for frameworks with suitable positions consistent across the network and methodologies to diminish latency, ensuring steady responses. These overhauls are basic for making HIoT systems strong and fit for dealing with extended loads, which is central for their wide gathering and convenience in grouped healthcare settings.

### 10.6.3 Interoperability and standardization goals

Interoperability and standardization are important for the steady blend of various HIoT devices and systems. The assessment highlights the prerequisite for communication standards and middleware applications to fuse communication between heterogeneous HIoT structures. Standardized APIs are essential to engage basic compromise of new devices and systems into existing HIoT establishments. Propelling interoperability and standardization is essential for making a firm and useful HIoT environment prepared for acclimating to new developments and devices.

## 10.7 CONCLUSION

Overall, IoT innovations in the medical services area involve a critical change in perspective that will affect patient care, healthcare organizations, and medical care communication overall. The movement and experience of healthcare could be different with IoT-enabled systems, like wearable sensors and telehealth organizations. By using consistent information, consistent association, and customized interventions, IoT empowers healthcare providers to make educated decisions, improve work processes, and achieve better results. Regardless, like any development, there are difficulties in executing IoT in the healthcare industry. Protecting patient insurance and keeping up with data integrity continues to depend on ensuring data security, interoperability, and regulatory consistency. Errors in admission to IoT-powered medical services arrangements must also be addressed to guarantee widespread access to fair care delivery. Overcoming these obstructions and understanding the most extreme limits of HIoT will require supportive assessment, progress, and key alliances. IoT-enabled healthcare courses of action, developments, examples, and future bearings will continue to be assembled from SLRs and reliable assessment surveys. Using the IoT's groundbreaking potential, the medical care industry can make a more interconnected, proficient, and patient-focused care environment that empowers individuals to live longer, better lives.

## REFERENCES

1. Ankrah, S.N., Burgess, T.F., Grimshaw, P., Shaw, N.E., 2013. Asking both university and industry actors about their engagement in knowledge transfer: what single-group studies of motives omit. *Technovation* 33 (2–3), 50–65.

2. Ardito, L., D'Adda, D., Messeni Petruzzeli, A., 2018. Mapping innovation dynamics in the internet of things domain: evidence from patent analysis. *Technol. Forecast. Soc. Chang.* 136, 317–330.
3. Ashton, K., 1999. An introduction to the Internet of Things (IoT). *RFID J.* 22 (7), 97–114.
4. Bandyopadhyay, D., Sen, J., 2011. Internet of things: Applications and challenges in technology and standardization. *Wirel. Pers. Commun.* 58 (1), 49–69.
5. Bhatt, Y., Bhatt, C., 2017. Internet of things in healthcare. In N. Dey, and A. S. Ashour (Eds.) *Internet of things and big data technologies for next generation HealthCare* (pp. 13–33). Springer, Cham.
6. Egham, 2017. Gartner says 8.4 billion connected "Things" will be in use in 2017, up 31 percent from 2016. *Gartner Newsroom*. Retrieved from http://www.gartner.com /newsroom.
7. Farahani, B., Firouzi, F., Chang, V., Badaroglu, M., Constant, N., Mankodiya, K., 2018. Towards fog-driven IoT eHealth: promises and challenges of IoT in medicine and healthcare. *Futur. Gener. Comput. Syst.* 78, 659–676.
8. Holler, J., Tsiatsis, V., Mulligan, C., Avesand, S., Karnouskos, S., Boyle, D., 2014. *From machine-to-machine to the Internet of Things: Introduction to a new age of intelligence*. Academic Press Inc.
9. Ceipek, R., Hautz, J., Petruzzelli, A.M., De Massis, A., Matzler, K., 2021. A motivation and ability perspective on engagement in emerging digital technologies: The case of internet of things solutions. *Long Range Plan.* 54 (5), 101991.
10. Salatino, A., Osborne, F., Motta, E., 2020, September. Researchflow: Understanding the knowledge flow between academia and industry. International Conference on Knowledge Engineering and Knowledge Management. Springer, Cham, pp. 219–236.
11. Chatterjee, S., Chatterjee, S., Choudhury, S., Basak, S., Dey, S., Sain, S., Sircar, S., 2017, October. Internet of things and body area network-an integrated future. 2017 IEEE 8th Annual Ubiquitous Computing, Electronics and Mobile Communication Conference (UEMCON). IEEE, pp. 396–400.
12. Aria, M., Cuccurullo, C., 2017. bibliometrix: An R-tool for comprehensive science mapping analysis. *J. Informetrics* 11 (4), 959–975.

Chapter 11

# Revolutionizing healthcare

## Cutting-edge technologies and their applications

*Silky Sharma, Nagaraj Subbarao, Shankar Kumar Jha, and Steve McKenna*

### 11.1 INTRODUCTION

The pivotal role of technology in healthcare profoundly shapes modern medical practices, fundamentally transforming how we diagnose, treat, and manage health conditions. Enhanced diagnostics are a key contribution, with sophisticated devices like MRI and CT scanners providing high-resolution images for early disease detection and precise abnormality identification. Artificial intelligence further augments this process by analyzing vast medical datasets to identify patterns beyond human observation, resulting in quicker diagnoses and better treatment outcomes. Technological advances revolutionize treatment methods, with minimally invasive robotic procedures reducing surgical trauma and recovery time. Gene therapy offers promising treatments at the genetic level, enhancing effectiveness and reducing physical demands on patients. Additionally, electronic health records (EHRs) streamline patient care by centralizing medical histories (Jensen, Jensen, & Brunak, 2012), facilitating informed decision-making, and eliminating the need for bulky medical records. Telemedicine expands access to care through remote consultations, benefiting individuals in remote areas or with limited mobility. Technology also empowers patients in health management. Mobile health apps enable monitoring of vitals, medication adherence, and appointment scheduling, while wearable devices provide real-time data on heart rate, sleep patterns, and activity levels. This fosters preventative healthcare practices and a sense of ownership over one's health.

In the modern world, today's significance of using technology in the healthcare industry helps in numerous ways, and these technological advances are transforming healthcare, offering promising benefits for society as a whole (refer to Table 11.1).

#### 11.1.1 The intention and scope of this chapter

The main aim of this chapter is to examine the latest developments and trends in healthcare technology and their impact on healthcare delivery,

 DOI: 10.1201/9781003634089-11

*Table 11.1* Healthcare technology and devices

| *Healthcare segment* | *Healthcare technology* | *Devices used* | *Outcome* |
|---|---|---|---|
| **Improved diagnostics** | High-resolution medical imaging | X-rays, CT scans, and MRIs aid | Early and accurate disease detection, facilitating timely interventions and better patient outcomes |
| **Enhanced treatment** | Innovations in minimally invasive procedures | Robotic-assisted surgery and gene therapy | Precise and effective treatment options, improving surgical accuracy and patient recovery |
| **Better patient care** | Electronic health records (EHRs) | Epic, Oracle Cerner, MEDITECH, CPSI, ambulatory or outpatient EHR systems | Improves care coordination and communication by providing efficient storage and retrieval of patient information |
| **Disease prevention and management** | Wearable devices and remote monitoring tools | Activity tracker, smart clothing, smart watches like Fitbit, Smart Jewellery such as AI-based Health and Fitness Rings, Bracelets and so on. | Promoting proactive health maintenance by self-tracking health vitals and managing chronic conditions effectively |

patient outcomes, and the future of medicine. It covers advancements in artificial intelligence (AI), machine learning (ML), telehealth, 3D printing, augmented reality (AR) and virtual reality (VR) in healthcare, blockchain technology, big data analytics, robotics, and automation, highlighting their influence on diagnostics, treatment, patient care, and public health.

The first part of this chapter outlines the history of technological advances in healthcare. This section traces significant technological milestones, from the discovery of X-rays in 1895 to contemporary innovations like robotic-assisted surgery, illustrating the rapid pace of advancement. In addition, it covers the phase of rapid advancement in technology related to healthcare that took place in the 19th and 20th centuries, such as the development of anesthesia, modern infectious disease control, and vaccinations. In the 20th century, in particular, there was an explosion of innovations such as the discovery of antibiotics like penicillin and the development of imaging technologies like MRI and CT scans that revolutionized diagnostics in healthcare. Innovations such as EHRs and telemedicine are also considered as digital innovations in healthcare.

The second part of the chapter investigates, in detail, a number of the latest healthcare technologies. These technologies, along with their applications, examples, and implementation, are described. The scope of this discussion is limited to the benefits and revolutionary impacts of these technologies, rather than a consideration of their limitations. The evolution of healthcare technologies is an ongoing process and constantly developing through research and practice in healthcare.

## 11.2 History of technological advances in healthcare

Technological advances in healthcare span centuries, and have consistently revolutionized diagnosis, treatment, and patient care. Ancient civilizations, such as the Egyptians, Greeks, and Romans, made significant contributions in developing surgical tools, herbal remedies, and observational techniques, laying the foundations for the future evolution of medical knowledge. The Hippocratic Oath from ancient Greece established early ethical principles for physicians.

The Renaissance period in Europe marked a resurgence of scientific inquiry and innovation in healthcare. Anatomical studies by Leonardo da Vinci and Andreas Vesalius provided unprecedented insights into human anatomy, improving diagnosis and surgical procedures. The 17th-century invention of the microscope by Antonie van Leeuwenhoek revolutionized microbiology, enabling the discovery of pathogens and advancing disease understanding. By the 18th century, efforts toward health technology assessment (HTA) began (Andrew, Milne, and Burls, 2003), evaluating the value of treatments and tests, a practice that continues to be essential today.

### *11.2.1 Phase of rapid advancement in technology related to healthcare*

The 19th and 20th centuries saw rapid advances in medical technology driven by scientific discoveries and industrialization in manufacturing for medical devices and support systems. The development of anesthesia, pioneered by William Morton and others, revolutionized surgery by alleviating pain and enabling complex procedures. Louis Pasteur's germ theory of disease laid the groundwork for modern infectious disease control and vaccination. The 20th century witnessed an explosion of technological and other innovations that transformed healthcare. The discovery of antibiotics, such as penicillin by Alexander Fleming, revolutionized the treatment of bacterial infections. Imaging technologies like X-rays, MRI, and CT scans revolutionized diagnostics, allowing for non-invasive visualization of internal structures.

The digital revolution of the late 20th and early 21st centuries offered opportunities for new developments in healthcare. EHRs, telemedicine, and wearable devices have enhanced communication, efficiency, patient monitoring, and the collection of enormous amounts of data for use in further research. AI and machine learning are increasingly being utilized for diagnostics, drug discovery, and personalized medicine, promising to further revolutionize healthcare delivery. Thus, the history of technological advances in healthcare is a long and continuous one, with some notable milestones including:

- **1895, X-ray discovery**: Wilhelm Röntgen's discovery of X-rays revolutionized medical imaging, allowing for the visualization of bones and internal structures (Mould, 1995; Pasveer, 2006).
- **1928, Penicillin discovery**: Alexander Fleming's discovery of penicillin ushered in the era of antibiotics, drastically reducing mortality rates from infectious diseases (Brown, 2005).
- **1953, DNA structure discovery**: James Watson and Francis Crick's discovery of the DNA double helix paved the way for advances in genetics and personalized medicine (Davies, 2002; Bansal, Kaushik, & Kukreti, 2022).
- **1971, First CT scan**: The invention of the CT scanner marked a significant leap in medical imaging, providing detailed cross-sectional views of the body (Rubin, 2014).
- **1990s, Minimally invasive surgery**: The development of laparoscopic surgery techniques allowed for smaller incisions and faster recovery times for patients (Ahmed et al., 2011).
- **2011**: Fingerprint sensing on mobile device (Bojinov et al., 2014).
- **2019**: Telehealth solutions, a high-quality video powered by 5G (Albreem, 2015) assist patients and clinicians in establishing a rapid and precise connection.

The history of technological advances in healthcare as given in Figure 11.1 highlights human ingenuity and the relentless pursuit of improvement in medical care. From ancient civilizations to the digital age, each era has progressed innovations in ways that have saved lives, alleviated suffering, and enhanced the quality of healthcare globally. As technology continues to evolve, the future of healthcare holds immense potential for further advances. Current applications of these technologies are revolutionizing patient treatment, surgeries, data management, and long-term health record tracking, providing personalized guidance and better control for future healthcare outcomes.

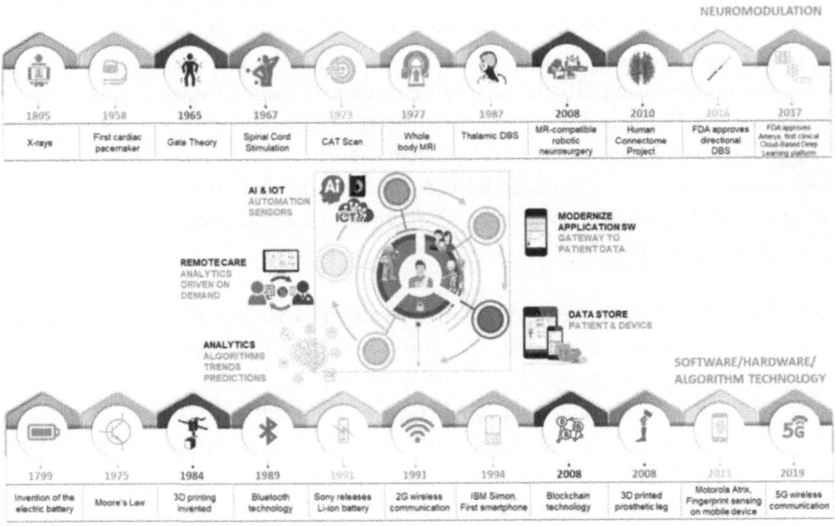


*Figure 11.1* Evolution of technology leading to the age of digital healthcare iterative advances. (Source: "Digital Health Integration with Neuromodulation Therapies: The Future of Patient-Centric Innovation in Neuromodulation," Scientific Figure on ResearchGate. Available from: https://www.researchgate.net/figure/Evolution-of-technology-leading-to-the-age-of-digital-healthcare-Iterative-advances-in_fig1_351700276.)

### *11.2.2 Revolutionizing healthcare technologies in the 21st century*

The COVID-19 pandemic compelled many industries, including education and healthcare, to undergo rapid changes leading to threat to the concept of Sharing Economy in special reference to global supply chains (Meahjohn & Persad, 2020) and unsustainable just-in-time production (Zhu, Chou, & Tsai, 2020). This pandemic also led to severe socio-economic implications (Nicola et al., 2020) and adverse effects on global supply chains in particular to inconsistencies in Labor and Material supply (Raj et al., 2022), and in accommodation sectors (Hossain, 2021). Similar shifts were seen in the supply chain, manufacturing, higher education, fintech, banking, and insurance sectors (Sharma et al. 2022). The COVID-19 pandemic accelerated the digital transformation of education services, establishing distance learning as the new norm (Kang, 2021). Leading software companies like Amazon, Apple, and Microsoft (CB Insights Report, 2022) are heavily investing in healthcare technology, and driving significant advances in healthcare systems. Although the healthcare sector utilized technology extensively before 2020, the pandemic heightened this reliance. The global market for health apps is projected to soar to $125 billion by 2028, up from $2.4 billion

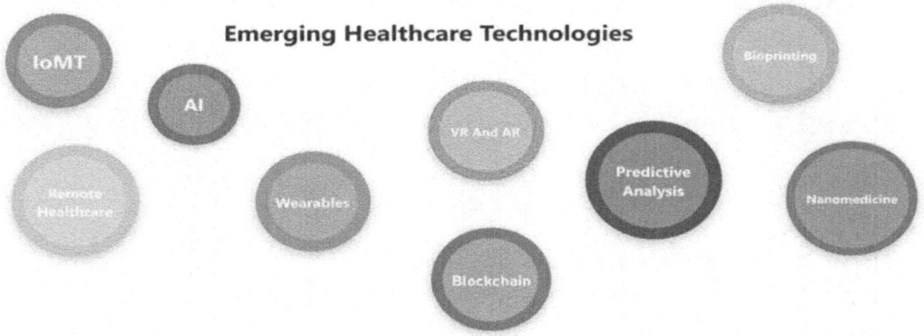


*Figure 11.2* Emerging healthcare technologies.

in 2017. According to "The 2021 Future of Healthcare Report," 80% of healthcare providers are now more inclined to invest in digital solutions and new technologies (as mentioned in Figure 11.2) rather than conventional approaches (HIMSS, 2021, p. 2).

Aside from advances in COVID-19-related healthcare technology, other areas of healthcare, such as disease diagnosis and early genetic disease detection, are rapidly integrating technology driven by technological innovation, evolving patient needs, and global health challenges. The healthcare landscape is undergoing a significant transformation driven by various emerging technologies as mentioned in Table 11.2, and these innovative technologies are able to provide numerous benefits to society at large.

Each of these areas of development and innovation in the healthcare sector are outlined in the remaining sections.

## 11.3 ARTIFICIAL INTELLIGENCE IN HEALTHCARE

A professor of medicine and engineering at the University of Southern California, Keck School of Medicine, and Viterbi School of Engineering, David B. Agus, MD shares

> Unlocking data [on health conditions] that historically we've made simple decisions about, AI allows us to get much deeper and look for associations the human brain isn't able to do … but a computer can.
>
> (Mack, n.d.)

AI has already shown its potential to transform healthcare through techniques like machine learning and deep learning to analyze data and make informed predictions and decisions. This potential and applications in healthcare are identified in Figure 11.3 and include:

*Table 11.2* Latest healthcare technology and their contribution

| *Healthcare technology* | *Contribution to the innovation in healthcare services or facilities* | | | |
|---|---|---|---|---|
| **Artificial intelligence (AI)** | Transforming diagnostics and drug discovery | Decision support systems | Personalized medicine approaches | (Mak, Wong, & Pichika, 2023; Magrabi et al., 2019) |
| **Telemedicine and remote patient monitoring** | Facilitating remote consultations | Improving access to care | Enabling chronic disease management | (Almathami, et al., 2020) |
| **Wearable health devices** | Empowering individuals to monitor their health metrics | Promoting preventive care | Early detection of potential health issues (Belciug & Gorunescu, 2020) | (Oldenburg et al., 2015; Agarwal et al., 2020; Li et al., 2016) |
| **Blockchain technology** | Enhancing data security | Ensuring privacy | Interoperability in healthcare data management | (Hussein et al., 2021; Bibhu et al., 2023; Yaqoob et al., 2022; Jabbar et al., 2020; Dagher et al., 2018) |
| **3D printing** | Revolutionizing medical device manufacturing | Enabling customization of implants and prosthetics | Bioprinting tissues and organs | (Datta & Barua, 2024) |
| **Robotics and automation** | Improving surgical precision and efficiency | Automating repetitive tasks | Facilitating remote surgery | (Andras et al., 2020) |
| **Personalized medicine and genomics** | Tailoring healthcare decisions | Customizing interventions to patients | Consideration for unique genetic makeup of individuals | (Ginsburg & Willard, 2009; Chan & Ginsburg, 2011) |
| **Augmented reality (AR) and virtual reality (VR)** | Improving medical training and education | Surgical preparation | Providing therapeutic solutions for pain management and tailoring mental health solutions | (Ayoub & Pulijala, 2019; Kakhi et al., 2022) |

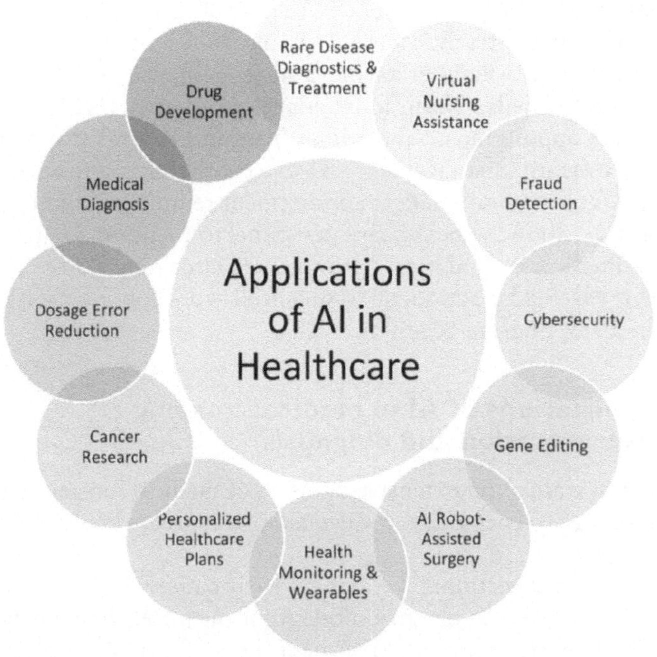


*Figure 11.3* Top applications of AI in healthcare.

**Improving diagnostic accuracy:** AI-powered diagnostic systems analyze medical images such as X-rays, CT scans, MRIs, and mammograms with high accuracy. By using deep learning algorithms producing vast datasets, these systems help radiologists identify abnormalities, tumors, fractures, and disease indicators, enhancing diagnostic precision and early disease detection, thus improving patient outcomes (Šimundić, 2009).

**Personalizing treatment plans:** AI algorithms analyze comprehensive patient data, including electronic health records (EHRs), genetic profiles, lifestyle factors, and treatment histories, to create personalized treatment plans. Machine learning methods predict individual responses to medications, identify optimal treatments, and suggest interventions tailored to a patient's unique characteristics, increasing treatment efficacy and reducing adverse effects (Ho et al., 2015b).

**Assisting in drug discovery and development:** AI accelerates drug discovery and development by analyzing vast biological and chemical data to identify potential drug targets, forecast molecular interactions, and optimize drug candidates. Machine learning models streamline drug screening, predict effectiveness and safety, and facilitate the repurposing of existing drugs, reducing the time and cost of traditional drug development (Mak, Wong, & Pichika, 2023).

**Enhancing administrative tasks:** AI automates administrative tasks, improving operational efficiency and reducing the burden on healthcare professionals. Natural language processing (NLP) algorithms automate appointment scheduling, insurance claims processing, and medical records management. AI-driven chatbots and virtual assistants handle patient queries, appointment reminders, and basic medical advice, allowing healthcare personnel to focus on complex patient care. Predictive analytics optimize resource distribution, forecast patient caseloads, and identify potential workflow obstacles (Duong et al., 2019; Sharma & Singh, 2021).

### 11.3.1 Applications of AI in medical imaging interpretation and diagnosis

AI algorithms, trained on extensive datasets of medical images, are achieving near-human-level accuracy in various critical areas:

- **Early cancer detection:** AI enhances early cancer diagnosis by analyzing medical scans to identify subtle signs of cancer that may be missed by human eyes, improving treatment outcomes (Bera et al., 2022).
- **Neurological condition diagnosis:** AI aids in diagnosing neurological disorders such as Alzheimer's and Parkinson's by carefully examining brain scans, potentially revolutionizing neurological care (Jiang et al., 2017).
- **Bone health assessment:** AI excels in analyzing bone scans, including X-rays and CT scans, to detect fractures, bone abnormalities, and osteoporosis. This capability accelerates diagnosis and treatment, reducing the time patients wait for care (George et al., 2023).

### 11.3.2 AI-powered decision support systems

Emerging AI-driven decision support systems are enhancing healthcare by offering several key functionalities for healthcare professionals to deal with real-time decisions for more accuracy, for risk assessments, and patients' genetic and medical history.

- **Real-time clinical decision support:** AI analyzes comprehensive patient data, including medical records, lab results, imaging scans, and vital signs, to assist healthcare professionals with accurate and timely diagnosis. These systems suggest potential diagnoses, recommend evidence-based treatments, and identify possible drug interactions, thus preventing adverse events (Ramírez, 2024; Kirkendall et al., 2019).

- **Risk assessment:** AI identifies patients at high risk for complications from procedures, medications, or conditions. By flagging these high-risk individuals, the system enables proactive interventions to mitigate risks and improve outcomes (Rana & Shuford, 2024).
- **Genetic and medical history analysis:** AI evaluates a patient's genetic information and medical history to identify relevant genetic markers and recommend personalized treatment plans. This supports personalized medicine, allowing for tailored therapies and improved patient care (ElKefi & Asan, 2021).

## 11.4 TELEMEDICINE AND REMOTE PATIENT MONITORING

Telemedicine is revolutionizing healthcare by using technology to provide remote medical services, overcoming geographical barriers (Table 11.3). It allows patients to consult doctors from home via video calls, secure messaging apps, and remote monitoring devices. This approach enhances healthcare access for those in remote locations or with mobility issues, eliminating the need for travel to a clinic.

A study undertaken in the Netherlands to assess the electronic patient records (EPRs) in healthcare (Michel-Verkerke, Stegwee, & Spil in 2015), resulted in researchers developing a six P's model of EPR use (Table 11.4) for ensuring the successful implementation of EPRs at a national level. In the model, the important users are the person (patient), professionals, and public. Against these users, the purpose, process, and prerequisites are mentioned for the successful implementation of ERPs nationwide.

Similarly to the Hitachi Social Innovation Project in Telemedicine, which is a new introduction to developing countries like India, the approach suggested from the Netherlands study is enabling advances in virtual patient

*Table 11.3* Evolution of telemedicine

| | |
|---|---|
| **Early stages (1950s–1970s)** | Telemedicine originated with the utilization of telephones and radio for consultations (Field & Grigsby, 2002; Armstrong & Haston, 1997; Brown & Hartley, 1992; Thrall & Boland, 1998; Haleem et al., 2021) in remote areas. |
| **Advancements (1980s–1990s)** | The ascent of video conferencing (Wosik et al., 2020; Rush et al., 2018; Winters & Winters, 2007) and electronic health records (EHRs) (Kane 2015; Shubber, Svensson, & Larsson, 2018) facilitated broader acceptance. |
| **Modern era (2000s–present)** | With the emergence of mobile health (mHealth) (Handel, 2011; Kumar et al., 2013; Luxton et al., 2011; Botha et al., 2018) or eHealth (Oh et al., 2005) technologies, high-speed internet, and advancements in wearables and remote monitoring tools, telemedicine has evolved into a more sophisticated system. |

*Table 11.4* Six P model of EPR use

| *Use(r)* | *Purpose (of using the EPR) (P4)* | *Process (how is the EPR used) (P5)* | *Prerequisite (what is essential for use) (P6)* |
|---|---|---|---|
| **Person (Patient) (P1)** | Health<br>Self-management | Communication | Privacy |
| **Professional (P2)** | Maintain records<br>Inform clinical decision-making | Provide care<br>Collaborate<br>Evaluation and research | Access to relevant data |
| **Public (P3)** | Health statistics<br>Quality assurance<br>Billing | Data retrieval<br>Benchmark | Data quality |

Source: Michel-Verkerke, Stegwee, and Spil (2015).

diagnosis, online prescription ordering, and remote patient care through telemedicine. At a micro level, such advances are offering patients affordable, accredited, and accessible healthcare, as well as helping healthcare to achieve macro-level goals (Figure 11.4) through P5 medicine, i.e. personal, participatory, preventive, precision, predictive (Longo et al., 2021) based on proactive approach, and primarily for all stakeholders.

The telemedicine market in the Indian healthcare industry is expected to reach US$5.4 billion by 2025 (Mandal, 2020) with a compound annual

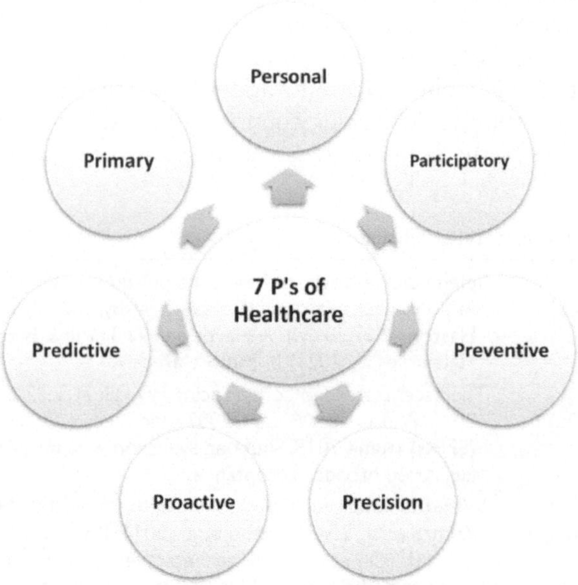


*Figure 11.4* Seven P's in Healthcare.

growth rate (CAGR) of 31% (Mandal, 2020). To tackle the huge patient database in India, companies like Hitachi, a Japanese multinational conglomerate, have come up with ambitious plans with its platform MGRM Net Telemedicine Solutions (Figure 11.5) that will help in enabling the digital healthcare of the future.

Telemedicine offers versatile applications across various healthcare settings (Figure 11.6):

- **Primary care:** Telemedicine enables patients to have routine check-ups with their primary care doctors without needing in-person visits. This enhances ongoing health monitoring and preventive care, allowing for remote discussions on medication adjustments, prescription renewals, management of concerns, and improving medication adherence (Haleem et al., 2021).
- **Chronic disease management:** Telemedicine integrates with wearable devices to monitor vital signs, blood glucose, blood pressure, and other metrics for chronic conditions such as diabetes and heart disease leading to lower mortality rate (Bashshur et al., 2014). Healthcare providers use virtual consultations to review patient conditions, adjust treatment plans, offer disease management education, and address any issues (Ezeamii et al., 2024). Chronic diseases account for more than 70% of all expenditure as well as deaths occurring among the patients (Bashshur & Shannon, 2009).
- **Mental health services:** Telemedicine enables remote therapy sessions with mental health professionals, providing convenient access to counselling and support for patients having chronic diseases (Wootton, 2012) related issues like anxiety, depression, stress, and PTSD. Patients can connect with psychiatrists, psychologists, or counselors via video or phone calls, receiving personalized treatment plans, medication management, and coping strategies tailored to their specific needs (Mehrotra et al., 2017).
- **Specialist consultations:** Telemedicine allows patients to connect with specialists regardless of their location, removing geographical barriers and reducing travel burdens. This enables timely consultations, second opinions, and expert advice without long-distance travel. Telemedicine promotes collaboration between primary care physicians and specialists, facilitating comprehensive and coordinated care for complex medical conditions, thereby enhancing patient outcomes and satisfaction (Neufeld et al., 2007).
- **Post-surgical care:** Healthcare providers can remotely evaluate surgical incisions, monitor vital signs, address pain management, and manage any complications or concerns, thus minimizing hospital readmissions and improving recovery outcomes. Telemedicine also enables patients to engage with physical therapists and rehabilitation specialists for guidance on exercises, mobility training, and recovery

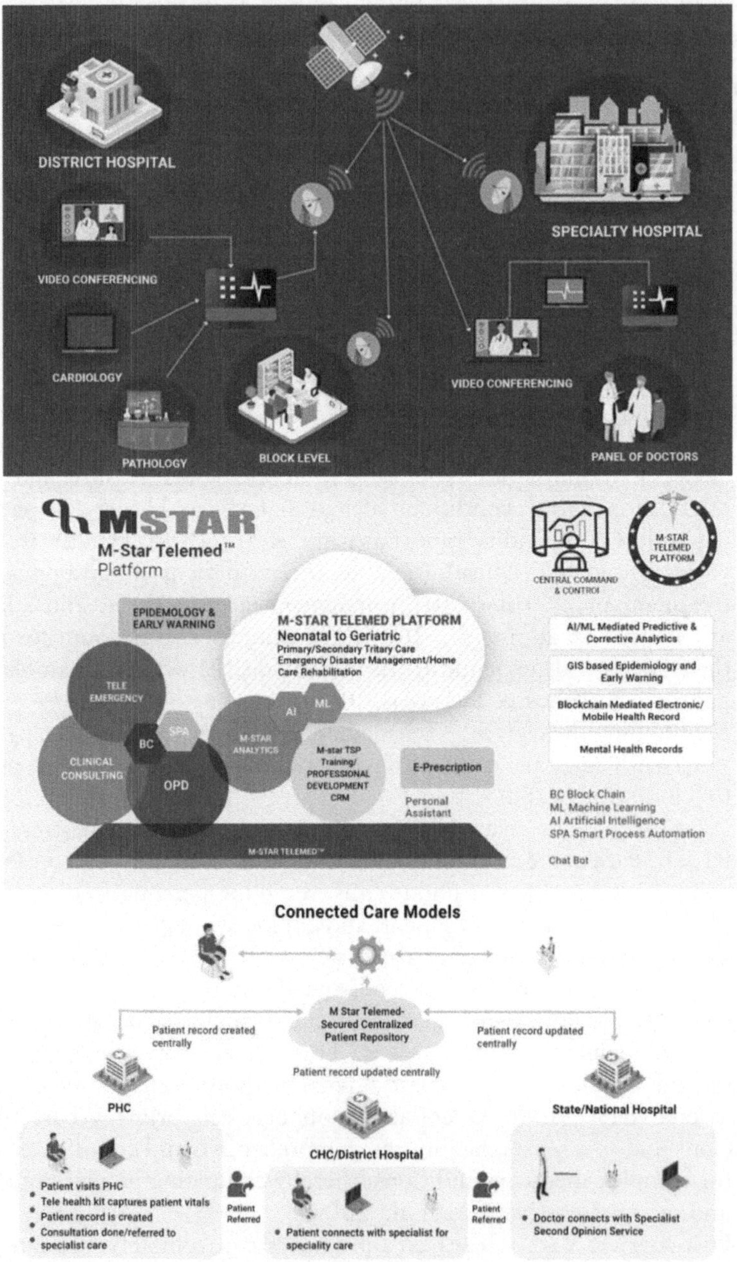


*Figure 11.5* Hitachi MGRM Net Telemedicine Solutions. (Source: Social Innovation Project – Hitachi.)

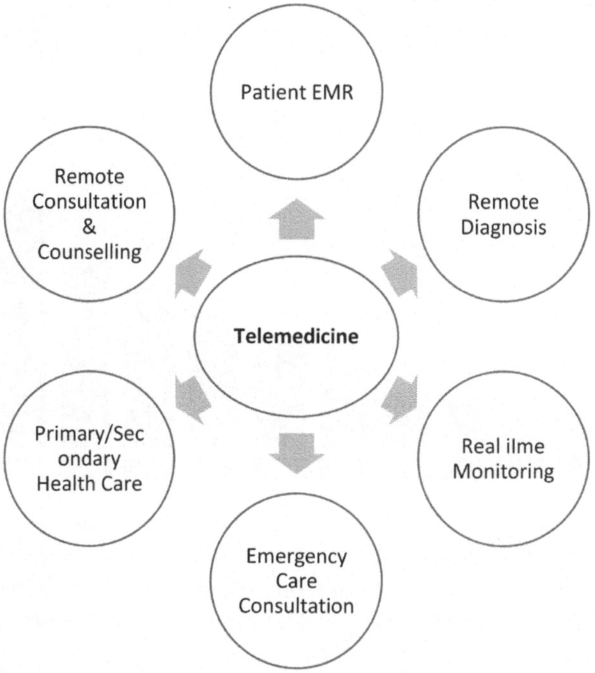


*Figure 11.6* Services offered by healthcare providers through telemedicine.

protocols, facilitating expedited rehabilitation and functional recovery (Awad, 2012).

## 11.5 WEARABLE HEALTH DEVICES

Wearable health devices are electronic gadgets with various sensors designed for comfortable use on the body (Lou et al., 2020; Dias & Paulo Silva, 2018; Majumder, Mondal, & Deen, 2017). These devices continuously collect and transmit health-related data, enabling individuals to monitor their well-being and fitness in real time. Equipped with multiple sensors, they discreetly gather data throughout the day.

The market for wearable health devices is driven by the rise in chronic diseases linked to lifestyle choices, increasing health awareness, an aging population, the growing acceptance of remote monitoring and home healthcare, and the emphasis on individualized patient care (Malasinghe, Ramzan, & Dahal, 2019). According to a November 2023 report by Precedence Research, the wearable medical devices market was valued at \$30 billion in 2022 and is projected to reach \$90.82 billion by 2027 and \$280.51 billion by 2032, with a CAGR of 25.1% (Figure 11.7).

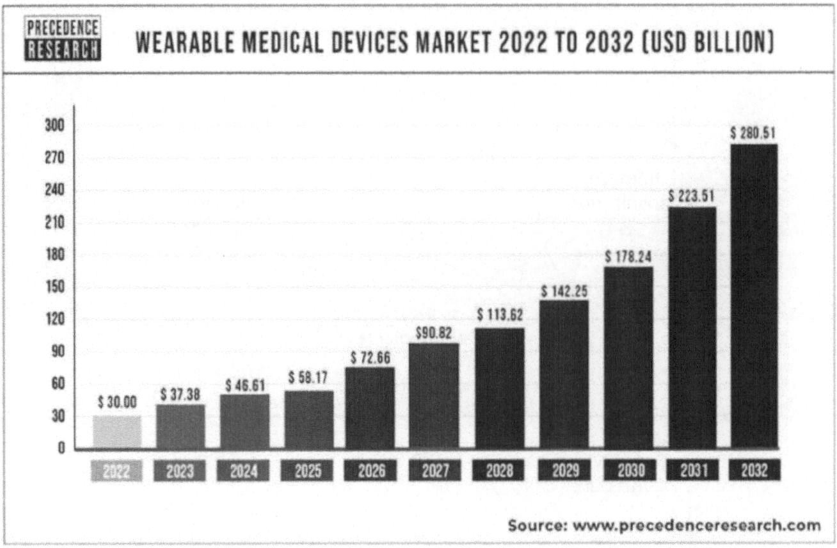


*Figure 11.7* Wearable medical devices market 2022 to 2032 (in USD billion). (Source: https://www.precedenceresearch.com/wearable-medical-device-market.)

Wearable health devices (Figure 11.8) available in the healthcare market include:

- **Fitness trackers:** These basic wearables monitor essential health metrics such as steps taken, distance traveled, calories burned, and sleep patterns, providing users with an overview of their physical habits. Advanced models include heart rate monitoring and GPS tracking, which aid in outdoor activities and performance monitoring (Henriksen et al., 2018). Fitness trackers offer real-time feedback on activity levels, helping users set and achieve fitness goals, and make informed decisions about their lifestyle and exercise routines, promoting overall health and well-being.
- **Smartwatches:** Combining traditional timekeeping with advanced computing capabilities, smartwatches track various health metrics, including heart rate, blood oxygen saturation ($SpO_2$), sleep quality, and even electrocardiograms (ECG) for detecting irregular heart rhythms. They also synchronize with smartphone apps for notifications, support contactless payments, music playback, navigation, and more. Users can customize watch faces and download additional apps, making smartwatches versatile tools for health monitoring and daily activities (Bender & Cappos, 2017).

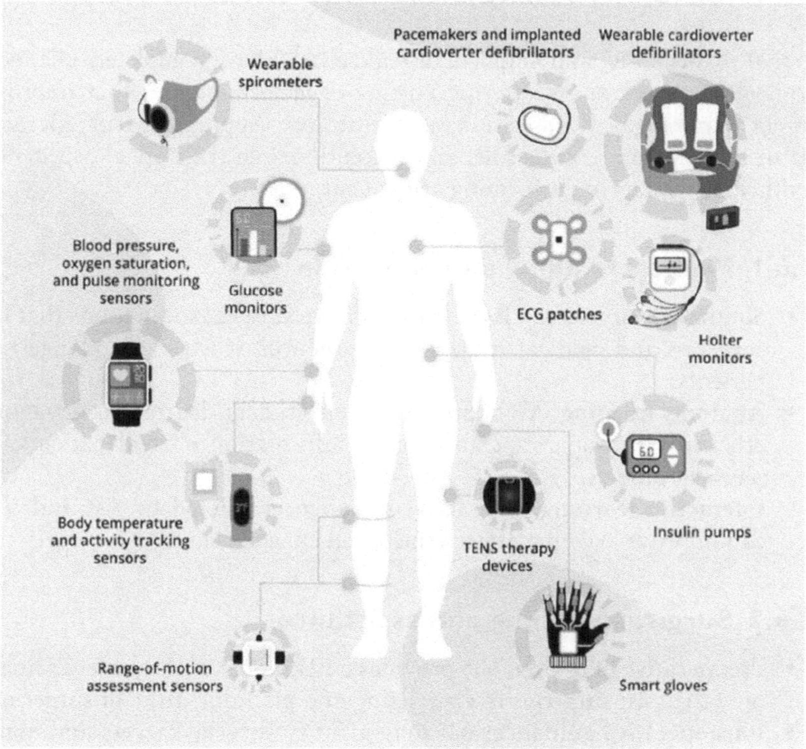


*Figure 11.8* Wearable devices in healthcare. ( Source: ScienceSoft | Healthcare,https://www.scnsoft.com/healthcare/wearables/examples-wearable-medical-devices_diagram.png.)

- **Smart clothing:** Integrating textile-based sensors, smart clothing monitors physiological signals such as heart rate, respiration, and body temperature. It benefits athletes by tracking performance metrics during training and holds promise in healthcare for monitoring patients' vital signs and movement during recovery, providing valuable data for treatment customization (Smith, Li, & Tse, 2023).
- **Advanced wearables:** These specialized devices monitor specific health conditions like blood pressure and blood glucose levels, and perform ECGs. Wearable blood pressure monitors and continuous glucose monitors provide real-time data for managing conditions like hypertension and diabetes, while portable ECG devices detect irregular heart rhythms, extending diagnostic capabilities outside clinical settings (Lin et al., 2010; Guzik & Malik, 2016).

## 11.6 AR AND VR IN HEALTHCARE INDUSTRY

Virtual reality (VR) and augmented reality (AR) have completely changed the healthcare sector by offering cutting-edge technologies that improve patient care, medical education, and training. Applications of AR and VR in healthcare are numerous and revolutionizing the critical aspects of healthcare, such as in performing critical surgeries.

### 11.6.1 Medical training and education

- **Simulated surgeries:** VR produces lifelike surgical simulations that let surgeons and medical students hone their craft without endangering patients.
- **Anatomy learning:** AR applications help students learn anatomy more efficiently by superimposing digital information on real patients or physical models.
- **Interactive learning:** Interactive experiences offered by AR and VR can improve learning effectiveness and engagement.

### 11.6.2 Surgical planning and assistance

- **Preoperative planning:** VR provides a 3D model of the patient's anatomy to assist surgeons in visualizing and planning difficult surgeries.
- **Intraoperative guidance:** AR may identify surgical targets and highlight blood vessels, among other important information, over a surgeon's field of vision during a procedure.
- **Minimally invasive surgeries:** By improving accuracy and shortening recovery periods, VR can assist surgeons with minimally invasive surgeries.

### 11.6.3 Patient care and rehabilitation

- **Pain management:** VR can be utilized to create immersive experiences that help patients forget about their pain while receiving medical care or undergoing rehabilitation.
- **Physical therapy:** Virtual reality enhances the effectiveness and engagement of rehabilitation by offering guided exercises in a simulated setting.
- **Mental health therapy:** By exposing patients to stimuli in a safe and supervised setting, VR is utilized in exposure therapy to treat PTSD, phobias, and anxiety disorders.

### 11.6.4 Medical imaging and diagnosis

- **Enhanced visualization:** AR improves medical imaging by directly superimposing diagnostic pictures (such as CT scans and MRIs) onto the patient's body, helping in precise diagnosis.
- **Telemedicine:** AR and VR provide remote diagnosis and consultation, enabling medical professionals to virtually assess patients and offer on-the-spot support.

### 11.6.5 Patient education and engagement

- **Patient education:** VR can be utilized to help patients better comprehend their treatment plan by providing them with an explanation of difficult medical processes.
- **Management of chronic diseases:** AR applications can help patients stick to their treatment plans and make lifestyle and pharmaceutical adjustments.

### 11.6.6 Teleoperated surgery

Utilizing virtual reality technology, surgeons can conduct surgeries from a distance by manipulating robotic tools. This can be extremely helpful in emergency scenarios or for granting access to specialized treatment in remote places. Conducting teleoperated surgeries (telesurgery) has its advantages such as better instruction, improved patient results, and improved experience. Authentic and enhanced instruction helps in safe surgery without putting patients at danger. Surgical results are enhanced by increased precision and planning. It leads to less discomfort and worry, and ensures greater comprehension of the processes. By enhancing patient care, training, and surgical results, the healthcare business is being transformed by the integration of AR and VR. AR and VR will probably become increasingly more essential to healthcare as technology develops, providing fresh opportunities to improve patient satisfaction and care quality.

## 11.7 BLOCKCHAIN TECHNOLOGY IN HEALTHCARE

The patient care process in the healthcare industry involves multiple stakeholders, including medical professionals, facilities, insurance providers, and governmental bodies, making it highly intricate (Blumenthal, 2011; Hansen & Baroody, 2020; Davidson et al., 2018; Ozdemir et al., 2011). This complexity, coupled with the sensitivity of medical data, has led to numerous breaches, such as the compromise of over 50.4 million patient records in 2021 (Protenus, Inc., 2022). Additionally, the World Health Organization estimates that up to 30% of medications in parts of Asia, Africa, and Latin America may be counterfeit (Sansone, Cuzin, & Jannini, 2021).

Blockchain technology offers a solution by facilitating secure communication among stakeholders without third-party involvement (Khan & Salah, 2018; Li et al., 2020; Tanwar, Parekh, & Evans, 2020). It creates a decentralized platform for storing medical records, providing patients with complete control over their health data while allowing medical professionals to access records from anywhere. For instance, Mike Gault, CEO of Guardtime, shared that Estonia's e-health foundation has partnered with his organization to store all health records on a secure, decentralized platform, improving patient care through easier access to medical records using Oracle technology (Guardtime blog, 2024).

The global blockchain market for healthcare is expected to grow at a CAGR of 76.30% from 2021 to 2028, reaching a projected value of $7308.32 million (Verified Market Research, 2022).

### 11.7.1 Applications in healthcare data management and interoperability

Blockchain holds immense potential to transform healthcare data management and interoperability (Yaqoob et al., 2022; Attaran, 2022).

- **Secure and efficient data sharing:** Blockchain technology enables secure and efficient healthcare data sharing, giving patients greater control over their medical information. Patients can use blockchain platforms to own their data and selectively grant access to healthcare providers, researchers, and other entities. Each access request is logged on the blockchain, ensuring transparency and data security. By eliminating centralized intermediaries and maintaining data integrity through cryptographic hashing, blockchain fosters trust among stakeholders and enables seamless data exchange across diverse healthcare systems (Singh et al., 2023).
- **Improved care coordination:** Blockchain simplifies the sharing and interoperability of healthcare data, enhancing care coordination and continuity across various healthcare environments. It allows real-time, secure access to and updating of medical records, enabling healthcare providers to make informed clinical decisions. This reduces administrative burdens, minimizes redundant tests and procedures, and improves patient care quality. Blockchain-based networks facilitate collaboration among multidisciplinary care teams, leading to better outcomes for patients with complex medical needs (Palas & Bunduchi, 2021).

- **Enhanced medication tracking:** Blockchain optimizes medication tracking and supply chain management, reducing the risk of counterfeit drugs and improving patient safety. By recording every stage of a medication's lifecycle on the blockchain, stakeholders can verify the authenticity and reliability of pharmaceutical products in real time. This transparent tracking system increases accountability, reduces medication errors, and combats counterfeit drugs. Blockchain platforms can also implement smart contracts to enforce regulatory compliance, manage recalls, and streamline inventory management (Li & Kassem, 2021; Wang et al., 2019).
- **Streamlined clinical research:** Blockchain creates a decentralized network for data exchange among researchers, clinicians, and patients, accelerating clinical research and innovation (see Figure 11.9). This framework ensures data privacy, integrity, and provenance while providing access to diverse datasets. Blockchain's transparency and auditability enhance research reproducibility, encourage collaboration, and drive data-driven insights. Smart contracts automate data sharing agreements, consent management, and royalty payments, simplifying administrative tasks and promoting collaborative research. This approach accelerates therapy development, improves patient outcomes, and advances healthcare (Bates et al., 2015).

## 11.8 THE INTEGRATION OF 3D PRINTING IN THE MEDICAL FIELD

3D printing, or additive manufacturing, is a computer-guided method that creates three-dimensional objects layer-by-layer from a digital blueprint. In healthcare, it has applications in drug delivery and medical stores (Trenfield et al., 2019; Datta & Barua, 2024).

### 11.8.1 Applications in medical device manufacturing and prosthetics

- **Custom prosthetics:** 3D printing enables the creation of customized prosthetic limbs, fingers, and facial features tailored to an individual's anatomy and functional needs. This approach improves comfort, fit, and functionality, enhancing mobility and quality of life for individuals with limb loss or differences. It also allows for rapid prototyping and iterative design enhancements, fostering innovative prosthetic solutions (Kesner & Howe, 2011).
- **Surgical instruments and implants:** 3D printing is increasingly used to produce surgical instruments, implants, and anatomical models for preoperative planning and simulation. Surgeons can use 3D-printed

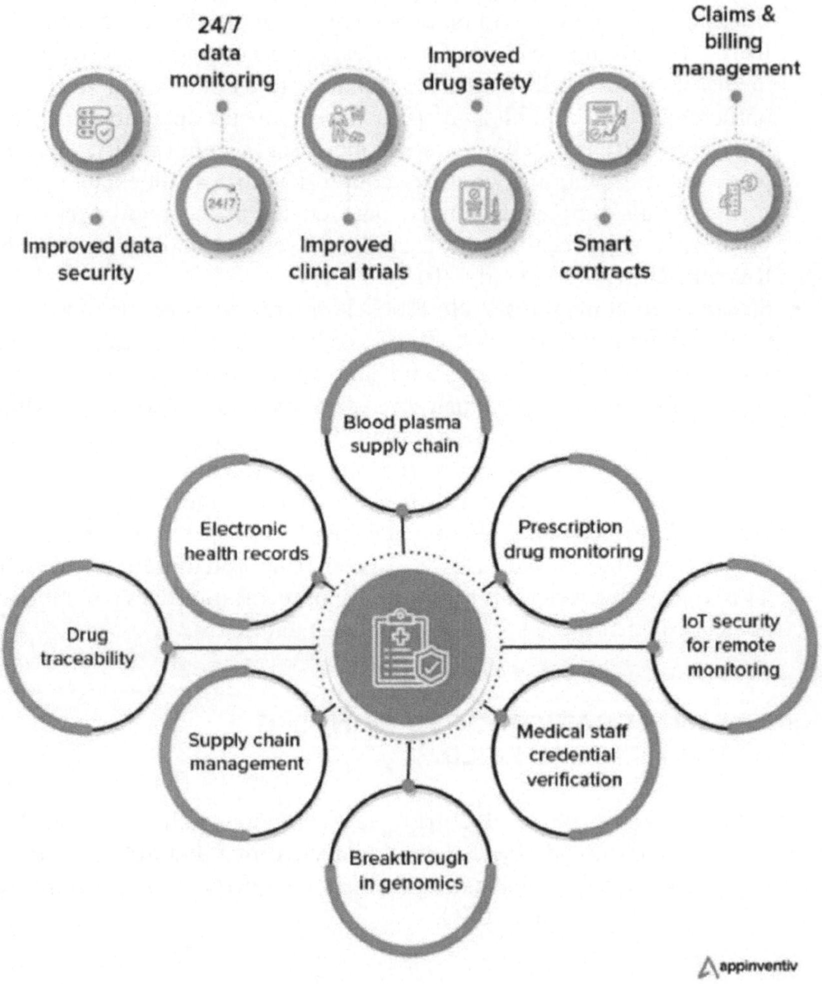


*Figure 11.9* Applications of blockchain in healthcare. (Source: Appinventiv, https://appinventiv.com/wp-content/uploads/2018/07/Ways-blockchain-is-transforming-the-healthcare-industry.webp.)

models of bones and organs to visualize procedures, practice techniques, and develop personalized treatment plans. These patient-specific models improve surgical outcomes by helping surgeons anticipate challenges and optimize approaches. Custom-made implants, such as orthopedic and dental prostheses, offer superior fit and performance compared to standard alternatives (Trenfield et al., 2019).

- **Manufacturing of medical devices:** 3D printing allows for the on-demand production of customized surgical instruments, splints, braces, and other medical devices. Unlike conventional manufacturing, which is labor-intensive and slow, 3D printing enables rapid prototyping, iterative refinement, and small-batch or just-in-time production. This flexibility helps healthcare providers address specific patient needs effectively and incorporate advanced materials and intricate designs to enhance device performance and functionality (Zhang et al., 2017).

### 11.8.2 Tailoring implants and tissues using 3D printing technology

One of the most promising applications of 3D printing in medicine involves customizing implants and tissues.

**Bioprinting:** Bioprinting is a specialized form of 3D printing that uses biocompatible materials, known as bioinks, to create tissues and potentially organs for transplantation. Unlike conventional 3D printing, which uses plastics or metals, bioprinting layers living cells to form three-dimensional tissue structures (see Figure 11.10). These engineered tissues mimic the intricate features and functions of natural tissues, offering promising prospects for tissue regeneration, organ transplantation, and personalized medical treatments (Gu et al., 2020; Patra & Young, 2016).

**Customized implants:** 3D printing in medicine allows for the creation of patient-specific implants, such as joint replacements, bone grafts, and dental implants, leading to better fit and improved long-term outcomes. Traditional implants come in standard sizes, which may not perfectly match

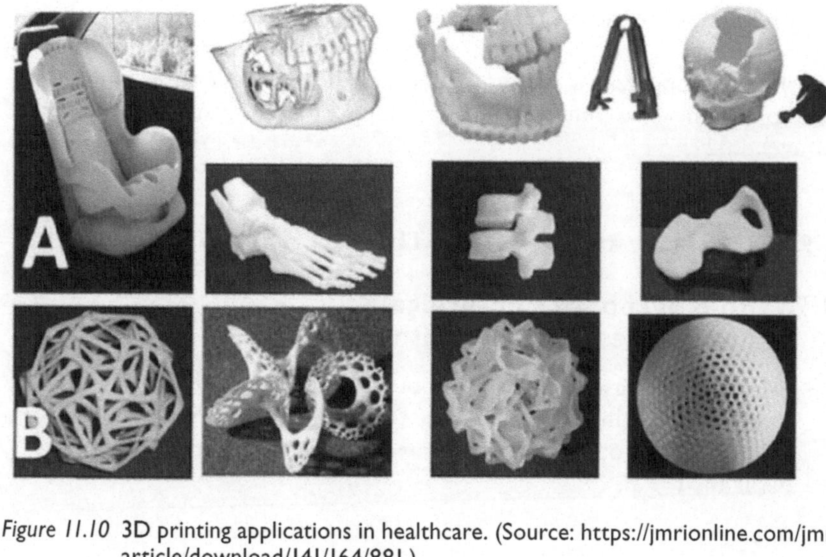


*Figure 11.10* 3D printing applications in healthcare. (Source: https://jmrionline.com/jmri/article/download/141/164/881.)

an individual's anatomy. With 3D printing, implants can be tailored to each patient's unique needs using data from medical imaging scans, anatomical measurements, and biomechanical assessments (Mobbs et al., 2017; Ho et al., 2015a).

### 11.8.3 Pros of 3D printing in healthcare

**Customization:** A major advantage of 3D printing in healthcare is its ability to produce personalized medical devices and implants that precisely match an individual's anatomy. Using patient-specific data from CT scans or MRIs, healthcare professionals can design and manufacture custom implants that fit perfectly, enhancing performance and comfort. This personalized approach leads to better patient outcomes and reduces the risk of complications (Guk et al., 2019).

**Reduced production time:** 3D printing can significantly reduce the manufacturing time for medical devices compared to traditional methods. Conventional manufacturing involves multiple stages, such as tooling, molding, and assembly, which are time-consuming and labor-intensive. In contrast, 3D printing allows for direct production from digital designs, eliminating the need for tooling and shortening production times. This rapid prototyping capability speeds up design iterations and the development of new medical devices and implants (Attaran, 2017; Liaw & Guvendiren, 2017).

**Complex structure creation:** 3D printing enables the fabrication of intricate and complex medical structures that are difficult or impossible to achieve with traditional methods. Unlike subtractive manufacturing, which removes material from a solid block, 3D printing builds objects layer by layer, allowing for the creation of complex geometries with internal cavities, lattice structures, and surface textures. This capability is especially useful in orthopedics, where implants with porous structures can be created to enhance osseointegration and support bone growth (Bozkurt & Karayel, 2021).

## 11.9 ROBOTICS AND AUTOMATION IN HEALTHCARE

### 11.9.1 Role of robotics in surgical procedures and rehabilitation

- **Minimally invasive surgery:** Robotic-assisted surgical systems enhance precision, flexibility, and control during complex procedures, surpassing traditional laparoscopic techniques (DiGioia III, Jaramaz, & Colgan, 1998).

- **Improved surgical outcomes:** These systems can lead to smaller incisions, reduced blood loss, faster recovery times, and better patient outcomes (Ostrowitz et al., 2009).
- **Rehabilitation assistance:** Robots are increasingly used in physical therapy to provide targeted assistance, improve range of motion, and enhance patient engagement (Weber & Stein, 2018; Zhang, Davies, & Xie, 2013).

### 11.9.2 Automation of repetitive tasks in healthcare facilities

- **Pharmacy automation:** Robotic systems improve medication dispensation by accurately administering medications, preparing IV solutions, labeling prescriptions, and tracking inventory, thereby reducing medication errors and increasing efficiency (Poon et al., 2006).
- **Laboratory automation:** Automated laboratory systems handle repetitive tasks like blood tests and analysis, speeding up turnaround times and improving accuracy. These systems manage various tests, including blood, urine analysis, microbiology cultures, and molecular diagnostics, with high throughput and precision (Markin & Whalen, 2000).
- **Administrative tasks:** Automation streamlines administrative tasks such as appointment scheduling, data entry, and insurance claim processing. Robotic process automation (RPA) software can handle repetitive tasks involving manual data entry, document processing, and rule-based decision-making, freeing up staff time for patient care (Hofmann, Samp, & Urbach, 2020; Ribeiro et al., 2021). An example illustration is given in Figure 11.11.

### 11.9.3 Enhancing precision and efficiency in medical interventions

- **Improved precision:** Robotic surgical systems provide unmatched precision and stability, minimizing human error and complications during surgery. These systems use robotic arms controlled by surgeons, offering precise movements and dexterity beyond traditional techniques (Moustris et al., 2011).
- **Enhanced efficiency:** Automation streamlines workflows, reduces processing times, and optimizes resource utilization, allowing healthcare professionals to focus on complex tasks requiring human expertise (Granlund & Wiktorsson, 2013; Zayas-Cabán et al., 2021).
- **Remote surgery:** Robotic systems enable remote surgery, allowing specialists to perform procedures in geographically distant locations via teleoperated systems, thus providing expert care to patients in remote or underserved regions (Laaki, Miche, & Tammi, 2019).

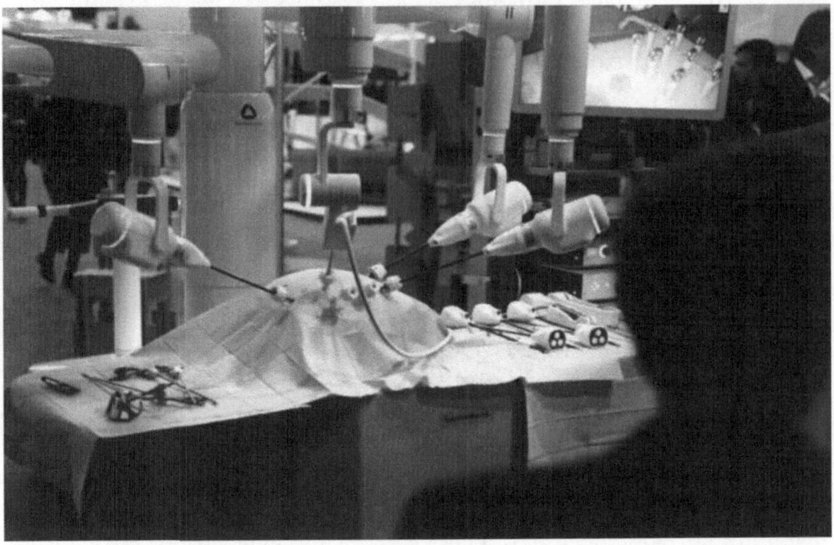

*Figure 11.11* Robotics in healthcare. (Photo: Thomas Coex/AFP via Getty Images, https://1734811051.rsc.cdn77.org/data/images/full/425697/spain-telecom-technology.jpg?w=820.)

## 11.10 CONCLUSION

The future of healthcare holds both promise and challenges. Technological advances, such as artificial intelligence, telemedicine, and personalized medicine, are already revolutionizing healthcare delivery, making it more efficient, accessible, and patient-centered (Li et al., 2021; Oates, Weston, & Jordan, 2000; Chawla and Davis, 2013). The integration of big data analytics and predictive modeling offers potential for proactive healthcare management and early disease detection (Dash et al., 2019; Wang, Kung, & Byrd, 2018).

However, significant challenges must be addressed, including data privacy and security (Chen & Zhao, 2012; Medaglia & Serbanati, 2010; Terzi, Terzi, & Sagiroglu, 2015), ethical implications of AI in healthcare (Schönberger, 2019), the digital gap (Chang et al., 2004), artificial intelligence and other technology adoption (Sharma et al., 2024), and disparities in access to advanced technologies (Khang et al., 2022). Another significant challenge is about convincing people that they really have a problem concerning them and convincing them about the right solution chosen (Dixon-Woods, McNicol, & Martin, 2012). Additionally, rising healthcare costs (Bodenheimer, 2005), an aging population (Dall et al., 2013), and the increasing burden of chronic diseases (Abegunde et al., 2007) demand innovative solutions and sustainable healthcare models.

The future of healthcare will be shaped by collaborative efforts among stakeholders, including healthcare providers, policymakers, technology developers, and patients (Gray & Purdy, 2018; Frow, McColl-Kennedy, & Payne, 2016). "Holistic Systems Approach" should be used to deal with the challenge of huge volumes of data representing a striking signal-to-noise (S/N) challenge (Hood, Balling, & Auffray, 2012). Regular reviews, critical evaluations, and support from leaders and senior management are essential to make emerging technologies user-friendly, especially in their nascent stages (Øvretveit et al., 2007). By embracing innovation while upholding ethical standards and prioritizing inclusivity and affordability, the healthcare industry can navigate future complexities and strive toward a healthier, more equitable world.

## REFERENCES

Abegunde, D. O., Mathers, C. D., Adam, T., Ortegon, M., & Strong, K. (2007). The burden and costs of chronic diseases in low-income and middle-income countries. *The Lancet*, *370*(9603), 1929–1938.

Agarwal, R., Dugas, M., Gao, G. G., & Kannan, P. K. (2020). Emerging technologies and analytics for a new era of value-centered marketing in healthcare. *Journal of the Academy of Marketing Science*, *48*(1), 9–23.

Ahmed, K., Wang, T. T., Patel, V. M., Nagpal, K., Clark, J., Ali, M., ... Paraskeva, P. (2011). The role of single-incision laparoscopic surgery in abdominal and pelvic surgery: A systematic review. *Surgical Endoscopy*, *25*, 378–396.

Albreem, M. A. (2015, April). 5G wireless communication systems: Vision and challenges. 2015 International Conference on Computer, Communications, and Control Technology (I4CT), Kuching, Malaysia. IEEE, pp. 493–497, doi: 10.1109/I4CT.2015.7219627.

Almathami, H. K. Y., Win, K. T., & Vlahu-Gjorgievska, E. (2020). Barriers and facilitators that influence telemedicine-based, real-time, online consultation at patients' homes: Systematic literature review. *Journal of Medical Internet Research*, *22*(2), e16407.

Andras, I., Mazzone, E., van Leeuwen, F. W., De Naeyer, G., van Oosterom, M. N., Beato, S., ... Mottrie, A. (2020). Artificial intelligence and robotics: A combination that is changing the operating room. *World Journal of Urology*, *38*, 2359–2366.

Andrew, S., Milne, R., & Burls, A. (2003, June 1). Health technology assessment: History and demand, *Journal of Public Health*, *25*(2), 98–101. https://doi.org/10.1093/pubmed/fdg022

Armstrong, I. J., & Haston, W. S. (1997). Medical decision support for remote general practitioners using telemedicine. *Journal of Telemedicine and Telecare*, *3*(1), 27–34.

Attaran, M. (2017). The rise of 3-D printing: The advantages of additive manufacturing over traditional manufacturing. *Business Horizons*, *60*(5), 677–688.

Attaran, M. (2022). Blockchain technology in healthcare: Challenges and opportunities. *International Journal of Healthcare Management*, *15*(1), 70–83.

Awad, S. S. (2012). Adherence to surgical care improvement project measures and post-operative surgical site infections. *Surgical Infections, 13*(4), 234–237.

Ayoub, A., & Pulijala, Y. (2019). The application of virtual reality and augmented reality in Oral & Maxillofacial Surgery. *BMC Oral Health, 19*, 1–8.

Bansal, A., Kaushik, S., & Kukreti, S. (2022). Non-canonical DNA structures: Diversity and disease association. *Frontiers in Genetics, 13*, 959258.

Bashshur, R. L., & Shannon, G. W. (2009). *History of telemedicine: Evolution, context, and transformation*. Mary Ann Liebert, Inc., Publishers.

Bashshur, R. L., Shannon, G. W., Smith, B. R., Alverson, D. C., Antoniotti, N., Barsan, W. G., ... Yellowlees, P. (2014). The empirical foundations of telemedicine interventions for chronic disease management. *Telemedicine and e-Health, 20*(9), 769–800.

Bates, S. E., Berry, D. A., Balasubramaniam, S., Bailey, S., LoRusso, P. M., & Rubin, E. H. (2015). Advancing clinical trials to streamline drug development. *Clinical Cancer Research, 21*(20), 4527–4535.

Belciug, S., & Gorunescu, F. (2020). *Intelligent decision support systems-a journey to smarter healthcare* (pp. 130–137). Springer International Publishing.

Bender, C. G., Hoffstot, J. C., Combs, B. T., Hooshangi, S., & Cappos, J. (2017, March). Measuring the fitness of fitness trackers. 2017 IEEE Sensors Applications Symposium (SAS) (pp. 1–6). IEEE.

Bera, K., Braman, N., Gupta, A., Velcheti, V., & Madabhushi, A. (2022). Predicting cancer outcomes with radiomics and artificial intelligence in radiology. *Nature Reviews Clinical Oncology, 19*(2), 132–146.

Bibhu, V., Das, L., Rana, A., Sharma, S., Salagrama, S. (2023). AI Model for Blockchain Based Industrial Application in Healthcare IoT. In B. Bhushan, A. K. Sangaiah, & T. N. Nguyen (Eds.), AI models for blockchain-based intelligent networks in IoT systems. Engineering Cyber-Physical Systems and Critical Infrastructures (Vol. 6). Springer. https://doi.org/10.1007/978-3-031-31952-5_8

Blumenthal, David. 2011. Implementation of the federal health information technology initiative. *New England Journal of Medicine, 365*(25), 2426–2431.

Bodenheimer, T. (2005). High and rising health care costs. Part 1: Seeking an explanation. *Annals of Internal Medicine, 142*(10), 847–854.

Bojinov, H., Michalevsky, Y., Nakibly, G., & Boneh, D. (2014). Mobile device identification via sensor fingerprinting. *arXiv preprint arXiv:1408.1416*.

Botha, A., Weiss, M., & Herselman, M. (2018). Towards a taxonomy of mHealth. International Conference on Advances in Big Data, Computing and Data Communication Systems (icABCD), Durban, South Africa.

Bozkurt, Y., & Karayel, E. (2021). 3D printing technology; methods, biomedical applications, future opportunities and trends. *Journal of Materials Research and Technology, 14*, 1430–1450.

Brown, K. (2005). *Penicillin man*. The History Press.

Carrasco Ramírez, J. G. (2024). AI in healthcare: Revolutionizing patient care with predictive analytics and decision support systems. *Journal of Artificial Intelligence General Science (JAIGS), 1*(1), 31–37. https://doi.org/10.60087/jaigs.v1i1.p37

Chan, I. S., & Ginsburg, G. S. (2011). Personalized medicine: Progress and promise. *Annual Review of Genomics and Human Genetics, 12*, 217–244.

Chang, B. L., Bakken, S., Brown, S. S., Houston, T. K., Kreps, G. L., Kukafka, R., ... Stavri, P. Z. (2004). Bridging the digital divide: Reaching vulnerable populations. *Journal of the American Medical Informatics Association*, *11*(6), 448–457.

Chawla, N. V., & Davis, D. A. (2013). Bringing big data to personalized healthcare: A patient-centered framework. *Journal of General Internal Medicine*, *28*, 660–665.

Chen, D., & Zhao, H. (2012, March). Data security and privacy protection issues in cloud computing. In *2012 international conference on computer science and electronics engineering* (Vol. 1, pp. 647–651). IEEE.

Dagher, G. G., Mohler, J., Milojkovic, M., & Marella, P. B. (2018). Ancile: Privacy-preserving framework for access control and interoperability of electronic health records using blockchain technology. *Sustainable Cities and Society*, *39*, 283–297.

Dall, T. M., Gallo, P. D., Chakrabarti, R., West, T., Semilla, A. P., & Storm, M. V. (2013). An aging population and growing disease burden will require a large and specialized health care workforce by 2025. *Health Affairs*, *32*(11), 2013–2020.

Dash, S., Shakyawar, S. K., Sharma, M., & Kaushik, S. (2019). Big data in healthcare: Management, analysis and future prospects. *Journal of Big Data*, *6*(1), 1–25.

Datta, S., & Barua, R. (2024). 3D printing in modern healthcare: An overview of materials, methods, applications, and challenges. In M. Garcia & R. de Almeida (Eds.), *Emerging technologies for health literacy and medical practice* (pp. 132–152). IGI Global Scientific Publishing. https://doi.org/10.4018/979-8-3693-1214-8.ch007

Davidson, Elizabeth, Aaron Baird, and Karl Prince. 2018. Opening the envelope of health care information systems research. *Information and Organization*, 28(3), 140–151.

Davies, K. (2002). *Cracking the genome: Inside the race to unlock human DNA*. JHU Press.

Dias, D., & Paulo Silva Cunha, J. (2018). Wearable health devices—vital sign monitoring, systems and technologies. *Sensors*, *18*(8), 2414.

DiGioia III, A. M., Jaramaz, B., & Colgan, B. D. (1998). Computer assisted orthopaedic surgery: Image guided and robotic assistive technologies. *Clinical Orthopaedics and Related Research®*, *354*, 8–16.

Dixon-Woods, M., McNicol, S., & Martin, G. (2012). Ten challenges in improving quality in healthcare: Lessons from the Health Foundation's programme evaluations and relevant literature. *BMJ Quality & Safety*, *21*(10), 876–884.

Duong, M. T., Rauschecker, A. M., Rudie, J. D., Chen, P. H., Cook, T. S., Bryan, R. N., & Mohan, S. (2019). Artificial intelligence for precision education in radiology. *The British Journal of Radiology*, *92*(1103), 20190389.

Ezeamii, V. C., Okobi, O. E., Wambai-Sani, H., Perera, G. S., Zaynieva, S., Okonkwo, C. C., Ohaiba, M. M., William-Enemali, P. C., Obodo, O. R., & Obiefuna, N. G. (2024). Revolutionizing healthcare: How telemedicine is improving patient outcomes and expanding access to care. *Cureus*, *16*(7), e63881. doi: 10.7759/cureus.63881. PMID: 39099901; PMCID: PMC11298029.

ElKefi, S., & Asan, O. (2021). How technology impacts communication between cancer patients and their health care providers: A systematic literature review. *International Journal of Medical Informatics*, *149*, 104430.

Field, M. J., & Grigsby, J. (2002). Telemedicine and remote patient monitoring. *JAMA*, *288*(4), 423–425.

Frow, P., McColl-Kennedy, J. R., & Payne, A. (2016). Co-creation practices: Their role in shaping a health care ecosystem. *Industrial Marketing Management*, *56*, 24–39.

George, A. H., Shahul, A., & George, A. S. (2023). Artificial intelligence in medicine: A new way to diagnose and treat disease. *Partners Universal International Research Journal*, 2(3), 246–259.

Ginsburg, G. S., & Willard, H. F. (2009). Genomic and personalized medicine: Foundations and applications. *Translational Research*, *154*(6), 277–287.

Granlund, A., & Wiktorsson, M. (2013). Automation in healthcare internal logistics: A case study on practice and potential. *International Journal of Innovation and Technology Management*, *10*(03), 1340012.

Gray, B., & Purdy, J. (2018). *Collaborating for our future: Multistakeholder partnerships for solving complex problems*. Oxford University Press.

Gu, Z., Fu, J., Lin, H., & He, Y. (2020). Development of 3D bioprinting: From printing methods to biomedical applications. *Asian Journal of Pharmaceutical Sciences*, *15*(5), 529–557.

Guk, K., Han, G., Lim, J., Jeong, K., Kang, T., Lim, E. K., & Jung, J. (2019). Evolution of wearable devices with real-time disease monitoring for personalized healthcare. *Nanomaterials*, *9*(6), 813.

Guzik, P., & Malik, M. (2016). ECG by mobile technologies. *Journal of Electrocardiology*, *49*(6), 894–901.

Haleem, A., Javaid, M., Singh, R. P., & Suman, R. (2021). Telemedicine for healthcare: Capabilities, features, barriers, and applications. *Sensors International*, 2, 100117.

Handel, M. J. (2011). mHealth (mobile health)—using apps for health and wellness. *EXPLORE: The Journal of Science and Healing*, 7(4), 256–261.

Hansen, S., & Baroody, A. J. (2020). Electronic health records and the logics of care: Complementarity and conflict in the US healthcare system. *Information Systems Research*, *31*(1), 57–75.

Henriksen, A., Haugen Mikalsen, M., Woldaregay, A. Z., Muzny, M., Hartvigsen, G., Hopstock, L. A., & Grimsgaard, S. (2018). Using fitness trackers and smartwatches to measure physical activity in research: Analysis of consumer wrist-worn wearables. *Journal of Medical Internet Research*, *20*(3), e110.

Ho, C. M. B., Ng, S. H., & Yoon, Y. J. (2015a). A review on 3D printed bioimplants. *International Journal of Precision Engineering and Manufacturing*, *16*, 1035–1046.

Ho, D., Wang, C. H. K., & Chow, E. K. H. (2015b). Nanodiamonds: The intersection of nanotechnology, drug development, and personalized medicine. *Science Advances*, *1*(7), e1500439.

Hofmann, P., Samp, C., & Urbach, N. (2020). Robotic process automation. *Electronic Markets*, *30*(1), 99–106.

Hood, L., Balling, R., & Auffray, C. (2012). Revolutionizing medicine in the 21st century through systems approaches. *Biotechnology Journal*, 7(8), 992–1001.

Hossain, M. (2021). The effect of the Covid-19 on sharing economy activities. *Journal of Cleaner Production, 280*, 124782.

Hussien, H. M., Yasin, S. M., Udzir, N. I., Ninggal, M. I. H., & Salman, S. (2021). Blockchain technology in the healthcare industry: Trends and opportunities. *Journal of Industrial Information Integration, 22*, 100217.

Jabbar, R., Fetais, N., Krichen, M., & Barkaoui, K. (2020, February). Blockchain technology for healthcare: Enhancing shared electronic health record interoperability and integrity. 2020 IEEE International Conference on Informatics, IoT, and Enabling Technologies (ICIoT). IEEE, pp. 310–317.

Jensen, P. B., Jensen, L. J., & Brunak, S. (2012). Mining electronic health records: Towards better research applications and clinical care. *Nature Reviews Genetics, 13*(6), 395–405.

Jiang, F., Jiang, Y., Zhi, H., Dong, Y., Li, H., Ma, S., ... Wang, Y. (2017). Artificial intelligence in healthcare: Past, present and future. *Stroke and Vascular Neurology, 2*(4).

Kakhi, K., Alizadehsani, R., Kabir, H. D., Khosravi, A., Nahavandi, S., & Acharya, U. R. (2022). The internet of medical things and artificial intelligence: Trends, challenges, and opportunities. *Biocybernetics and Biomedical Engineering, 42*(3), 749–771.

Kane, Gerald C. 2015. How digital transformation is making health care safer, faster and cheaper. *MIT Sloan Management Review*, 57(1).

Kang, B. (2021). How the COVID-19 pandemic is reshaping the education service. In J. Spohrer & N. Leitner (Eds.), *The future of service post-COVID-19 pandemic, volume 1: Rapid adoption of digital service technology* (pp. 15–36). Springer. https://doi.org/10.1007/978-3-030-82498-2_2

Kesner, S. B., & Howe, R. D. (2011). Design principles for rapid prototyping forces sensors using 3-D printing. *IEEE/ASME Transactions on Mechatronics, 16*(5), 866–870.

Khan, M. A., & Salah, K. (2018). IoT security: Review, blockchain solutions, and open challenges. *Future Generation Computer Systems, 82*, 395–411.

Khang, A., Ragimova, N. A., Hajimahmud, V. A., & Alyar, A. V. (2022). Advanced technologies and data management in the smart healthcare system. In *AI-centric smart city ecosystems* (pp. 261–270). CRC Press.

Kirkendall, E. S., Ni, Y., Lingren, T., Leonard, M., Hall, E. S., & Melton, K. (2019). Data challenges with real-time safety event detection and clinical decision support. *Journal of Medical Internet Research, 21*(5), e13047.

Kumar, S., Nilsen, W., Pavel, M., & Srivastava, M. (2013). Mobile health: Revolutionizing healthcare through transdisciplinary research. *Computer*, 46(1), 28–35.

Laaki, H., Miche, Y., & Tammi, K. (2019). Prototyping a digital twin for real time remote control over mobile networks: Application of remote surgery. *Ieee Access, 7*, 20325–20336.

Li, H., Jing, W., Gao, Y., & Shi, Y. 2016. Examining individuals' adoption of healthcare wearable devices: An empirical study from privacy calculus perspective. *International Journal of Medical Informatics*, 88, 8–17.

Li, J. P. O., Liu, H., Ting, D. S., Jeon, S., Chan, R. P., Kim, J. E., ... Ting, D. S. (2021). Digital technology, tele-medicine and artificial intelligence in ophthalmology: A global perspective. *Progress in Retinal and Eye Research, 82*, 100900.

Li, J., & Kassem, M. (2021). Applications of distributed ledger technology (DLT) and Blockchain-enabled smart contracts in construction. *Automation in Construction*, *132*, 103955.

Li, X., Jiang, P., Chen, T., Luo, X., & Wen, Q. (2020). A survey on the security of blockchain systems. *Future Generation Computer Systems*, *107*, 841–853.

Liaw, C. Y., & Guvendiren, M. (2017). Current and emerging applications of 3D printing in medicine. *Biofabrication*, *9*(2), 024102.

Lin, C. T., Chang, K. C., Lin, C. L., Chiang, C. C., Lu, S. W., Chang, S. S., ... Ko, L. W. (2010). An intelligent telecardiology system using a wearable and wireless ECG to detect atrial fibrillation. *IEEE Transactions on Information Technology in Biomedicine*, *14*(3), 726–733.

Longo, U. G., Carnevale, A., Massaroni, C., Lo Presti, D., Berton, A., Candela, V., Schena, E., & Denaro, V. (2021). Personalized, predictive, participatory, precision, and preventive (P5) medicine in rotator cuff tears. *Journal of Personalized Medicine*, *11*(4), 255. https://doi.org/10.3390/jpm11040255

Lou, Z., Wang, L., Jiang, K., Wei, Z., & Shen, G. (2020). Reviews of wearable healthcare systems: Materials, devices and system integration. *Materials Science and Engineering: R: Reports*, *140*, 100523.

Luxton, D.D., McCann, R. A., Bush, E., Mishkind, M. C., & Reger, G. M. (2011). mHealth for mental health: Integrating smartphone technology in behavioral healthcare. *Professional Psychology: Research and Practice*, *42*(6), 505–512.

Mack, J. (n.d.). *How artificial intelligence is impacting the health care field*. University of San Diego. Retrieved April 2, 2025, from https://onlinedegrees.sandiego.edu/ai-healthcare/

Magrabi, F., Ammenwerth, E., McNair, J. B., De Keizer, N. F., Hyppönen, H., Nykänen, P., ... Georgiou, A. (2019). Artificial intelligence in clinical decision support: Challenges for evaluating AI and practical implications. *Yearbook of Medical Informatics*, *28*(01), 128–134.

Majumder, S., Mondal, T., & Deen, M. J. (2017). Wearable sensors for remote health monitoring. *Sensors*, *17*(1), 130.

Mak, K. K., Wong, Y. H., & Pichika, M. R. (2023). Artificial intelligence in drug discovery and development. In H. G. Vogel & J. Maas (Eds.), *Drug discovery and evaluation: Safety and pharmacokinetic assays* (pp. 1–38). Springer. https://doi.org/10.1007/978-3-030-73317-9_92-1

Malasinghe, L. P., Ramzan, N., & Dahal, K. (2019). Remote patient monitoring: A comprehensive study. *Journal of Ambient Intelligence and Humanized Computing*, *10*, 57–76.

Mandal, S. (2020). *Why telemedicine is the next big opportunity in Indian healthtech*. Inc42. https://inc42.com/datalab/telemedicine-market-opportunity-in-indian-healthtech/

Markin, R. S., & Whalen, S. A. (2000). Laboratory automation: Trajectory, technology, and tactics. *Clinical Chemistry*, *46*(5), 764–771.

Meahjohn, I., & Persad, P. (2020). The impact of COVID-19 on entrepreneurship globally. *Journal of Economics and Business*, *3*(3), 1165–1173. https://doi.org/10.31014/aior.1992.03.03.272

Medaglia, C. M., & Serbanati, A. (2010). An overview of privacy and security issues in the internet of things. The Internet of Things: 20th Tyrrhenian Workshop on Digital Communications, New York. Springer, pp. 389–395.

Mehrotra, A., Huskamp, H. A., Souza, J., Uscher-Pines, L., Rose, S., Landon, B. E., ... Busch, A. B. (2017). Rapid growth in mental health telemedicine use among rural Medicare beneficiaries, wide variation across states. *Health Affairs*, *36*(5), 909–917.

Michel-Verkerke, M. B., Stegwee, R. A., & Spil, T. A. (2015). The six P's of the next step in electronic patient records in the Netherlands. *Health Policy and Technology*, *4*(2), 137–143.

Mobbs, R. J., Coughlan, M., Thompson, R., Sutterlin, C. E., & Phan, K. (2017). The utility of 3D printing for surgical planning and patient-specific implant design for complex spinal pathologies: Case report. *Journal of Neurosurgery: Spine*, *26*(4), 513–518.

Mould, R. F. (1995). The early history of x-ray diagnosis with emphasis on the contributions of physics 1895–1915. *Physics in Medicine & Biology*, *40*(11), 1741.

Moustris, G. P., Hiridis, S. C., Deliparaschos, K. M., & Konstantinidis, K. M. (2011). Evolution of autonomous and semi-autonomous robotic surgical systems: A review of the literature. *The International Journal of Medical Robotics and Computer Assisted Surgery*, 7(4), 375–392.

Neufeld, J. D., Yellowlees, P. M., Hilty, D. M., Cobb, H., & Bourgeois, J. A. (2007). The e-Mental Health Consultation Service: Providing enhanced primary-care mental health services through telemedicine. *Psychosomatics*, *48*(2), 135–141.

Nicola, M., Alsafi, Z., Sohrabi, C., Kerwan, A., Al-Jabir, A., Iosifidis, C., ... Agha, R. (2020). The socio-economic implications of the coronavirus pandemic (COVID-19): A review. *International Journal of Surgery*, *78*, 185–193.

Oates, J., Weston, W. W., & Jordan, J. (2000). The impact of patient-centered care on outcomes. *Family Practice*, *49*(9), 796–804.

Oh, H., Rizo, C., Enkin, M., & Jadad, A. (2005). What is eHealth (3): A systematic review of published definitions. *Journal of Medical Internet Research*, *7*(1), e1.

Oldenburg, B., Taylor, C. B., O'Neil, A., Cocker, F., & Cameron, L. D. (2015). Using new technologies to improve the prevention and management of chronic conditions in populations. *Annual Review of Public Health*, *36*, 483–505.

Ostrowitz, M. B., Eschete, D., Zemon, H., & DeNoto, G. (2009). Robotic-assisted single-incision right colectomy: Early experience. *The International Journal of Medical Robotics and Computer Assisted Surgery*, *5*(4), 465–470.

Øvretveit J, Scott, T., Rundall, T. G., Shortell, S. M., & Brommels, M. (2007, October). Improving quality through effective implementation of information technology in healthcare. International Journal for Quality in Health Care, *19*(5), 259–266. doi: 10.1093/intqhc/mzm031. Epub 2007 Aug 23. PMID: 17717038.

Ozdemir, Z., Barron, J., & Bandyopadhyay, S. (2011). An analysis of the adoption of digital health records under switching costs. *Information Systems Research*, 22(3), 491–503.

Palas, M. J. U., & Bunduchi, R. (2021). Exploring interpretations of blockchain's value in healthcare: A multi-stakeholder approach. *Information Technology & People*, *34*(2), 453–495.

Pasveer, B. (2006). Representing or mediating: A history and philosophy of X-ray images in medicine. In L. Pauwels (Ed.), *Visual cultures of science: Rethinking representational practices in knowledge building and science communication* (pp. 41–62). Dartmouth College Press.

Patra, S., & Young, V. (2016). A review of 3D printing techniques and the future in biofabrication of bioprinted tissue. *Cell Biochemistry and Biophysics*, *74*, 93–98.

Poon, E. G., Cina, J. L., Churchill, W., Patel, N., Featherstone, E., Rothschild, J. M., ... Gandhi, T. K. (2006). Medication dispensing errors and potential adverse drug events before and after implementing bar code technology in the pharmacy. *Annals of Internal Medicine*, *145*(6), 426–434.

Preston, J., Brown, F. W., & Hartley, B. (1992). Using telemedicine to improve health care in distant areas. *Psychiatric Services*, *43*(1), 25–32.

Raj, A., Mukherjee, A. A., de Sousa Jabbour, A. B. L., & Srivastava, S. K. (2022). Supply chain management during and post-COVID-19 pandemic: Mitigation strategies and practical lessons learned. *Journal of Business Research*, *142*, 1125–1139.

Rana, M. S., & Shuford, J. (2024). AI in Healthcare: Transforming Patient Care through Predictive Analytics and Decision Support Systems. *Journal of Artificial Intelligence General Science (JAIGS)* *1*(1).

Ribeiro, J., Lima, R., Eckhardt, T., & Paiva, S. (2021). Robotic process automation and artificial intelligence in industry 4.0–a literature review. *Procedia Computer Science*, *181*, 51–58.

Rubin, G. D. (2014). Computed tomography: Revolutionizing the practice of medicine for 40 years. *Radiology*, *273*(2S), S45–S74.

Rush, K. L., Howlett, L., Munro, A., & Burton, L. (2018). Videoconference compared to telephone in healthcare delivery: A systematic review. *International Journal of Medical Informatics*, *118*, 44–53.

Sansone, A., Cuzin, B., & Jannini, E. A. (2021). Facing counterfeit medications in sexual medicine. A systematic scoping review on social strategies and technological solutions. *Sexual Medicine*, *9*(6), 100437–100437.

Schönberger, D. (2019). Artificial intelligence in healthcare: A critical analysis of the legal and ethical implications. *International Journal of Law and Information Technology*, *27*(2), 171–203.

Sharma, S., & Singh, G. (2021). Comparison of voice based virtual assistants fostering indian higher education – a technical perspective. 2021 International Conference on Technological Advancements and Innovations (ICTAI), Tashkent, Uzbekistan, 2021, pp. 162–167, doi: 10.1109/ICTAI53825.2021.9673307.

Sharma, S., Singh, G., Sharma, C.S., et al. (2024). Artificial intelligence in Indian higher education institutions: A quantitative study on adoption and perceptions. *International Journal of System Assurance Engineering and Management*. https://doi.org/10.1007/s13198-023-02193-8

Sharma, S., Srivastav, S., Gupta, A., & Manglick, A. (2022). Application of technology and innovation in Fintech and its adaptability in India. 2022 2nd International Conference on Innovative Practices in Technology and Management (ICIPTM), Gautam Buddha Nagar, India, 2022, pp. 305–311. doi: 10.1109/ICIPTM54933.2022.9753933

Shubber, M., Svensson, A., & Larsson, L. (2018). Acceptance of video conferencing in healthcare planning in hospitals. AMCIS 2018 Proceedings, pp. 1–10.

Šimundić, A. M. (2009). Measures of diagnostic accuracy: Basic definitions. *Ejifcc*, *19*(4), 203.

Singh, Y., Jabbar, M. A., Kumar Shandilya, S., Vovk, O., & Hnatiuk, Y. (2023). Exploring applications of blockchain in healthcare: Road map and future directions. *Frontiers in Public Health*, *11*, 1229386.

Smith, A. A., Li, R., & Tse, Z. T. H. (2023). Reshaping healthcare with wearable biosensors. *Scientific Reports*, *13*(1), 4998.

Tanwar, S., Parekh, K., & Evans, R. (2020). Blockchain-based electronic healthcare record system for healthcare 4.0 applications. *Journal of Information Security and Applications*, *50*, 102407.

Terzi, D. S., Terzi, R., & Sagiroglu, S. (2015, December). A survey on security and privacy issues in big data. 2015 10th International Conference for Internet Technology and Secured Transactions (ICITST). IEEE, pp. 202–207.

Thrall, J. H., & Boland, G. (1998, April). Telemedicine in practice. In *Seminars in nuclear medicine* (Vol. 28, No. 2, pp. 145–157). WB Saunders.

Trenfield, S. J., Awad, A., Madla, C. M., Hatton, G. B., Firth, J., Goyanes, A., ... Basit, A. W. (2019). Shaping the future: Recent advances of 3D printing in drug delivery and healthcare. *Expert Opinion on Drug Delivery*, *16*(10), 1081–1094. https://doi.org/10.1080/17425247.2019.1660318

Wang, S., Ouyang, L., Yuan, Y., Ni, X., Han, X., & Wang, F. Y. (2019). Blockchain-enabled smart contracts: Architecture, applications, and future trends. *IEEE Transactions on Systems, Man, and Cybernetics: Systems*, *49*(11), 2266–2277.

Wang, Y., Kung, L., & Byrd, T. A. (2018). Big data analytics: Understanding its capabilities and potential benefits for healthcare organizations. *Technological Forecasting and Social Change*, *126*, 3–13.

Weber, L. M., & Stein, J. (2018). The use of robots in stroke rehabilitation: A narrative review. *NeuroRehabilitation*, *43*(1), 99–110.

Winters, J. M., & Winters, J. M. (2007). Videoconferencing and telehealth technologies can provide a reliable approach to remote assessment and teaching without compromising quality. *Journal of Cardiovascular Nursing*, *22*(1), 51–57.

Wootton, R. (2012). Twenty years of telemedicine in chronic disease management–an evidence synthesis. *Journal of Telemedicine and Telecare*, *18*(4), 211–220.

Wosik, J., Fudim, M., Cameron, B., Gellad, Z. F., Cho, A., Phinney, D., ... Tcheng, J. (2020). Telehealth transformation: COVID-19 and the rise of virtual care. *Journal of the American Medical Informatics Association*, *27*(6), 957–962.

Yaqoob, I., Salah, K., Jayaraman, R., & Al-Hammadi, Y. (2022). Blockchain for healthcare data management: opportunities, challenges, and future recommendations. *Neural Computing & Applications 34*, 11475–11490. https://doi.org/10.1007/s00521-020-05519-w

Zayas-Cabán, T., Haque, S. N., & Kemper, N. (2021). Identifying opportunities for workflow automation in health care: Lessons learned from other industries. *Applied Clinical Informatics*, *12*(03), 686–697.

Zhang, M., Davies, T. C., & Xie, S. (2013). Effectiveness of robot-assisted therapy on ankle rehabilitation–a systematic review. *Journal of Neuroengineering and Rehabilitation*, *10*, 1–16.

Zhang, Y., Zhang, F., Yan, Z., Ma, Q., Li, X., Huang, Y., & Rogers, J. A. (2017). Printing, folding and assembly methods for forming 3D mesostructures in advanced materials. *Nature Reviews Materials*, *2*(4), 1–17.

Zhu, G., Chou, M. C., & Tsai, C. W. (2020). Lessons learned from the COVID-19 pandemic exposing the shortcomings of current supply chain operations: A long-term prescriptive offering. *Sustainability*, *12*(14), 5858.

## WEBSITES

CB Insights Report. (2022). The big tech in healthcare report how Amazon, Google, Microsoft, Apple, & Oracle are fighting for the $11T market. https://runwise.oss-accelerate.aliyuncs.com/sites/15/2023/08/CB-Insights_Big-Tech-In-Healthcare-2022-1.pdf

Digital health integration with neuromodulation therapies: The future of patient-centric innovation in neuromodulation - scientific figure on researchgate. Retrieved September 3, 2024, from https://www.researchgate.net/figure/Evolution-of-technology-leading-to-the-age-of-digital-healthcare-Iterative-advances-in_fig1_351700276

HIMSS. (2021). The 2021 future of healthcare report. https://www.himss.org/sites/hde/files/handout-FutureOfHealthcareReport-EMC-0821-FINAL_156.pdf

Kennedy, Lauren Paige. (2018). How artificial intelligence helps in health care. Medically Reviewed by Arefa Cassoobhoy, MD, MPH, https://www.webmd.com/a-to-z-guides/features/artificial-intelligence-helps-health-care

Protenus, Inc. (2022, March 10). Hacking incidents dominate health data breaches according to new breach barometer report. https://www.globenewswire.com/news-release/2022/03/10/2400998/0/en/Hacking-Incidents-Dominate-Health-Data-Breaches-According-to-New-Breach-Barometer-Report.html

Verified Market Research Report. (2022, April 6). Blockchain in healthcare market size worth $ 7308.32 Million, globally, by 2028 at 76.30% CAGR: Verified market research report. https://www.prnewswire.com/news-releases/blockchain-in-healthcare-market-size-worth--7308-32-million-globally-by-2028-at-76-30-cagr-verified-market-research-301518876.html

https://assets.delveinsight.com/blog/wp-content/uploads/2022/02/09180614/Applications-of-AI-in-Healthcare.jpg,

https://guardtime.com/blog/estonian-ehealth-partners-guardtime-blockchain-based-transparency

https://guardtime.com/blog/estonian-ehealth-partners-guardtime-blockchain-based-transparency#:~:text=Estonian%20eHealth%20Foundation%20uses%20Oracle,lifecycle%20management%20of%20patient%20records.

https://inc42.com/datalab/telemedicine-market-opportunity-in-indian-healthtech/

https://journals.sagepub.com/doi/10.1177/0972063421995025

https://scholar.google.co.in/scholar?q=research+paper+on+technology+in+healthcare&hl=en&as_sdt=0&as_vis=1&oi=scholart#d=gs_qabs&t=1711338288285&u=%23p%3DS1EL07OFhgMJ

https://social-innovation.hitachi/en-in/knowledge-hub/techverse/healthcare-with-telemedicine/-/media/Project/Hitachi/SIB/en-IN/knowledge-hub/hitachi-voice/healthcare-with-telemedicine/images

https://www.delveinsight.com/blog/top-applications-of-artificial-intelligence-in-healthcare

https://www.ibm.com/topics/healthcare-technology#:~:text=Healthcare%20technology%20is%20any%20technology,designed%20to%20support%20healthcare%20organizations

https://www.ncbi.nlm.nih.gov/pmc/articles/PMC5787626/

https://www.precedenceresearch.com/wearable-medical-device-market

https://www.researchgate.net/publication/333689726_The_Impact_of_Technology_Trends_on_Healthcare_Systems_A_Study_on_Opportunities_and_Threats

https://www.simplilearn.com/how-has-technology-improved-our-lives-article#:~:text=By%20seeping%20into%20every%20aspect,by%20facilitating%20more%20advanced%20features

https://www.valuecoders.com/blog/blockchain-ml/reshaping-medical-supply-management-with-blockchain/#:~:text=According%20to%20PR%20Newswire%2C%20the,technology%20in%20the%20healthcare%20sector

Chapter 12

# Speech emotion recognition in mental health

## A novel approach using machine learning

*Meghali Das and Garima Srivastava*

## 12.1 INTRODUCTION

According to Patel (2014) observing and managing mental health is vital for improving physical health and promoting safety in neighborhoods and relationships. In recent years, the interplay between mental and physical health has increasingly been recognized as essential for holistic well-being. Mental health, encompassing emotional, psychological, and social well-being, plays a pivotal role in shaping one's overall health status. Beyond its direct impact on cognitive and emotional functioning, mental health influences various aspects of physical health. This interconnectedness underscores the significance of addressing mental well-being as a fundamental component of promoting and maintaining optimal physical health. By understanding and nurturing mental health, individuals can effectively enhance their resilience, manage chronic conditions, and adopt healthier lifestyles, thereby fostering a comprehensive approach to wellness. According to Zhou (2019), globally, the number of people suffering from mental diseases is increasing. In 2016, the Institute for Health Metrics and Evaluation (IHME) reported that more than 1 billion people worldwide were diagnosed with mental disorders. The World Health Organization (WHO) reported a 25% increase in symptoms of anxiety and depression during the COVID-19 pandemic's initial stages through the first phase of the COVID-19 epidemic, particularly among the youth. At the same time, inadequate mental health care has led to an increase in suicide rates.

Speech is a key mode of communication that conveys information and a wide range of emotions. Knowing how to interpret the emotions portrayed by speech is critical for efficient communication because emotions reflect intents, attitudes, and sentiments. Speech emotion identification using machine learning aims to link the divide between what people say and the feelings that they convey. This technology has received increased attention in a variety of fields, including interaction between humans and computers, healthcare, social robots, and entertainment. Speech emotion recognition (SER) using machine learning (ML) represents a transformative approach

 DOI: 10.1201/9781003634089-12

with profound implications for mental health assessment and treatment. Emotions play a pivotal role in our psychological well-being, influencing everything from daily interactions to the manifestation and management of mental health conditions. Traditional methods of assessing emotional states in clinical settings often rely on subjective self-reports or observations, which can be limited by biases and inconsistencies. In contrast, the integration of ML techniques into SER offers a promising avenue for more objective and scalable emotional assessment. By analyzing acoustic features extracted from speech signals, ML algorithms can discern subtle patterns and nuances in emotional expression that may not be readily apparent to human observers. This capability opens up new possibilities for enhancing diagnostic accuracy, monitoring treatment progress, and personalizing therapeutic interventions in mental health care. According to Pourebrahim (2021), the capacity to effectively perceive and interpret sentiments in speech has many practical uses. By taking account of speech signal characteristics and using the Gaussian mixture algorithm to generate a classifier, emotions are identified in this work. The Gaussian mixture model algorithm leverages the statistical properties of Gaussian distributions to create a probabilistic classifier for emotion recognition based on speech parameters. By modeling each emotional state as a mixture of Gaussian components in the feature space, GMMs provide a flexible framework for capturing complex patterns and variability in speech data, making them suitable for diverse applications in emotion recognition systems.

In order to judge the emotion of a user in a voice signal, acceptable characteristics must be carefully chosen such that the features contain information about emotions. There are several characteristics in a speech signal, such as spectral features, prosodic features, and temporal aspects. SER heavily relies on spectral characteristics due to their ability to capture crucial acoustic features that convey emotional states in speech signals. Spectral characteristics, such as pitch, formants, and spectral energy distribution, provide detailed information about the frequency content and modulation patterns of speech. These features reflect variations in vocal tract configurations, pitch dynamics, and intensity levels that accompany different emotional expressions like happiness, sadness, anger, and neutrality. By extracting and analyzing these spectral features, SER systems can effectively discern subtle nuances in speech patterns associated with various emotions, enabling accurate classification and interpretation of emotional states in diverse contexts and across different speakers. The emphasis on spectral characteristics underscores their pivotal role in enhancing the robustness, accuracy, and applicability of SER technologies in fields ranging from human–computer interaction to psychological assessment and beyond. In strained speaking, the vocal cord spectrum is modulated, changing the entire spectrum.

## 12.2 LITERATURE REVIEW

The finest features of emotion recognition through voice have been assessed in the study of Sawit Kasuriya et al. (2019). In the experiment, they've been able to extract 152 features. Two databases have been used; one has an interactive sentiments database in English, and the other contains a multilingual emotional tag corpus that is verbalized in Thai. Hidden Markov model (HMM) classification is used to train the extracted features. However, this model does not achieve a performance of more than 69%.

Soujanya Poria (2018) believes that a measure of the state of consciousness can be useful in sentiment examination. They used both speech and text features as well as visual imagery in order to determine the state of human consciousness. A new methodology for the analysis of feelings has been suggested in this paper. Based on the results of the pragmatic analysis, the researcher concluded that the voice attribute "pitch" is crucial in identifying emotions in speech.

Chen et al. (2012) used a three-layered emotion recognition system from speech in an effort to enhance speech emotion recognition that is independent of speakers. Using the Fisher rate, this method uses a coarse-to-fine classification system to identify the right feature. An input parameter for a multiple-layered support vector machine (SVM)-based classifier is the Fisher percentage output. Also, four comparative trials are organized and the number of attributes is reduced using principal component analysis (PCA) and an artificial neural networks (ANN), respectively. PCA + SVM, Fisher + ANN, PCA + ANN, and Fisher + SVM are the four comparison experiments. The conclusion is that Fisher outperforms PCA in dimension reduction, while SVM outclasses ANN in classification when it comes to speaker-independent emotion recognition. Three levels had individual recognition rates of 86.5%, 68.5%, and 50.2% in the Beihang University database of emotional speech (BHUDES).

Nwe et al. (2003) recommended another framework for the feeling order of expression waves. The classifier and speech signals were described by the procedure using discrete HMM and short time log frequency power coefficients (LFPCs). This strategy ordered the feeling into six distinct classes, then, at that point, utilized the private dataset to prepare and test the new framework. LFPCs are contrasted with mel-frequency cepstral coefficients (MFCCs) and linear prediction cepstral coefficients (LPCCs) to assess the proposed method's efficacy. The results show that the best classification accuracy was 96% and the average was 78%, respectively. Additionally, the results demonstrate that LFPC outperforms standard features as a feature for emotion classification.

New modulation spectral features (MSFs) for human speech emotion recognition were proposed by Wu et al. (2011). Utilizing a modulation filterbank and an auditory filterbank for the purpose of speech decomposition, an appropriate feature was extracted from an auditory-inspired long-term spectro-temporal. Rather than relying solely on conventional short-term spectral features, this approach produced acoustic frequency and temporal modulation frequency components that could be used to convey crucial data. SVMs equipped with a radial basis function (RBF) are used in the classification process. In order to evaluate MSFs, Berlin and Vera am Mittag (VAM) are utilized. In comparison to MFCCs and perceptual linear prediction coefficients (PLPCs), the experimental results show that the MSFs perform well. Recognition performance is significantly improved when MSFs are used to augment prosodic features. Additionally, a classification recognition rate of 91.6% is achieved overall.

Narayanan (2005) proposed using speech signals from a call center application to recognize domain-specific emotions. Recognizing pessimistic and non-gloomy inclination (for example outrage and cheerfulness) are the primary focal points of this examination. Various sorts of data, including acoustic, lexical, and talk, are utilized for feeling acknowledgment. To get data on emotion information at the language level, information-theoretic contents of emotional salience are also presented. Both k-nearest neighbor (KNN) and direct discriminant classifiers are utilized to work with various sorts of features. The results of the experiment show that combining acoustic and language data produces the best results. Results exhibited by joining three data sources rather than one source, arrangement exactness increases by 40.7% for guys and 36.4% for females. Male accuracy ranges from 1.4% to 6.75%, while female accuracy ranges from 0.75% to 3.96%.

Lee et al. (2011) address various levels of computational structures to distinguish feelings. The input speech signal is mapped in one of the corresponding emotion classes using this technique, which employs layers of binary classifications. The fundamental idea is that the various levels in the tree address simplest tasks first to lessen error propagation. AIBO and USC IEMOCAP information bases are utilized to assess the grouping technique. The absolute result improves the accuracy archives by 72.44% to 89.58% over the baseline SVM. The outcome demonstrates the detailed progressive technique is effective for ordering close to home discourse in different data sets.

A multidimensional model based on emotion primitives for speech emotion recognition was proposed by Grimm et al. (2007). Valence, activation, and dominance are the three estimates of emotion primitives that were combined to create the three dimensions. These factors are assumed to have values in the span [–1, +1]. In order to evaluate the emotion primitives and achieve best inter-evaluator agreement, a text-free, image-based method was developed. Fuzzy logic and a rule-based estimator are used to extract acoustic features such as energy, spectral specifications, and pitch specifications. The draws closer are approved by testing two EMA (electromagnetic graphic articulatory) and VAM datasets, which are acted feeling and unconstrained discourse feeling. Both datasets are from German television talk shows. Finally, KNN was used as a classifier to map the emotion primitives to a particular emotion category. The total recognition rate of KNN can reach 83.5%.

KNN and SVM are two classification algorithms that Dorota Kamińska et al. (2012) presented as a way to recognize emotion/feeling from voice. The tests were implemented with tenfold cross-validation. The tests were run on two dissimilar datasets. One dataset features professional actors, whereas the other features writers who speak naturally. They came to the conclusion that professional actors' speech was very accurate after comparing these two datasets.

A technique to gauge the severity of Parkinson's disease based on the level of deterioration of speech was developed by Zoltan Galaz (2016). Parkinson's has an impact on phonation, fluency, and pronunciation of speech. Using the guided regularized random forest technique, speech characteristics from 42 voice samples were retrieved for the tests.

By examining cognitive qualities, P. R. Chaudhari and J. S. R. Alex (2016) examined how to comprehend an individual's emotions/feelings and determine the utterance mood. Long-term voice recordings were applied in this model to examine how the human mind is functioning. To categorize emotional states, they created a statistical model. In the literature, writers have employed the main standard feature extraction methods—MFCC prosody elements and LPCC method for feature extraction separately—to identify speech emotions.

## 12.3 METHODOLOGY

The system proposes to combine prosodic features that are capable of providing a great deal of information about emotions in speech signals. One of the difficult tasks is to select the best characteristics that will allow you to see a person's mental state. The parameters to be taken into account in this model are the formants, pitch, root mean square (RMS) energy, and zero crossing rates. Using the Telugu Speech Corpus (IITKGP-SESC) benchmark dataset, classification models are developed using GMM classifiers.

### 12.3.1 Pattern recognition in emotion recognition

Pattern recognition in emotion recognition refers to the process of identifying and categorizing emotional states based on patterns observed in various sources of data, such as facial expressions, voice tone, gestures, and textual content. In essence, pattern recognition in emotion recognition involves the systematic extraction of features, detection of meaningful patterns, classification into emotional categories, and adaptation to various contextual factors. These processes enable machines to comprehend and react to human emotions more effectively, facilitating applications in fields like virtual reality, human–computer interaction, healthcare, and customer service. Here's how pattern recognition is involved in this process:

1. **Feature extraction:** Emotion recognition systems first extract relevant features from the input data, such as facial landmarks, voice pitch, intensity of gestures, or linguistic patterns in text. These features are extracted because they are known to correlate with specific emotional states.
2. **Pattern matching:** Once features are extracted, the system compares them against known patterns or models of emotions. These models could be based on empirical data (e.g., databases of facial expressions linked to emotions) or learned through machine learning algorithms.
3. **Classification:** The separated traits are then classified into specific emotional categories such as sad, happy, and angry based on the patterns recognized. Machine learning techniques such as SVMs, neural networks, or decision trees are commonly used for this classification task.
4. **Feedback and learning:** Many emotion recognition systems are devised in a manner that can enhance their performance in time with the help of responses received on their classifications. This feedback helps refine the patterns and models used for recognition, leading to better accuracy and reliability.
5. **Integration of multiple modalities:** Emotion recognition often involves combining data from multiple modalities (e.g., facial expressions and voice tone) to improve accuracy. Pattern recognition techniques are used to combine and interpret these different sources of information.
6. **Real-time recognition:** In applications where real-time emotion recognition is required (e.g., human–computer interaction, virtual assistants), efficient pattern recognition algorithms are essential for quick and accurate identification of emotions.

**Contextual understanding:** Advanced emotion recognition systems also consider contextual factors that influence emotions, such as cultural norms, situational cues, and individual differences. Pattern recognition helps in adapting to these contextual variations.

Feature extraction, training, as well as testing are the three fundamental working procedures in the pattern recognition issue of emotion identification from speech as shown in Figure 12.1.

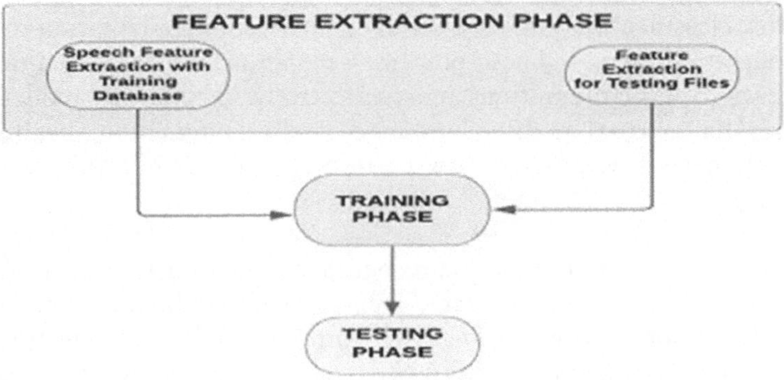


*Figure 12.1* System model for emotion recognition.

### 12.3.2 Data collection

It is a significant task to collect suitable databases in the emotion recognition system through speech. It is a pivotal undertaking in the development of emotion recognition systems focused on speech. The quality and diversity of the databases gathered directly impact the system's ability to accurately interpret and classify emotional states from speech signals. An essential aspect of this task involves selecting datasets that encompass a wide range of emotional expressions across various demographic groups, including differences in age, gender, cultural background, and linguistic diversity. This diversity ensures that the system can effectively generalize its learning and accommodate the nuanced means that emotions are expressed through speech in different contexts and among different populations.

Furthermore, meticulous attention is paid to the annotation and labeling of collected speech data with emotional categories. Clear and consistent labeling is crucial to training machine learning algorithms effectively. It ensures that the models can learn to distinguish between subtle variations in speech patterns associated with different emotions, thereby enhancing the system's accuracy and robustness. Ethical considerations also play a significant role in this process, ensuring that data collection practices respect participant privacy, obtain informed consent, and uphold principles of fairness and generality. Ultimately, by meticulously curating and annotating diverse datasets, developers lay the basis for emotion recognition systems that are both reliable in performance and sensitive to the complexities of human emotional expression through speech.

The main aim is to ensure that existing emotional speech data collection records are updated as soon as possible. A brief discussion will be given of the number of emotional states, languages, numbers of speakers, and types of speech. The type of database that will be used in the system has an extremely important effect on the effectiveness of voice emotion/feeling identification. The Danish emotional corpus database was used by some of the researchers for emotional identification from speech stated by Jianfeng Zhao et al. (2019). The primary source for this system is an acted-affect Telugu voice database. It uses the IIT-KGP Speech Corpus. We looked at 15 semantically neutral Telugu sentences in order to analyze emotions. In a single session, one artist had to talk 15 words in four different emotions. There were ten sessions taken into account for the preparation of the database. For recording the conversations, man and woman speakers between 30 and 35 years of age were taken into consideration.

### 12.3.3 Feature extraction

Emotion recognition systems extract relevant features from input data sources. For example, from facial expressions, features might include the position of facial landmarks like eyes and mouth, or changes in skin coloration. From voice tone, features could be pitch, intensity, and rhythm. Textual content might be analyzed for specific words or linguistic patterns associated with emotions. In the realm of voice tone analysis, systems extract features such as pitch (the highness or lowness of the voice), intensity (the strength or volume of the voice), and rhythm (the pattern of speech or pauses). These acoustic features are pivotal in detecting nuances in vocal expression associated with different emotions. For example, a higher pitch and faster rhythm might indicate excitement or happiness, while a lower pitch and slower rhythm might suggest sadness or contemplation.

Textual content is another valuable source for emotion recognition systems, where algorithms analyze specific words, phrases, or linguistic patterns that correlate with particular emotional states. Sentiment analysis techniques can detect emotional cues from written text, considering factors like the use of emotive language, word choice, and grammatical structure. This textual analysis complements other modalities like facial expressions and voice tone, providing a comprehensive understanding of emotional contexts in applications ranging from customer feedback analysis to mental health monitoring.

The feature extraction procedure is the most vital step in the emotion identification system; choosing the appropriate features is essential for accurate categorization. The voice features are calculated from the signal's quick Fourier transform. With a window size of 20 ms and a shift of 15 ms, every frame is analyzed (Figure 12.2).

For instance, suppose that the entire voice signal lasts for 2 seconds.
Speech signal is denoted by S.
Size of frame = 20 ms, Frame shift = 15 ms
Sample frequency = 18000 per sec
Samples in total speech signal T = 2 × 18000 = 36000
Number of samples in one frame n = (20/1000) × 18000 = 360

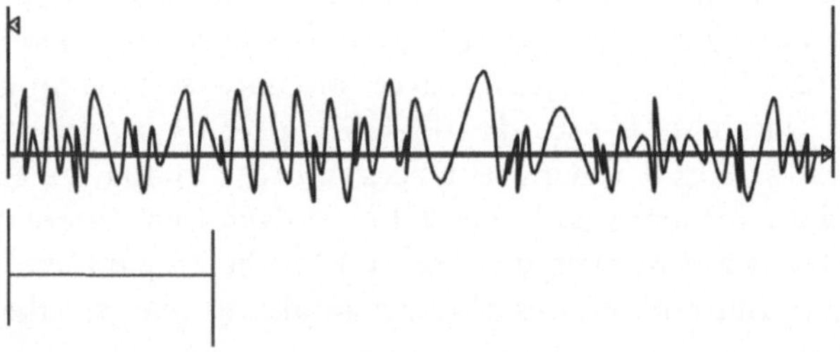

*Figure 12.2* Speech signal frames.

Separated by samples m = (15/1000) × 18000) = 270
Step size S = n – m
S = 360 – 270 = 90
Total number of frames in speech signal = (T/S) – 1
= (36000/90) – 1
= 399 frames in a speech of 2 seconds

The primary objective for this system is the extraction of dependable characteristics. In the feature extraction stage, two datasets will be extracted: the training dataset as well as the testing dataset. The training dataset contains the data, and the features extracted in the testing dataset will be provided to the classification prototype to determine the emotion in a test signal that was provided to the model to test. Formants, pitch, root mean square, and zero crossing rate, prosodic qualities that are more dependable in extracting information from voice signals, were used to build the system.

### 12.3.4 Training phase

The training phase in pattern recognition for emotion recognition systems is pivotal for teaching algorithms to discern and classify emotional states based on extracted features from input data. This phase begins with the careful selection and extraction of relevant features from diverse sources such as facial expressions, voice tone, gestures, and textual content. These features serve as the foundation for machine learning algorithms to learn and distinguish patterns associated with different emotions. During training, labeled datasets play a crucial role, where each data instance is paired with an emotional label (e.g., happy, sad, angry). The algorithm iteratively adjusts its parameters to minimize errors and improve its ability to accurately predict emotional states from new, unseen data.

Various machine-learning techniques can be employed during the training phase, depending on the complexity and nature of the data. Neural networks, SVMs, and ensemble methods are commonly utilized to handle the multidimensional and often nonlinear relationships between extracted features and emotional expressions. The effectiveness of the training phase is assessed through validation metrics like accuracy and F1-score on a separate validation set, ensuring the ability of the model to simplify beyond the data that is employed for training. This iterative process of training, evaluation, and refinement is essential for developing robust emotion recognition systems capable of interpreting and responding to human emotions across different contexts and applications, from healthcare to human–computer interaction.

According to Liu et al. (2019), in order to train the extracted features and generate class models, a classifier algorithm should be used in the training phase. The prosodic features that are extracted from speech signals are used to train the Gaussian mixture model (GMM) and build emotion systems. B. W. Schuller (2018) said that the arrangement of data locus in the input feature area is known to be captured by GMMs. It is an important but technically challenging problem to determine the ideal integer of components from the Gaussian model. We have analyzed a range of Gaussian components, including 2, 4, 8, 16, 32, 64, 128, and 256. In order to be able to represent as one feature of various emotions, the voice files of the training dataset are merged into one voice signal and sent to an extraction stage so that each emotion can have its own individual clusters based on anger, fear, happiness, or neutral. In the file, each cluster is kept as a single variable. The GMM classifier is used for training the extracted elements and generates a class model (Figure 12.3).

## 12.3.5 Testing phase

The testing phase in pattern recognition for emotion recognition systems is a critical stage where the performance of the trained model is evaluated on fresh, unseen data to assess the accuracy and generalization capability. During this phase, the model is presented with a separate set of data that

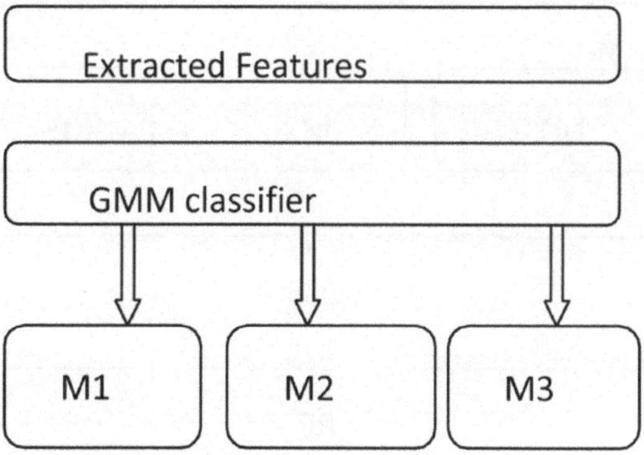


*Figure 12.3* Training classifier for different emotions.

it has not encountered during training. This dataset, known as the test set, is annotated with emotional labels to measure how well the model can correctly predict emotions based on the extracted features from input data such as gestures, facial expressions, voice tone, and textual content.

The key objective of the testing phase is to determine the model's effectiveness in real-world scenarios by evaluating criteria like recall, accuracy, F1-score, and precision. The standards give comprehension about the ability of the model to accurately categorize emotional states across distinct contexts and individuals. The successful testing phase confirms the model's generalization ability, ensuring that it can reliably recognize emotions beyond the specific instances it was trained on. Continuous testing and validation are crucial to refine and improve the model's performance, enabling emotion recognition systems to meet the accuracy and reliability requirements demanded by applications in fields like healthcare, education, and human–computer interaction.

The feature extraction is from a voice signal, each of which is tested for emotional state using the speech files from the testing dataset. Each speech file is 30 seconds long, but it has other elements (Figure 12.4).

### 12.3.6 Experimental setup

In this study MATLAB will be used to carry out the experiments. It is a highly recognized programming language in the software industry. According to

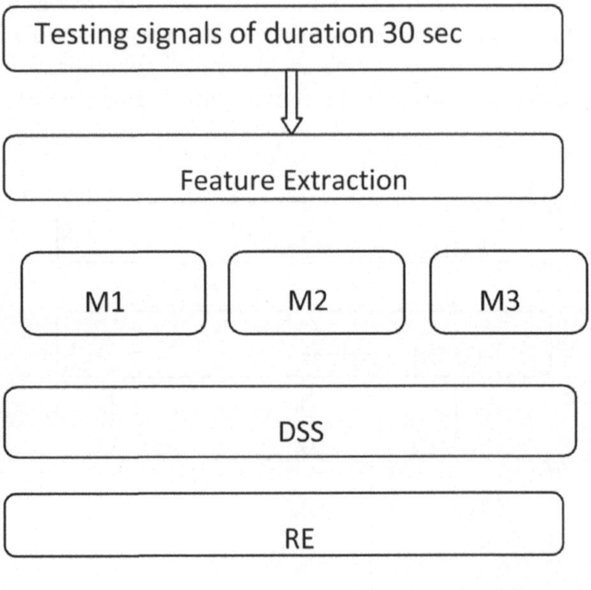


*Figure 12.4* Testing phase.

Peerzade (2018), it provides a user-friendly environment where solutions have already been mentioned in familiar mathematics notation. MATLAB, short for Matrix Laboratory, is a powerful and widely used programming environment and language specifically designed for numerical computing, data analysis, and visualization. Developed by MathWorks, MATLAB is renowned for its versatility in handling complex mathematical operations, matrix manipulations, and algorithm implementations across various scientific and engineering disciplines. Its intuitive syntax and extensive library of built-in functions make it an ideal choice for researchers, engineers, and data scientists seeking to prototype and deploy applications in fields such as signal processing, image processing, and machine learning.

According to Swain et al. (2018), the input speech signal was to be 30 seconds long. This was applicable for both the man and woman datasets. The speech signal was segmented into frames. Each frame yielded prosodic information. The GMM classifier is trained using the features extracted, and models for emotions fear, anger, neutral, and happy are generated. For the test phase, an input signal of 30 seconds of speech testing signal is used to perform emotion tests and prosodic features are produced. A comparison of evaluation metrics will be made with the extracted features from the test signal. On the basis of four prosodic groups, we chose the following parameters: energy, the basic frequency, formant frequencies, and zero crossing based on the acoustic association discussed in the literature on automated emotion recognition from the preceding section. Contours represent the energy, basic frequency, and formant frequencies.

According to Hirst and de Looze (2021), the normal frequency of a man's speech signal, which is marked with the number F0, is referred to as pitch. For the fact that this feature depends on vocal fold anxiety, it has information about emotion. The normal frequencies of the human voice are between 50 and 500 Hz (Figure 12.5).

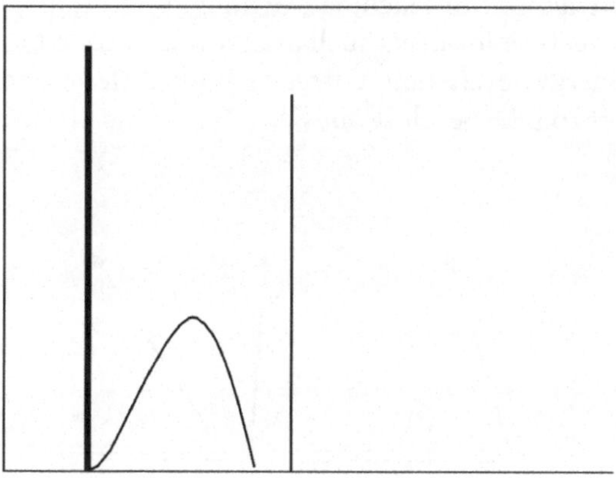

*Figure 12.5* Pitch of the voice signal.

The formant attribute plays a crucial part in the identification of a person's emotion. The other uppermost frequencies are known as formants in the frequency spectrum, apart from the first frequency. The formants are at a similar spectrum in neutral emotion.

According to Heracleous et al. (2017), the zero crossing rate features inform users how frequently the voice signal's amplitude passes over a value of zero. The rate at which zero crossings take place is a basic indicator of a signal's regularity content (Figure 12.6).

It is said by Kavita Bhatnagar et al. (2017) that the RMS energy is a very important aspect of an audio signal that is used for estimating the consecutive allocation of energy. It represents the effective or average power contained in the signal by calculating the square root of the arithmetic mean of the squares of the signal values over a specified time window.

In the context of audio signals, RMS energy serves several important purposes:

1. **Energy estimation:** RMS energy provides a reliable estimate of the total energy present in the signal during a specific time interval. This is particularly useful for tasks such as detecting speech activity in audio recordings or identifying segments of music with varying levels of intensity.
2. **Dynamic range measurement:** It helps in assessing the varying bounds of the audio wave, which refers to the difference between the sharpest and softest measures of the wave. High RMS values indicate louder sections, while lower RMS values correspond to quieter sections.
3. **Normalization:** RMS energy normalization is often used in audio processing tasks to ensure consistent signal levels across different recordings or segments. By normalizing based on RMS energy, audio engineers can adjust the amplitude of the signal without introducing distortion or compromising the signal-to-noise ratio.
4. **Feature extraction:** In machine learning applications, RMS energy is a valuable feature for tasks such as emotion recognition, where variations in energy levels may correlate with different emotional states conveyed through speech or music.

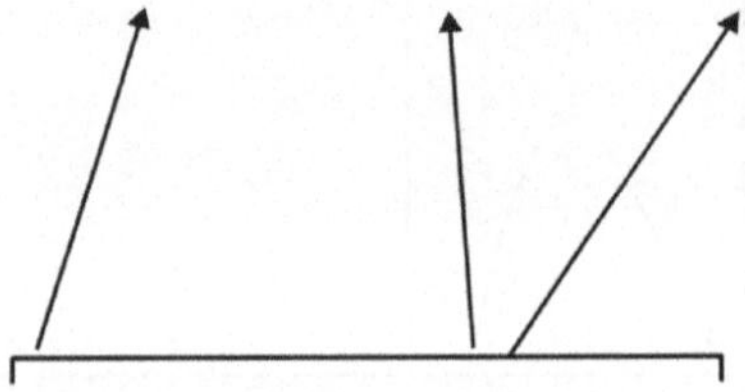

*Figure 12.6* Zero crossing rate.

5. **Segmentation:** RMS energy is also employed in audio segmentation tasks to identify boundaries between different segments based on changes in signal energy levels. This aids in dividing longer audio recordings into meaningful sections for further analysis or processing.

Overall, RMS energy provides critical insights into the temporal distribution of energy within an audio signal, making it an indispensable tool in various audio processing applications ranging from speech and music analysis to sound quality assessment and beyond. Its simplicity and effectiveness make it a widely used metric in both research and practical audio engineering contexts.

Considering the size of the frame as 20 ms and the frame shift as 15 ms, all the characteristics that were previously described are taken out using the framing and windowing procedures, which provide additional information about the audio signal without sacrificing any available information in the speech. As the prosodic features have the data of an accent of a person along with word stress, they are the greatest features for determining the emotion.

## 12.4 EXPERIMENTAL RESULTS

According to Shaw et al. (2016), there are two types of emotion recognition from speech systems: automatic text-dependent and automatic text-independent emotion detection.

In text-dependent systems, the analysis of emotions is based on the content of the speech itself, where the linguistic content plays a crucial role. These systems typically rely on extracting features such as pitch, intonation, speech rate, and linguistic content (e.g., choice of words, sentence structure) to infer emotions. The recognition process often involves analyzing how these features correlate with known emotional patterns or models, which are trained using labeled datasets where emotions are explicitly linked to speech content. Text-dependent systems are particularly useful in applications where the context or content of speech is known or controlled, such as in scripted dialogues or specific command-based interactions with virtual assistants.

On the other hand, text-independent emotion recognition systems focus on analyzing emotional states solely based on acoustic properties of speech, independent of the linguistic content. These systems extract features such as prosody (e.g., pitch, rhythm, stress), spectral characteristics (e.g., formants, energy distribution), and non-verbal vocal cues (e.g., sighs, laughter) from the speech signal. Unlike text-dependent systems, text-independent approaches do not rely on understanding the semantic meaning or content of the speech. Instead, they detect emotional cues based on the acoustic and paralinguistic features present in the speech waveform itself. This makes text-independent systems more suitable for applications where spontaneous or natural speech is involved, such as in conversational interfaces, sentiment analysis from customer service calls, or emotional state monitoring in healthcare settings.

Both types of emotion recognition systems have their strengths and are chosen based on the specific requirements of the application, the availability of training data, and the desired level of control over speech content and context. Advances in machine learning and signal processing techniques continue to enhance the accuracy and applicability of both text-dependent and text-independent emotion recognition systems in various real-world scenarios.

The same voice cues are utilized in the training and testing phases of automated text-dependent emotion recognition systems. In Table 12.1, a man speech signal with a duration of 30 seconds is used as input for the feature extraction phase, and a man speech signal with a duration of 3 seconds is assessed in the testing phase. F0 is the metric pitch, FT is the formant, RMS is the root mean square, and ZC is the zero crossing rate. It has been discovered that combining formant, RMS, and ZC yields greater accuracy (see Tables 12.1–12.4 and Figures 12.7–12.10).

As formants contain a large amount of information on the speech signal's peak value, it is found to be more accurate than any other feature (Trigeorgis et al., 2016). The place where the resonance of the vocal cord is located in the frequency domain depends on the shape and physical dimensions of the vocal range that helps to identify an emotion. Formants and their combinations have a greater accuracy compared to individual characteristics, as can be seen in Table 12.3.

## 12.5 CONCLUSION AND FUTURE SCOPE

The primary objective of emotion identification through speech analysis is to accurately discern individuals' emotional states based on distinctive speech patterns. Key parameters such as zero crossing rate, pitch, formant frequencies, and root mean square play crucial roles in categorizing sentiments like happiness, neutrality, sadness, and anger. These parameters are essential for creating distinct classes that represent different emotional reactions. In this context, Gaussian mixture model (GMM) classifiers are utilized to train on these extracted speech features, leveraging statistical modeling to identify patterns indicative of specific emotions.

In a specific experimental analysis conducted using the IITKGP-SESC Telugu speech corpus dataset, the system demonstrated promising results with an average accuracy of 91.65% when using formant parameters alone. This achievement underscores the system's effectiveness in accurately

*Table 12.1* Recognition of emotion from speech with man training and testing dataset

| *Training dataset: Dataset with man voice* | | | | | | | | | | | | | | | |
|---|---|---|---|---|---|---|---|---|---|---|---|---|---|---|---|
| *Testing: Man audio of length 3 sec* | | | | | | | | | | | | | | | |
| *Emotions (%)* | *F0* | *FT* | *ZC* | *RMS* | *F0 + FT* | *F0 + ZC* | *F0+ RMS* | *FT + ZC* | *FT + RMS* | *ZC + RMS* | *F0 + FT + ZC* | *F0 + ZC + RMS* | *FT + ZC + RMS* | *F0 + FT + RMS* | *F0 + FT + Z C + RMS* |
| Anger | 99 | 99 | 99 | 99 | 99 | 99 | 99 | 99 | 99 | 99 | 99 | 99 | 99 | 100 | 100 |
| Fear | 51 | 15.66 | 99 | 15.66 | 100 | 99 | 84.33 | 98 | 84.33 | 65.66 | 99 | 99 | 85.33 | 100 | 100 |
| Happy | 34.33 | 34.33 | 34.33 | 34.33 | 99 | 34.33 | 99 | 99 | 99 | 34.33 | 99 | 99 | 67.66 | 50 | 83.33 |
| Neutral | 67.66 | 65.66 | 65.66 | 65.66 | 34.33 | 35.33 | 84.33 | 65.66 | 85.33 | 99 | 99 | 99 | 85.33 | 66.66 | 33.33 |

*Table 12.2* Recognition of emotion from speech using training with man dataset and testing with woman dataset

| | | | | | | | | | | | | | | |
|---|---|---|---|---|---|---|---|---|---|---|---|---|---|---|
| | *Training dataset: Man audio dataset* | | | | | | | | | | | | | | |
| | *Testing: Woman audio signals* | | | | | | | | | | | | | | |
| *Emotions (%)* | *F0* | *FT* | *ZC* | *RMS* | *F0 + FT* | *F0 + ZC* | *F0 + RMS* | *FT + ZC* | *FT + RMS* | *ZC + RMS* | *F0 + FT + ZC* | *F0 + ZC + RMS* | *FT + ZC + RMS* | *F0 + FT + RMS* | *F0 + FT + Z C + RMS* |
| Anger | 34.33 | 49 | 82.33 | 34.33 | 83.33 | 100 | 33.33 | 33.33 | 83.33 | 33.33 | 33.33 | 33.33 | 100 | 100 | 83.33 |
| Fear | 100 | 33.33 | 33.33 | 33.33 | 33.33 | 33.33 | 33.33 | 16.66 | 33.33 | 33.33 | 33.33 | 33.33 | 33.33 | 33.33 | 33.33 |
| Happy | 33.33 | 100 | 33.33 | 16.66 | 33.33 | 33.33 | 16.66 | 83.33 | 66.66 | 100 | 100 | 100 | 33.33 | 33.33 | 33.33 |
| Neutral | 33.33 | 33.33 | 83.33 | 100 | 16.66 | 33.33 | 100 | 33.33 | 33.33 | 33.33 | 33.33 | 33.33 | 16.66 | 16.66 | 66.66 |

*Table 12.3* Recognition of emotion from speech with woman training and testing dataset

| *Training dataset: Woman audio dataset* | | | | | | | | | | | | | | | |
|---|---|---|---|---|---|---|---|---|---|---|---|---|---|---|---|
| *Testing: Woman audio signals* | | | | | | | | | | | | | | | |
| *Emotions (%)* | *F0* | *FT* | *ZC* | *RMS* | *F0 + FT* | *F0 + ZC* | | *FT + ZC* | *FT + RMS* | *ZC + RMS* | *F0 + FT + ZC* | *F0 + ZC + RMS* | *FT + ZC + RMS* | *F0 + FT + RMS* | *F0 + FT + ZC + RMS* |
| Anger | 65.66 | 99 | 65.66 | 99 | 100 | 100 | 100 | 100 | 100 | 100 | 100 | 100 | 100 | 100 | 100 |
| Fear | 33.33 | 33.33 | 33.33 | 33.33 | 100 | 100 | 33.33 | 100 | 100 | 100 | 100 | 100 | 100 | 100 | 100 |
| Happy | 33.33 | 33.33 | 100 | 33.33 | 83.33 | 83.33 | 33.33 | 100 | 100 | 83.33 | 100 | 83.33 | 83.33 | 50 | 100 |
| Neutral | 100 | 33.33 | 66.66 | 100 | 100 | 100 | 100 | 100 | 100 | 100 | 100 | 100 | 100 | 83.33 | 100 |

*Table 12.4* Recognition of emotion from speech using training with woman dataset and testing with man dataset

| | *Training dataset: Woman audio dataset* | | | | | | | | | | | | | | |
|---|---|---|---|---|---|---|---|---|---|---|---|---|---|---|---|
| | *Testing: Man audio signals* | | | | | | | | | | | | | | |
| *Emotions (%)* | *F0* | *FT* | *ZC* | *RMS* | *F0 + FT* | *F0 + ZC* | *F0 + RMS* | *FT + ZC* | *FT + RMS* | *ZC + RMS* | *F0 + FT + ZC* | *F0 + ZC + RMS* | *FT + ZC + RMS* | *F0 + FT + RMS* | *F0 + FT + ZC + RMS* |
| Anger | 34.33 | 99 | 35.33 | 34.33 | 34.33 | 34.33 | 35.33 | 35.33 | 35.33 | 34.33 | 34.33 | 34.33 | 34.33 | 34.33 | 34.33 |
| Fear | 99 | 84.33 | 64.66 | 34.33 | 84.33 | 34.33 | 34.33 | 99 | 99 | 99 | 34.33 | 51 | 65.66 | 34.33 | 51 |
| Happy | 84.33 | 34.33 | 65.66 | 34.33 | 51 | 99 | 34.33 | 84.33 | 34.33 | 85.33 | 64.66 | 35.33 | 35.33 | 34.33 | 34.33 |
| Neutral | 34.33 | 34.33 | 99 | 99 | 84.33 | 34.33 | 99 | 34.33 | 34.33 | 99 | 99 | 99 | 99 | 99 | 65.66 |

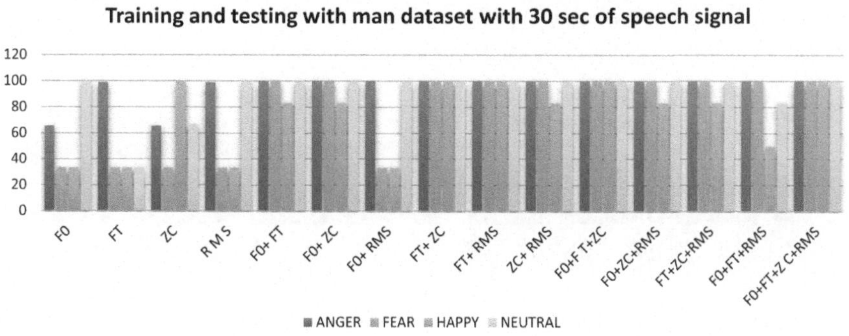


*Figure 12.7* Man training and testing dataset.

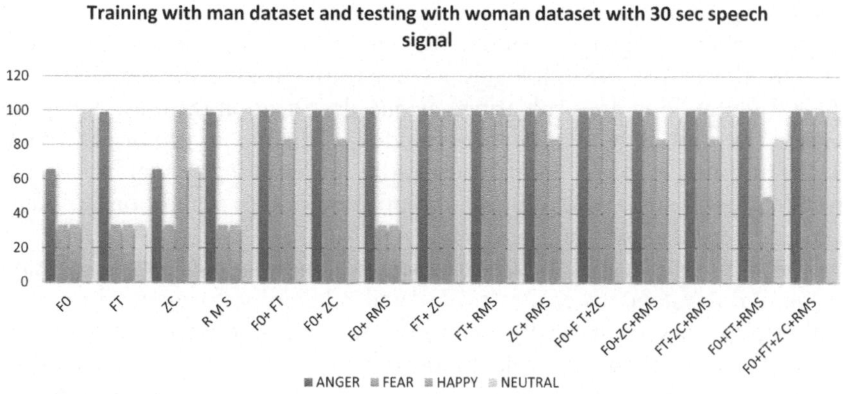


*Figure 12.8* Training with man dataset and testing with woman dataset.

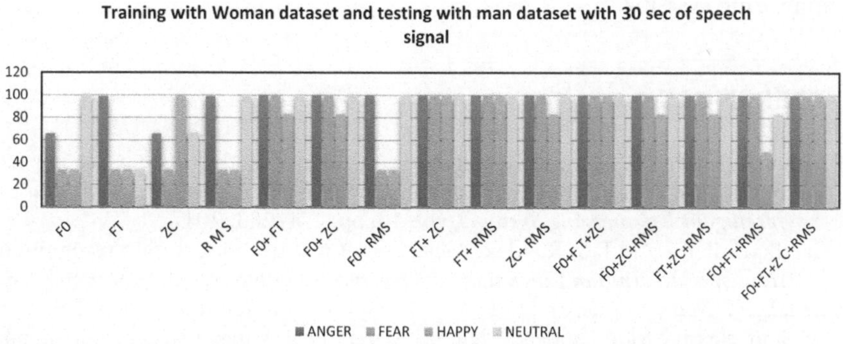


*Figure 12.9* Training with woman dataset and testing with man dataset.

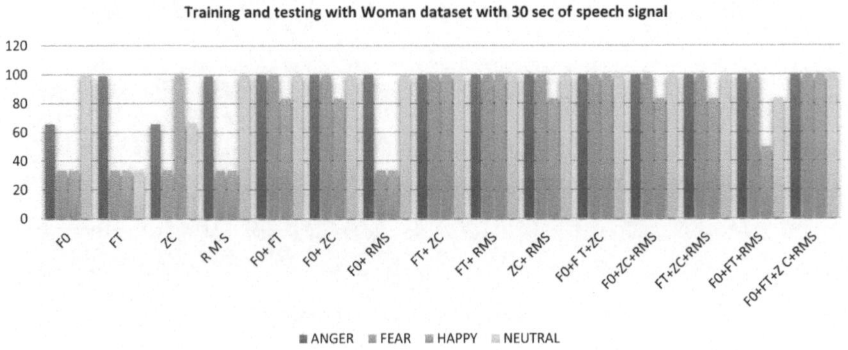


*Figure 12.10* Woman training and testing dataset.

classifying emotions based on the nuanced speech characteristics specific to the Telugu language context. To further enhance performance and explore alternative methodologies, a comparative study will be undertaken. This study will involve evaluating various classification techniques beyond GMM, as well as hidden Markov models and support vector machines. These techniques offer different strengths in handling complex patterns within speech signals, aiming to optimize emotion recognition accuracy across diverse datasets and real-world applications.

The overarching goal of this comparative analysis is to refine emotion recognition systems to ensure robust and reliable performance in practical settings. By systematically comparing and potentially combining different approaches, the study seeks to identify the most effective strategies for improving accuracy and generalizability across varying speech datasets and real-world scenarios. This approach not only contributes to advancing the field of emotion recognition technology but also holds significant implications for applications ranging from virtual assistants to emotional health monitoring systems.

## REFERENCES

Bhatnagar, K., and S. C. Gupta. "Extending the neural model to study the impact of effective area of optical fiber on laser intensity," *International Journal of Intelligent Engineering Systems*, vol. 10, pp. 274–283, 2017.

Chaudhari, P. R., and J. S. R. Alex. "Selection of features for emotion recognition from speech", *Indian Journal of Science and Technology*, vol. 9, no. 39, 2016.

Chen, L., X. Mao, Y. Xue, and L. L. Cheng. "Speech emotion recognition: Features and classification models," *Digital Signal Processing*, vol. 22, no. 6, pp. 1154–1160, December 2012.

Galaz, Z., J. Mekyska, and Z. Smékal. "Degree of Parkinson's disease severity estimation based on speech signal processing," *39th International Conference on Telecommunications and Signal Processing (TSP)*, 503–506, 2016.

Grimm, M., K. Kroschel, E. Mower, and S. Narayanan. "Primitives-based evaluation and estimation of emotions in speech," *Speech Communication*, vol. 49, no. 10–11, pp. 787–800, October 2007.

Heracleous, P. Yasuda, K., F. Sugaya, A. Yoneyama, and M. Hashimoto. "Speech emotion recognition in noisy and reverberant environments," *Proceedings of the 2017 Seventh International Conference on Affective Computing and Intelligent Interaction (ACII)*, San Antonio, TX, USA, pp. 262–266, 23–26 October 2017.

Hirst, D. J., and C. de Looze. "Measuring speech. Fundamental frequency and pitch," *Cambridge Handbook of Phonetics*, vol. 1, 2021.

Kamińska, D., and A. Pelikant. "Spontaneous emotion recognition from speech signal using multimodal classification," *Informatyka Automatyka Pomiary w Gospodarce i Ochronie Środowiska, vol.* 2, no. 3, pp. 36–39, 2012.

Kasuriya, S., T. Theeramunkong, C. Wutiwiwatchai, and P. Sukhummek. "Developing a Thai emotional speech corpus from Lakorn (EMOLA)," *Language Resources and Evaluation*, vol. 53, no. 1, pp. 17–55, 2019.

Lee, C.-C., E. Mower, C. Busso, S. Lee, and S. Narayanan. "Emotion recognition using a hierarchical binary decision tree approach," *Speech Communication*, vol. 53, no. 9–10, pp. 1162–1171, November 2011.

Liu, Z.-T., et al. "Speaker-Independent Speech Emotion Recognition Based on CNN-BLSTM and Multiple SVMs," *International Conference on Intelligent Robotics and Applications*, Springer, Cham, 2019.

Narayanan, S. S. "Toward detecting emotions in spoken dialogs," *IEEE Transactions on Speech and Audio Processing*, vol. 13, no. 2, pp. 293–303, March 2005.

Nwe, T. L., S. W. Foo, and L. C. De Silva. "Speech emotion recognition using hidden Markov models," *Speech Communication*, vol. 41, no. 4, pp. 603–623, November 2003.

Patel, V. "Why mental health matters to global health," *Transcultural Psychiatry*, vol. 51, no. 6, pp. 777–789, 2014.

Peerzade, G. N., R. Deshmukh, and S. A. Waghmare. "A review: Speech emotion recognition," *International Journal of Computer Science and Engineering*, vol. 6, pp. 400–402, 2018.

Poria, S., N. Majumder, D. Hazarika, E. Cambria, A. Gelbukh, and A. Hussain. "Multimodal sentiment analysis: Addressing key issues and setting up the baselines," *IEEE Intelligent Systems*, vol. 33, no. 6, pp. 17–25, 2018.

Pourebrahim, Y., et al. "Semi-supervised parallel shared encoders for speech emotion recognition," *Digital Signal Processing*, vol. 118, 2021.

Schuller, B. W. "Speech emotion recognition: Two decades in a nutshell, benchmarks, and ongoing trends," *Communication ACM*, vol. 61, no. 5, pp. 90–99, 2018.

Shaw, A. Vardhan, R. K. Saxena, and S. Saxena. "Emotion recognition and classification in speech using artificial neural networks," *International Journal of Computer Applications*, vol. 145, pp. 5–9, 2016.

Swain, M., A. Routray, and P. Kabisatpathy. "Databases, Features and Classifiers for Speech Emotion Recognition: A Review," *International Journal of Speech Technology*, vol. 21, pp. 93–120, 2018.

Trigeorgis, G., F. Ringeval, R. Brueckner, E. Marchi, M. A. Nicolaou, B. Schüller, and S. Zafeiriou. "Adieu features? End-to-end speech emotion recognition using a deep convolutional recurrent network," *Proceedings of the IEEE International Conference on Acoustics, Speech and Signal Processing (ICASSP)*, Shanghai, China, 20–25 March 2016.

Wu, S., T. H. Falk, and W.-Y. Chan. "Automatic speech emotion recognition using modulation spectral features," *Speech Communication*, vol. 53, no. 5, pp. 768–785, May 2011.

Zhao, J., et al. "Speech emotion recognition using deep 1D & 2D CNN LSTM networks", *Biomedical Signal Processing and Control*, vol. 47, pp. 312–323, January 2019.

Zhou, T. H., G. L. Hu, and L. Wang. "Psychological disorder identifying method based on emotion perception over social networks," *International Journal of Environmental Research and Public Health*, vol. 16, no. 6, p. 953, 2019.

# Index

## A

## D



## E



## F

## G



## H



## I



## K

## L



## M



## N



## O



## P



## R

## S



## T

## U



## V



## W



## X